W9-AKT-360

Hand Function In The Child

Foundations for Remediation

Hand Function in the Child

Foundations for Remediation

Edited by

Anne Henderson, Ph.D., O.T.R.
Professor Emeritus
Department of Occupational Therapy
Boston University/Sargent College of Allied Health Professions
Boston, Massachusetts

Charlane Pehoski, Sc.D., O.T.R.
Director
Occupational Therapy
Shriver Center
Waltham, Massachusetts;
Adjunct Associate Professor
Boston University
Boston, Massachusetts

with 17 contributors
with 128 illustrations

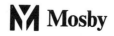 Mosby

An Affiliate of Elsevier

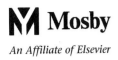

Mosby

An Affiliate of Elsevier

Editor: Martha Sasser
Editorial Assistant: Amy Dubin
Project Manager: John Rogers
Senior Production Editor: Helen Hudlin
Designer: Renée Duenow
Manufacturing Supervisor: John Babrick
Cover illustration: Mark Swindle

Copyright © 1995 by Mosby

All rights reserved. No part of this publication may be reproduced,
stored in a retrieval system, or transmitted, in any form or by any
means, electronic, mechanical, photocopying, recording, or otherwise,
without prior written permission from the publisher.

Permissions may be sought directly from Elsevier's Health Sciences Rights
Department in Philadelphia, USA: phone: (+1)215-238-7869, fax: (+1)215-238-2239,
email: healthpermissions@elsevier.com. You may also complete your request on-line via
the Elsevier Science homepage (http://www.elsevier.com), by selecting 'Customer Support'
and then 'Obtaining Permissions'.

Printed in the United States of America

Mosby
11830 Westline Industrial Drive
St. Louis, Missouri 63146

Library of Congress Cataloging-in-Publication Data

Hand function in the child: foundations for remediation / edited by
  Anne Henderson, Charlane Pehoski: with 17 contributors.
      p.   cm.
  Includes bibliographical references and index.
  ISBN 0-8016-6917-0
    1. Movement disorders in children.   2. Hand—Movements.   3. Motor
ability in children.   4. Occupational therapy for children.
  I. Henderson, Anne.   II. Pehoski, Charlane.
    [DNLM: 1. Hand—in infancy & childhood.   2. Hand—physiology.
  3. Motor Skills—in infancy & childhood.   4. Occupational Therapy—
  methods.   WE 830 H23092 1994]
  RJ496.M68H36   1994
  618.92'097575—dc20
  DNLM/DLC

04 05 06 07 08   9 8 7 6

Contributors

Mary Benbow, M.S., O.T.R.
Private Consultant and
International Lecturer
La Jolla, California

Jane Case-Smith, Ed.D, O.T.R.
Assistant Professor
Division of Occupational Therapy
School of Allied Medical Professions
The Ohio State University
Columbus, Ohio

Sharon A. Cermak, Ed.D, O.T.R., F.A.O.T.A.
Professor of Occupational Therapy
Department of Occupational Therapy
Boston University/Sargent College of Allied
Health Professions
Boston, Massachusetts

Sandra J. Edwards, M.A., O.T.R.
Associate Professor
Occupational Therapy Department
Western Michigan University
Kalamazoo, Michigan

Ann-Christin Eliasson, O.T.
Occupational Therapist
Institution of Woman and Child Health
Karolinska Institute
Stockholm, Sweden

Charlotte E. Exner, Ph.D, O.T.R., F.A.O.T.A.
Chairperson and Associate Professor
Occupational Therapy Department
Towson State University
Towson, Maryland

Judith E. Freeman, M.A., O.T.R.
Senior Occupational Therapist
Easter Seal Society of Ventura County
Infant Development Program
Ventura, California;
Instructor, California Lutheran University
Department of Special Education
Thousand Oaks, California

Ilene M. Goldkopf, O.T.R., B.C.P.
Private Practice;
Co-Founder, Pocket Full of Therapy
Morganville, New Jersey

Anne Henderson, Ph.D., O.T.R., F.A.O.T.A.
Professor Emeritus
Department of Occupational Therapy
Boston University/Sargent College of Allied
Health Professions
Boston, Massachusetts

Mary K. Lafreniere, M.S., O.T.R.
Occupational Therapist
Hospital for Special Care
New Britain, Connecticut

Elizabeth A. Murray, Sc.D., O.T.R., F.A.O.T.A.
Assistant Director of Occupational Therapy
Shriver Center
Waltham, Massachusetts;
Assistant Professor of Occupational Therapy
Boston University/Sargent College of Allied
Health Professions
Boston, Massachusetts

Charlane Pehoski, Sc.D., O.T.R., F.A.O.T.A.
Director, Occupational Therapy
Shriver Center
Waltham, Massachusetts;
Adjunct Associate Professor
Boston University
Boston, Massachusetts

Birgit Rösblad, Ph.D., P.T.
Physical Therapist
Department of Psychology
University of Umeå
Umeå, Sweden

Janet M. Stilwell, M.S., O.T.R.
Associate Professor of Clinical Occupational
Therapy
Department of Occupational Therapy
Louisiana State University Medical Center
New Orleans, Louisiana

James W. Strickland, M.D.
Chairman, Department of Hand Surgery
St. Vincent Hospital of Indianapolis;
Clinical Professor
Department of Orthopaedic Surgery
Indiana University School of Medicine
Indianapolis, Indiana

Michelle V. Tobias, O.T.R., B.C.P.
Private Practice;
Co-Founder, Pocket Full of Therapy
Morganville, New Jersey

Jenny Ziviani, Ph.D., O.T.
Senior Lecturer
Occupational Therapy Department
The University of Queensland
St. Lucia, Queensland, Australia

*This book
is dedicated to
James J. Papai*

Preface

. . . [M]an through the use of his hands, as they are
energized by mind and will, can influence the state
of his own health. (Reilly, 1962, p. 2)

The hand is our primary means of interaction with the physical environment, both through the dexterous grasp and manipulation of objects and as the enabler of multiple tool functions. The enormous variety of actions accomplished by our hands ranges from the practical to the creative. The hand is incredibly versatile. It can be a platform, a hook, or a vise. It can hold a football, a hammer, or a needle. It can explore objects, express emotion, or communicate language.

The hand is the subject of this book, most specifically the hand as a tool for action, as an organ of accomplishment. The motor functions of the hand are some of the most complex and advanced of all human motor skills. Hand use is voluntary, under the control of the conscious mind, and is regulated by feedback from sensory organs. The complexity of skilled hand use is shown by the long developmental period needed for its perfection. The ability to manipulate objects with the efficiency and precision of an adult continues to improve throughout late childhood and early adolescence.

The plan for this book grew out of the recognition that, although the treatment of hand dysfunction has been a critical area of occupational therapy practice since the beginning of the profes-

sion, for many years the professional literature in pediatrics placed a greater emphasis on the neurophysiology and development of gross motor abilities than on manipulative skills. A renewed attention to manipulative abilities, beginning about 15 years ago, was spearheaded by the writings of therapists such as Rhoda Erhart, Reggie Boehm, and Charlotte Exner, and professional literature on the developmental treatment of hand skills has since increased. During a similar period there has been increasing research attention in the fields of neurophysiology and psychology to the motor skills of the hand. Although there are many unresolved issues about hand development and dysfunction in childhood, it seemed timely to review that which is currently known.

This book is intended for the professional and student interested in the current research and treatment of problems in children's hand skills. The text is organized around themes from neurobehavior and development, drawing together information that is pertinent to the understanding of dysfunction of the hand in children and as a guidance to intervention. Hand function is reviewed from the perspectives of neurophysiology, neuropsychology, cognitive psychology, developmental psychology, and therapeutic intervention.

The text is organized into three sections, each of which presents several dimensions of hand function. Section I includes chapters on the biologic and psychologic foundations of hand

Reilly, M. (1962). Occupational therapy can be one of the great ideas of 20th century medicine. *American Journal of Occupational Therapy, 16,* 1–9.

function. The first chapter describes the cortical control of skilled hand use and identifies the properties of that control that are different from the control of gross motor skills. The second chapter presents the anatomic structure and function of the hand facilitating the varied functions. Two chapters on the sensory guidance of hand function follow, one on touch and proprioception and the other on vision. The other two chapters in Section I review knowledge from several branches of psychology, including the perceptual functions of the hand and the role of cognition in hand activity.

Section II focuses on development in both general and specific areas of hand skill. Two chapters in this section focus on the development of basic skills. The first reviews research on the development of grasp, release, and bimanual skills in infancy and the second the development of object manipulation. Other chapters cover specific and complex skill areas of graphic skill and self-care and the development of hand dominance.

Section III provides knowledge from selected pediatric clinical practice areas. Two of the five chapters describe dysfunction and treatment of special populations with cerebral palsy and Down syndrome. Another chapter presents the principles and practice of the remediation of hand skill problems, while a fourth focuses on the specific area of teaching handwriting. The remaining chapter identifies the many toys that are the natural media for the treatment of hand dysfunction in children.

Despite the acceleration of research in the last decade, the study of the development of hand use and the treatment of hand dysfunction in children is still in its infancy. It is our hope that assembling this information on hand skills will stimulate interest in the development of research programs that will increase the body of knowledge about normal and deviant hand skill development and the efficacy of intervention.

This text was written primarily for pediatric occupational therapists and could serve as a graduate level text or as a reference book in entry level education. However, we anticipate that it will be of value for anyone working with toddlers and children, including preschool and elementary teachers, special educators, early intervention providers, and other therapists.

Anne Henderson
Charlane Pehoski

Acknowledgments

The editors wish first to acknowledge with gratitude the time and expertise donated by each of the contributors to this volume. This text was fostered by a series of workshops for occupational therapists and physical therapists funded by the Maternal and Child Health Bureau, U.S. Department of Health and Human Services, Department of Public Health. The workshops were sponsored by the Occupational Therapy and Physical Therapy Departments at the University of Illinois at Chicago between 1988 and 1991. Several of the contributors to this book participated in task groups on hand function, motivated by the need to review information that would be of value for children with special needs.

The production of this text has been supported in part by the Shriver Center University-Affiliated Program and by the Neurobehavioral Rehabilitation Research Center of the Occupational Therapy Department of Boston University/Sargent College of Allied Health Professions. The Neurobehavioral Rehabilitation Research Center is a center for scholarship and research that is jointly funded by Boston University and the American Occupational Therapy Foundation/American Occupational Therapy Association. The Shriver Center University-Affiliated Program is funded by the Maternal and Child Health Bureau and the Administration on Developmental Disabilities of the Department of Public Health.

We thank our student assistants, Diana Bertozzi, Kendra Cermak, Kathleen Garrett-Subasic, and Randi Scheiner, for the performance of a variety of useful tasks along the way, and we thank David Ritchie for his cheerful service in the typing of portions of the manuscript.

Contents

S E C T I O N III
Therapeutic Intervention

Hand Function
in the Child

Foundations for Remediation

Foundations of Hand Skills

1

Cortical Control of Skilled Movements of the Hand

Charlane Pehoski

When we watch an infant pick up a pellet or a 3-year-old child trying to button his shirt, we are seeing the result of one of Nature's truly remarkable evolutionary feats, the performance of the human hand. The ability to use the hand with dexterity and skill has reached its highest level in humans and is the result of major changes in the central nervous system control of the extremities. Even the evolution of fingers does not result in skilled movements if the necessary central nervous system mechanisms are not present. For example, the rhesus monkey has the ability to pick up a small object between the index finger and the thumb, but the squirrel monkey, in which the shape of the hand and the fingers is almost identical, can pick up small objects only by closing the total hand around them. The rhesus monkey possesses the central nervous system control mechanisms that make this refined task possible, whereas the squirrel monkey does not (Lawrence and Hopkins, 1976).

In discussing the evolution of digital dexterity, Heffner and Masterton (1983) point out the increasing influence of the neocortex over the hand. This includes an extension of cortical control beyond cervical levels, which they suggest freed the forelimbs and hands from locomotor functions. They also point to the increase in the overall size of the corticospinal tracts and a reduction in the number of synapses between the cortex and the motor neurons in the spinal cord with evolution. This latter concept is particularly important, and we will return to it later. Lawrence and Kuypers

(1968b) suggest that the brainstem motor pathways function as the basic system by which the brain exerts control over movement, particularly for the maintenance of erect posture, the integration of the movements of the trunk and limbs, and for progression in space. A cortical system adds to these functions the independent control of the hands and the ability to move individual fingers, allowing refined tasks such as picking up a small object between the thumb and index finger.

Therefore small, delicate movements of the hand have evolved through an increase in the cortical motor control over these movements. But skilled movements also require sensory feedback. It should, therefore, not be surprising that cortical motor mechanisms are intimately connected with sensory structures and that the importance of this linkage has grown along with the increase in control of the distal extremity. With the increasing importance of sensory input to skilled movements, the cortical areas involved with the integration of sensory information have expanded, particularly the posterior parietal lobe. In addition, if you have a long leverlike arm and attach to it a hand in which the fingers can each move independently, the number of possible movements this structure can perform is phenomenal. Neural mechanisms are thus necessary to plan and sequence these movements to meet the demands of the intelligence driving them. In this chapter we review four aspects of cortical control of the hand: motor mechanisms, sensory mechanisms, cortical integration of sensory information, and the planning and sequencing of these complex acts at the cortical level.

CORTICAL MOTOR MECHANISMS CONTROLLING SKILLED HAND USE

Lemon (1990) made a statement that is very important to the understanding of the central nervous system control over movements of the upper extremity: ". . . the control of manipulation and of reach are mainly dependent on two different groups of descending fiber systems" (p. 1285). The man who is credited with the notion of such a *dual* motor system is Henricus Kuypers. When we observe the well-organized movements of a person reaching, grasping, and manipulating an object, the fact that these actions are under the control of different motor pathways is not apparent. Possibly for this reason Kuypers and his colleagues' early experimental results were questioned by physiologists of the time. One of Kuypers's classic studies

was the observation of the motor behavior of monkeys after selected lesions of the various descending motor pathways (Lawrence and Kuypers, 1968a,b). In this work he and Lawrence demonstrated the necessary role of the pyramidal tract in the control of individual finger movements. Lemon (1990) indicates that, after the publication of this work, a well-known physiologist of the time stated that monkeys do just what they like with their hands, pyramids or no pyramids. This physiologist turned out to be wrong. Without the pyramidal tract animals lose the capacity of individual, dexterous movements of the hand. As will be seen, no other motor pathway can substitute for this function.

If it is true that there is a dual motor system, it should be reflected in how we view the hand. In the motor development of the infant, controlled reach is achieved before refined pincer grasp or manipulation. This does not necessarily mean that there is *one* motor system developing in a proximal-to-distal direction. Research into the control of postural and limb muscles would indicate that the control of the shoulder and the skilled control of the hand are maturing together but at different rates. The phylogenetically older system controlling the shoulder matures first, and the comparatively newer system controlling the hand develops later.

Termination of Long Fiber Tracts in the Spinal Cord

Some of the early work of Kuypers and his colleagues examined the termination of the long fiber tracts on the motor neurons in the spinal cords. The alpha motor neuron is the final common pathway to the muscles, and any central nervous system control over the muscles must synapse at this point. The motor neurons in the ventral horn of the spinal cord are not randomly distributed but are clustered into cell columns, a medial cell column that contains the motor neurons for the trunk, shoulder girdle, and hips, and a lateral cell column that contains the motor neurons for the distal extremities (Figure 1-1). The long fiber tracts synapsing on these columns are different. Input to the medial cell column comes from subcortical structures (e.g., vestibulospinal tract and reticulospinal tract). In the monkey, input to the distal extremities comes from the cortex as well as through the subcortical rubrospinal path (Kuypers, 1981). In this chapter we discuss only the cortical input through the pyramidal tract. It

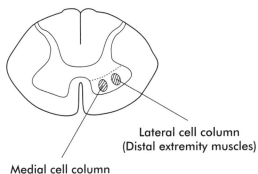

Lateral cell column
(Distal extremity muscles)

Medial cell column
(Trunk and girdle muscles)

Figure 1-1. Anterior gray area of the spinal cord, indicating the two cell columns containing the alpha motor neurons for the distal extremities and for the trunk, shoulder, and hip girdle.

would therefore appear that the mechanisms controlling more proximal movements, such as those supporting the trunk or controlling the shoulder, are different from those controlling the distal extremity, and, as we shall see, this is particularly true for skilled use of the hand.

To explore further the concept of a dual motor system, Lawrence and Kuypers (1968a,b) separately lesioned the subcortical motor pathways and the pyramidal pathways. What they found was that animals who had the subcortical pathways lesioned had difficulty maintaining erect posture and were unsteady when walking. But when these animals were required to use refined hand movements to pick up small bits of food, no detectable impairment was noted in the agility and speed of these movements.

When the pyramidal tracts were lesioned, the animals were still able to swing, climb, and jump. In general, the postural system of these animals appeared to be intact, but the hand was significantly affected. Although the hand was used in climbing, the animals never regained the ability to perform individual finger movements. Small pieces of food were picked up by action of all the fingers together, and a precision grip between the thumb and index finger was not seen. Lesion studies appear to support the hypothesis regarding a dual motor system, one system serving postural and axial movements and the other serving the muscles of the distal extremities and providing speed and dexterity to movements.

A second question that was asked was whether any other tracts could substitute for the pyramidal tract in the control of hand movements. The previously discussed experiments had been done

on adult animals where recovery from a lesion might be less dramatic than might be found in younger animals. Therefore Lawrence and Hopkins (1976) lesioned the pyramidal tracts in monkeys 5 days to 4 weeks of age and observed their development when compared to normal peers. What they found was that, for about the first 6 months of life, the experimental animals were able to do all the motor activities of their peers. They could jump, climb, and swing, although the quality of their movements made them stand out from other animals (i.e., apparently they were clumsier). It was only when the control animals began to develop a refined pincer grasp that the experimental animals looked markedly different. For the animals with complete lesions of the pyramidal tract, the ability to "fractionate" the fingers to produce a neat pincer grasp never developed during their 2 to 3 years of survival. This was true despite attempts to train the animals to use the radial fingers. Of interest was the fact that in one animal found later to have a few corticospinal fibers remaining, a pincer grasp did develop but only after training that forced the animal to use the radial fingers. Lawrence and Hopkins (1976) thus concluded that no other fiber tracts could substitute for the action of the pyramidal tract. When it is severed in adult and infant monkeys, refined movements of the hand never develop.

The most significant difference in the young experimental and control animals in the Lawrence and Hopkins (1976) study was the loss of individual finger movements. Since this difference did not appear until several months after birth, it would seem that the mechanisms controlling individual use of the fingers are not present at birth. Like human infants, neonate monkeys first pick up small objects using a mass grasp, where all fingers and the thumb tend to move as a unit. It is not until later in development that a neat pincer grasp is seen, where the index finger alone is opposed to the thumb and the remaining fingers bend out of the way. As indicated, pincer grasp never developed in the animals with complete pyramidal lesions. This level of control appears to be specifically related to a subset of pyramidal fibers, those with *direct* monosynaptic corticospinal connections on the motor neurons of the distal limbs.

The ventral horn of the spinal cord is divided into two main sections, an interneuron zone and the motor neuronal pool, mentioned previously. Both of these sections show the separation of postural, shoulder, and hip muscles from the distal muscles of the extremities. Almost all descending

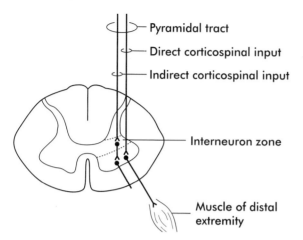

Figure 1-2. Termination of the pyramidal tract in the spinal cord. The diagram shows a single fiber that synapses in the interneuronal zone and then makes connection with a muscle through the interneuron. Also shown is a fiber within the pyramidal tract that makes a direct connection to a motor neuron of a distal limb muscle.

motor fibers first terminate in the interneuronal zone, so that there is at least one interneuron between the descending motor fiber and the motor neuron. A very important exception is the direct corticospinal fibers to alpha motor neurons of the distal extremity (Figure 1-2). In monkeys with dexterous hands these connections are largely concerned with the control of the muscles acting on the hand and the fingers (Lemon, Bennett, and Werner, 1990). These direct connections are thought to provide the ability to move the hand with skill. Also, in monkeys the connections of these direct fibers are not present at birth, but instead develop in parallel with the emergence of a neat pincer grasp (Kuypers, 1962). There is no reason to believe that the emergence of a neat pincer grasp in human infants is not also related to the same phenomenon.

Involvement of the Primary Motor Cortex

It is not just the pyramidal tract that is needed for skilled movements of the hand but the motor cortex as well. Lesions of this cortex in infant monkeys also result in a lack of precision grip (Passingham, Perry, and Wilkinson, 1978).

Muir and Lemon (1983) looked specifically at neurons in the primary motor cortex that had direct input to motor neurons of the hand (i.e., neurons with direct corticospinal connections to motor neurons of the hand). In this study they trained monkeys to squeeze two different manipulanda.

One required the animal to use a precision grip, and the other required the use of a mass grasp. During these activities the authors also monitored the EMG action of selected hand muscles. They found that the neurons from the motor cortex with direct input to hand muscles were preferentially related to the precision grip. That is, even though similar muscles were active in both grip patterns, the cortical neurons under study were much less active during the mass grasp pattern. As the authors explain, a precision grip requires the muscles to be used in a "fractionated" manner. When the EMG activity of hand muscles in monkeys and humans was studied using the same two manipulanda, the activation of the muscles involved in the precision grip task was quite varied, both with respect to the precise time of onset and the time course of activity during the task. In contrast, when the animal used a mass grasp, all of the muscles were coactivated (Muir, 1985). Muir states, "It is this fractionation of muscle excitation in space and time that has been suggested to be the special contribution of the corticomotoneuronal neurons of the precentral gyrus" (p. 163). This delicacy in the selection and timing of muscle input provides an important basis for skilled movements of the hand.

It is also interesting to note that Nudo et al. (1992) found a difference in the complexity of the topography of the primary motor cortex in the preferred hand of monkeys when compared with the nonpreferred hand. The authors indicate that the "greater complexity of movements represented in the dominant hemisphere would manifest a greater repertoire of more refined movement combinations" (p. 2945). That is, handedness would appear to have a neurophysiologic correlate, at least in the primary motor cortex of monkeys.

In summary, the motor cortex contains neurons that make direct connections to the muscles of the hand through the pyramidal tract. This input is thought to underlie the ability to delicately control the muscles of the hand so that the fingers can be moved individually or in combinations with both speed and accuracy. This is the basis not only for a precision grip but also for all in-hand manipulation tasks. Without this input, refined movements of the hand never develop or are lost.

MECHANISMS OF THE PRIMARY SOMATOSENSORY CORTEX INVOLVED WITH SKILLED HAND USE

Sensory feedback is critical during the acquisition of new tasks and is also important in most everyday activities. At an unconscious level we are acutely aware of this. For example, we automatically take off a glove when looking for a coin in our pocket or when picking up a coin from a table. Imagine how awkward it would be to accept change from a salesperson and then put it into a coin purse with gloves on. Manipulation tasks such as these are heavily dependent on sensory guidance from receptors in the hand. Vision is also important. Vision guides the hand into space, prepares the hand for grasp (Jeannerod, 1984), and can help determine the direction of manipulation. But it is information from the hand itself that guides the fingers around an object for grasp or guides the movement of an object within the hand. Somatosensory input also lets us grade our grip to both the weight of an object and its frictional characteristics (Westling and Johansson, 1984). Without this input the actions of the hand are severely limited. Vision can only partially substitute for this loss. It should be noted that there are movements that do not depend on continuous sensory feedback. An example is the highly skilled movements of a musician, where sensory feedback would be too slow to update the ongoing activity. But most everyday activities depend on sensory guidance.

There are reports in the literature of patients who have lost sensory input from the hand through a severe sensory neuropathy (Rothwell et al., 1982; Sanes et al., 1985). The subjects in these reports had difficulty in maintaining a limb posture or a constant force output. Activities of daily living were disturbed, and actions such as buttoning or the manipulation of coins in the hand were extremely difficult.

The hand is privileged in the number of sensory receptors located in the skin as well as in its muscles. For example, despite their small size, the intrinsic muscles of the hand contain more muscle spindle receptors than many muscles of the trunk and limbs (Cooper, 1960). Muscle spindle receptors are thought to provide information necessary to correct small errors in movement (Devandan, Ghosh, and John, 1983). The intrinsic muscles of the hand are known to be critical for refined, controlled movements. In addition, the hand is also richly endowed with tactile receptors. The human fingertips are also broad, allowing a greater sensory surface (Napier, 1962). This is an important component of human grip.

Dorsal Column Pathway

The dorsal column pathway carries the discrete somatosensory information necessary for tactile

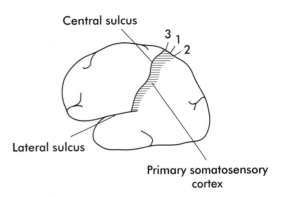

Figure 1-3. Diagram of the left cerebral hemisphere, showing the primary somatosensory cortex and areas *3, 1,* and 2.

perception as well as skilled motor actions. It has evolved in parallel with the pyramidal path and, like this motor pathway, it reaches its highest level of development in the human (Mountcastle, 1984). Information carried in this system can register small movements of joints and provide knowledge of the exact location of a stimulus on the skin. The information in the dorsal columns travels through two relay stations on its way to the cortex: the nucleus cuneatus and gracilis form the first relay, and the thalamus the second. One of the major destinations for this information in the cortex is the primary somatosensory area, which lies posterior to the central sulcus (Figure 1-3).

Primary Somatosensory Cortex

When information arrives through the dorsal columns, it is coded for discrete sensory modalities (e.g., touch, joint rotation) and for the exact location on the body that was stimulated. But this information does not remain in isolated bits. Rather, there is further processing of this information as it travels posterior through the three cytoarchitectonic divisions of the somatosensory area (i.e., areas 3, 1, and 2). In this respect, area 3 can be considered the primary receiving area, whereas area 2 is more of an association area (Iwamura et al., 1985). The neurons in area 2 have larger receptive fields than those in area 3 and also respond to complex input such as a somasthetic stimulus moving in a particular direction or to the feel of edges. These neurons also appear to represent functional surfaces; for example, one neuron might respond to input anywhere on the palm of the hand (Iwamura et al., 1985).

Of interest is the fact that the functional organization of the somatosensory cortex at any given time appears to reflect the behavioral experience of an animal (Recanzone et al., 1992); that is, experiments that have manipulated the sensory input to the primary sensory cortex in monkeys have resulted in either an expansion (Jenkins et al., 1990; Recanzone et al., 1992; Spinelli, Jensen, and DiPrisco, 1980) or a reduction (Allard et al., 1991) in the representation of selected skin surfaces. For example, Recanzone et al. (1992) trained two groups of monkeys to place their hands on a mold of the hand. The purpose of the mold was to keep the hand in the same position so a vibratory stimulus could be given to a small site on one of the fingers. One group of animals was trained to lift the hand when they perceived changes in the vibratory input. In other words, these monkeys were to attend to and then make an adaptive response to this tactile stimulus. Another group of monkeys also received the vibratory stimulus but were trained to lift the hand to changes in an auditory stimulus. These animals therefore received the vibratory stimulus in a passive manner and were not required to act on the input. When the area in the sensory cortex representing the stimulated portion of skin in these animals was mapped, both the control and the experimental animals showed an increase in the representation of this skin area. But the increase in the animals who had been passive recipients of the vibratory stimulus was very modest. What the authors suggest is that attention influences cortical reorganization and that stimulation alone is far less effective in driving cortical reorganization than an active response to the stimulus. In other words, being engaged in the activity and making an adaptive response based on the sensory input was the most effective means of driving the cortical changes seen in this study. There is also evidence in the literature that skilled use of the hand over the life of a human may result in changes in the primary sensory cortex, such as an increase in dendritic branching (Scheibel et al., 1990).

The primary sensory cortex is thus dynamic and changes in its organization. This information has clinical implications. Often children with poor hand skills avoid fine motor tasks. Even though they would appear to need more practice in this area, they may be receiving less input than their peers. They need help in becoming actively engaged in skilled motor tasks with the hands.

Somatosensory Cortex and Motor Functions

Given the intimate relationship between skilled movements of the hand and somatosensory feedback, it should not be surprising that the motor cortex receives somatosensory input from the periphery.

Area 2 sends information through corticocortical pathways to the primary motor area. In addition, the primary motor area receives somatosensory input from the thalamus (Asanuma and Mackel, 1989). Therefore many neurons in the primary motor cortex that are involved with the initiation of muscle responses also respond to somatosensory feedback from the periphery. Neurons in the hand and the shoulder area of the primary motor cortex differ in the form of sensory information represented in these areas. As might be expected, cutaneous modalities are particularly well represented in the hand area of the motor cortex although neurons also respond to joint rotation and deep pressure over muscles of the hand. This cutaneous information is almost exclusively from the palmar surface of the hand and the fingers, or those surfaces that will come in contact with an object when it is grasped. In contrast, neurons representing the more proximal forelimb muscles have only small representation of tactile input but primarily respond to joint movements or muscle palpation (Lemon, 1981; Rosen and Asanuma, 1972).

Asanuma and Arissian (1984) suggest that one of the roles of somatosensory input to the motor cortex is to assist in the learning of skilled motor tasks through cortical peripheral loops. They indicate:

> When a subject is trained to pursue a specific movement, the practice produces vigorous circulation of impulses in particular corticoperipheral loops related to that movement. Repeated practice results in an increased efficiency of synaptic transmission in these loops, resulting in the increased excitability of related cortical neurons (p. 224).

In an experiment to look at the effect of stimulation of the sensory cortex on the firing of motor neurons in the primary motor cortex, Sakamoto, Porter, and Asanuma (1987) found that electrical simulation of the sensory cortex produced changes in synaptic transmission in motor neurons; that is, this passive excitation of the motor cortex through the electrical stimulation of the sensory cortex had an effect on the future firing of the motor neurons. The type of changes observed have been equated with the development of "memories" in other parts of the central nervous system (e.g., hippocampus). The authors suggest that area 2 of the sensory cortex receives specific input during a particular movement and that by repeating the movement, area 2 sends repetitive impulses to the motor cortex neurons resulting in the changes in synaptic transmission thought to be related to motor memory. As demonstrated in cats (Sakamoto, Arissian, and Asanuma, 1989), when the primary sensory cortex was removed, the animals were significantly delayed in learning a new motor task. Also of interest is the fact that, once the task had been learned, lesions of the sensory cortex did not impair the skill, suggesting that input from the sensory cortex contributes to the learning but not retention of motor skills.

Of interest from a therapeutic point of view is that the experimental animals in the previous experiment who had the primary sensory cortex removed *did* learn the task and improved their performance with practice although they never achieved the accuracy of the control animals. Asanuma and Arissian (1984) indicate that:

... there is a possibility that functional recovery following injury to a part of the central nervous system can be improved by reinforcing a remaining input of similar function by electrical/or chemical as well as *natural stimulation* [italics added] during the recovery period (p. 225).

Therefore practice is necessary for skilled motor learning as well as the recovery of function following injury. This would appear to be particularly true of the hand where refined, controlled movements are necessary to produce a skilled performance.

INTEGRATION OF SENSORY AND MOTOR INFORMATION IN THE POSTERIOR PARIETAL LOBE

Thus far we have examined the relatively simple aspects of the control of skilled motor movements of the hand, input from the direct corticospinal fibers, and the integration of information from the motor cortex with somatosensory information. But it is likely that, when a child performs a task as complicated as learning to tie shoes, a greater cortical area is involved than discussed so far. One of these areas is the large expanse of cortex posterior to the primary sensory cortex, the posterior parietal lobe (Figure 1-4).

Integration of Sensory Information

The posterior parietal lobe in the monkey receives somatosensory input from the primary sensory cortex, visual information from part of the visual cortex, and, less commonly discussed, input

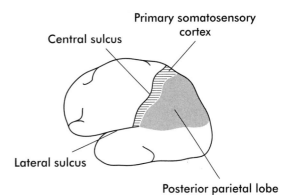

Figure 1-4. Diagram of the left cerebral hemisphere showing the location of the primary somatosensory cortex and the posterior parietal area.

from part of the auditory cortex (Stein, 1989). It is therefore a polysensory receiving area. But it should also be noted that much of this information comes from areas of the cortex where integration of that sensory modality has already taken place. For example, Jones and Powell (1970) indicated that the posterior parietal cortex receives already processed input from the primary somatosensory cortex and that the parietal lobe itself represents the highest order processing of this information. Neurons in this area therefore respond to complex combinations of information. For instance, a single neuron might respond not to one but to a combination of joint movements (Duffy and Burchfiel, 1971). As Sakata and Iwamura (1978) have pointed out in reference to Gibson's work, the movement of one joint is meaningless unless it is related to all the movements above it. This form of polysensory convergence is common in the posterior parietal lobe. For example, Mountcastle et al. (1975) found a "visual tracking" neuron in a monkey that also responded to passive stimulation of the skin.

Representation of Motor Acts

In a now classic article, Mountcastle et al. (1975) also reported that some neurons in the parietal lobe responded to motor acts. They referred to these as either arm extension neurons, since these neurons responded when a monkey reached for a desired object, or hand manipulation neurons, since they responded when an animal moved the fingers to pick up an object. An example of a hand manipulation neuron is a cell that fires strongly when an animal attempts to get a sunflower seed out of the examiner's hand.

Taira et al. (1990) have specifically studied neurons in the posterior parietal cortex as monkeys performed four different manipulation tasks (e.g., pulling a lever, pushing a button, pulling a knob, and pulling a recessed knob requiring isolation of the index finger and thumb). They found that there was a strong preference among different cells for specific objects. They also found that many of the hand movement neurons decreased their firing in the dark and therefore suggested that the difference in firing rates between the dark and light situations was probably due to some visual input to these cells. They called these units *visual and motor neurons* and suggested that they are concerned with the visual guidance of hand movements and with matching the movement to the spatial characteristics of the object.

Also of interest was the finding that these movement-related neurons respond to planned, goal-directed activities. They did not fire if the animal reached out to push the examiner away or attempted to use a pincer grasp to pinch the examiner rather than using the same movements to pick up a small piece of food. Furthermore, neurons in this area were undrivable when the animal was drowsy or asleep, and visual neurons discharged at very low rates when the animal was resting quietly; but the rate of discharge increased sharply when the animal began to visually explore the environment (Mountcastle et al., 1975). Many of these neurons therefore seem strongly related to goal-directed activities. In contrast, neurons in the primary motor cortex fire whenever the animal makes a voluntary movement whether to scratch, to push the examiner away, or to reach for a desired object.

Deficits in Humans

The research studies that have been mentioned so far were conducted on monkeys. In humans, the parietal area is more complex. For example, the area is larger and demonstrates hemispheric specialization. Furthermore the right parietal cortex is thought to be specialized for constructional tasks such as block designs and the spatial aspects of drawing. Lesions of the right parietal cortex often result in hemineglect of the left side of space (Stein, 1989).

The right parietal cortex has been referred to as an area of sensorimotor integration (Pause et al., 1989). Given its complexity, it is not surprising that the deficits demonstrated by persons with lesions in this area are also complex. Deficits

include the inability to localize visual targets, disturbances in spatial attention, loss of spatial memories, and the inability to represent the spatial relations in drawings or constructional tasks (Anderson, 1988). In adults these problems may also include dysgraphia, dyslexia, and dyscalculia (Stein, 1989).

The posterior parietal cortex has a specific relationship to performance of the hand. For example, Pause et al. (1989) studied the tactile and manipulation responses of nine patients with lesions confined to the posterior parietal lobes. The subjects were divided by the location of the lesion into those where the lesion was confined to the anterior portion of the lobe (two subjects) or the posterior area (three subjects) and those with combined lesions (four subjects). The subjects were given tasks to test their simple somatosensory abilities (e.g., localization of a spot touched, joint position sense), complex somatosensory abilities (e.g., the recognition of surface textures, recognition of common objects). In addition, recordings were made of each subject's hand movements. The authors found a difference in the performance of these patients depending on where the lesion was in the parietal cortex. As an example, the two subjects who had lesions in the anterior portion demonstrated disturbance in both simple and complex somatosensory functions but did not show the same disturbance in manipulation seen in the subjects with more posterior lesions. Subjects with posterior lesions had more difficulty with the more complex somatosensory tasks and also with complex exploratory and manipulative finger movements. Subjects with combined lesions had difficulty with both the motor and the sensory tests.

An example of the problems many of these patients faced is illustrated in Figure 1-5. This figure represents a woman with a lesion in the parietal lobe studied by Jeannerod, Michel, and Prablanc (1984). The subject is attempting to crumple a sheet of paper with her normal left hand and also with the involved right hand. Note the problems she appears to be having in guiding her right hand around the object. This problem in the control of the hand is apparent even though the subject had an intact motor system.

In summarizing their findings on the sensory and motor disturbances of their patients with parietal lobe lesions, Pause et al. (1989) state:

> The parietal lobe is not only involved in the elaboration and further processing of somatosensory information, but also in the conception and generation of those

RH   LH

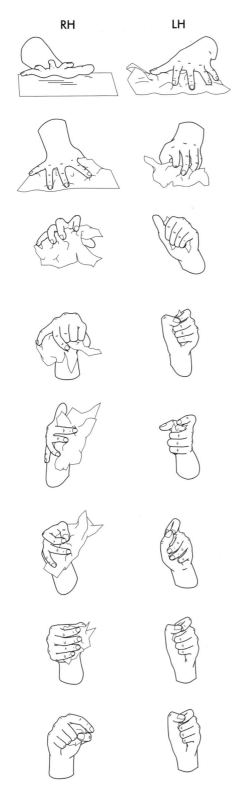

Figure 1-5. Schematic of a woman with a lesion in the parietal lobe attempting to crumple a sheet of paper with her left hand (*LH*) and involved right hand (*RH*).

(From Jeannerod, M., Michel, F., & Prablanc, C. [1984]. The control of hand movements in a case of hemianaesthesia following a parietal lesion. *Brain, 107,* 899-920.)

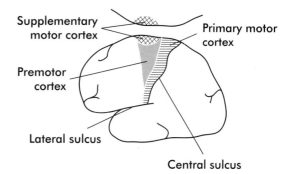

Figure 1-6. Diagram of the left cerebral hemisphere, illustrating location of the primary motor cortex, supplementary motor cortex, and the premotor areas.

motor programs required to collect this information. This illustrates an important aspect of sensorimotor integration, the dependence of feature extraction on purposive action (p. 1622).

The parietal lobe therefore seems to be involved in higher order sensory processing necessary for the guidance of motor acts. As we shall see, the area anterior to the primary motor cortex may be more related to the sequencing or planning of motor movement based on sensory information.

INFORMATION PROCESSING IN THE MOTOR ASSOCIATION CORTEX

When a child learns to write his name, he is taxing all the structures necessary for skilled action of the hand. The child must possess the distal control necessary to perform the small finger/thumb movements that guide the pencil. The child must develop a somatosensory template for the grasp of the pencil that includes not only the pencil position but also the force of grasp. Visual spatial skills are necessary to guide the placement of the letters and regulate their size. The child must also develop a motor plan for the formation of the letters. This plan is generally first developed from an external cue such as a visual model and later internalized so it can be produced from memory and eventually performed automatically. This section discusses additional structures that appear to be involved in the formation of these plans, specifically two cortical areas—the supplementary motor cortex and the premotor cortex (Figure 1-6).

It has been suggested that the premotor area and supplementary motor area play different roles in the structuring of skilled movements. The premotor area, particularly the inferior part, seems to generate movement sequences based on sensory input, whereas the supplementary motor area appears to respond to internally generated movements (Matelli et al., 1986). To test this hypothesis Mushiake, Inase, and Tanji (1991) looked at the firing of neurons in both the supplementary motor cortex and the premotor cortex during the execution of two different sequencing tasks by monkeys. In one task the monkeys were trained to touch three out of four pads placed in front of the animals on a panel. The sequence the monkeys were to use in touching the three pads was provided by lighting up the pads one by one in a random order. The monkey was to imitate this order. Therefore the sequence to be used was triggered by the visual input.

In the second task the animals were taught two fixed sequences so that no visual input assisted in the task. Two different auditory signals indicated to the animal which condition he was to follow. The authors found that more than half the neurons monitored in the premotor area were preferentially or exclusively active in relation to the visually triggered task, whereas more than half the neurons monitored in the supplementary cortex were active when the monkey had to remember the motor sequence and was not assisted by any external signals. Of interest was the fact that, to demonstrate this relative preference of the supplementary motor area and the premotor area, a complex task was necessary, which required the correct sequential ordering of individual motor components. When following visual information, the premotor cortex was preferentially active. When relying on a motor sequence stored in memory, the supplementary motor area was preferentially active.

That the supplementary motor area may be involved with motor patterns stored in memory is also seen in a study by Roland et al. (1980). They monitored the cerebral blood flow in human subjects as they executed a learned finger sequence. When the subject was asked to actually perform the sequence, the cerebral blood flow in both the supplementary motor area and premotor area increased (although the increase was greater in the supplementary motor area). But when the subject was asked just to *think* about the sequence and not move the fingers, the supplementary motor area of both hemispheres showed an increase. No changes were seen in the premotor area.

Rizzolatti and Gentilucci (1988) have suggested that the inferior premotor area contains a "vocabulary of elementary motor acts" connected to a specific aim or purpose. This area has also been found to contain a separate representation for proximal arm movements (Gentilucci et al., 1988) and another for hand and mouth movements (Rizzolatti et al., 1988). Neurons in these areas are related to a particular aim or goal of the animal, not to elementary acts. As an example, a grasping neuron in the hand/mouth area might fire to grasping with the mouth or with either hand. This neuron, then, appears to be related to the intent of the action—grasping—and not specific muscle groups. There are also neurons related to a particular type of grasp. The most representative grasps in this area were those involving delicate finger movements. Movements of the whole hand were represented the least (Rizzolatti et al., 1988). This area is reciprocally connected with areas of the posterior parietal lobe, and the authors point out that in many respects neurons in the two areas have some similar responses. It should also be noted that the premotor area is connected to the prefrontal cortex, whose role in the planning of sequential tasks has also been demonstrated.

SUMMARY AND THERAPEUTIC IMPLICATIONS

One of the marvels of evolution in humans is the skilled action of the hand. This ability is the result of cortical mechanisms that control these actions. Without the cortical organization observed in the human, the delicate movements of the hand would be lost and object manipulation would be severely impaired. We have discussed four aspects of cortical control over the actions of the hand: primary motor mechanisms, sensory mechanisms, the integration of sensory information, and the sequencing or planning of movements. Several points are important to emphasize with reference to the material reviewed:

- The ability to produce individual finger motions absolutely depends on the pyramidal tract and the primary motor cortex. Direct synapse of corticospinal fibers with motor neurons of the hand is critical. This input is felt to provide the ability to move individual fingers with speed and dexterity.
- The central nervous system control of the hand is therefore different from that of the shoulder, trunk, or other proximal movements. Even in the premotor area the shoulder and hand are represented separately. The separation of the control of the shoulder from that of the hand should not be surprising since the function of these two body parts is quite dif-

ferent. The primary purpose of the arm is to *place* the hand in a position of function. The purpose of the hand is to *act* on the environment. Central nervous system mechanisms have been designed to complement both these functions.

• Most everyday movements of the hand require sensory feedback. For example, tactile input regulates the force of grasp and controls for the slippage of objects. The representation of a body part in the primary somatosensory cortex depends on use. The greater the use, the more likely that the body part will have a larger representation and/or more dendritic branching. Information arriving in the primary sensory cortex has also been found to assist in the development of motor memories. Sensory feedback therefore is vital for the development and ongoing monitoring of most skilled function.

• Complex acts such as learning to write or learning to tie shoes also require the integration of sensory information. Both visual and tactile inputs are important. Vision helps define the spatial aspects of a task (e.g., the placement of letters on a line or spacing between words), and somatosensory feedback is necessary to guide the manipulative movements. The coordination of this sensory information with respect to goal-directed activities appears to be one of the roles of the posterior parietal cortex.

• Besides the sensory guidance of movements, complex acts also require the planning or correct sequencing of movements. This function is felt to be related to at least two motor association cortexes, the premotor and supplementary motor areas. Of interest is the finding that one may be more related to sequencing movements based on visual input and the other to action committed to memory.

• We outlined the pattern of cortical organization that is necessary for the execution of skilled motor acts. Cortical motor commands are passed down via the pyramidal tract, and discriminative sensory information about the movement is returned via the dorsal columns. At the cortical level, besides the primary motor and sensory cortexes, we have two main association areas that assist in processing sensory information and in the development of motor commands. One is the posterior parietal lobe, which appears to play a major role in somatosensory and visual guidance,

and the other is the premotor and supplementary motor areas, which appear to assist in providing motor commands for the sequencing of movements.

• It should also be noted that this chapter has not dealt with the problem of spasticity. None of the subjects (animal or human) in the studies mentioned in this chapter presented with this disability. When a child's motor movements are compromised by spasticity, the model of skilled motor performance presented here is no longer applicable, and intervention needs to be considered from a different perspective. Furthermore, it should be noted that this chapter has concentrated only on the cortical control over movements; other structures such as the basal ganglia and the cerebellum are also involved.

It is hoped that this information will be helpful in providing hypotheses on which therapeutic intervention for the child with poor or clumsy hand skills can be based. Remediation of the hand needs to be thought of differently from remediation of the shoulder. When a child has difficulty in both areas, they should be addressed in parallel, not sequentially. Activities that improve the shoulder may not have the same therapeutic effect on the hand. For example, one common activity used to increase the stability of the shoulder musculature is to have the subject bear weight on the arms. This may be an appropriate activity for the shoulder given the supportive function of the arm and the fact that shoulder motions may be more influenced by proprioceptive feedback. Weight-bearing may also have therapeutic value for the hand, particularly for the child with spasticity (Barnes, 1986, 1989), but this should not be the extent of the therapy to improve hand function. The hand needs to *act*. Its function is to perform goal-directed activities. In research studies with monkeys, mass grasp patterns did not activate neurons with direct connections to motor neurons of the distal extremity. Remediation of skilled hand use must involve practice in these activities. Skill requires practice. In animals with damaged motor and sensory structures the functions improved but *only after practice*. Left on their own, these skills did not appear.

Last, children with poor hand skills often avoid or are so poor at fine motor tasks that they may actually get less practice than their peers. As pointed out, at least one cortical area adapts the representation of a body part based on use. In addition, skill requires attention to the activity and is facilitated when there is an interest in the outcome. Children with poor hand skills may need help in selecting and adapting activities to meet their level of performance and interest. Being able to provide activities that challenge the child within the scope of his/her abilities and elicit the child's enthusiastic cooperation is the art of therapy.

REFERENCES

Allard, T., Clark, S.A., Jenkins, W.M., & Merzenich, M.M. (1991). Reorganization of somatosensory area 3b representations in adult owl monkey after digital syndactyly. *Journal of Neurophysiology, 66,* 1048-1058.

Anderson, R.A. (1988). Visual and visual-motor functions of the posterior parietal cortex. In P. Rakic, & W. Singer (Eds.). *Neurobiology of the neocortex.* London: John Wiley & Sons.

Asanuma, H., & Arissian, S. (1984). Experiments on functional role of peripheral input to motor cortex during voluntary movement in the monkey. *Journal of Neurophysiology, 52,* 212-227.

Asanuma, H., & Mackel, R. (1989). Direct and indirect sensory input pathways to the motor cortex: Its structure and function in relation to learning of motor skills. *Japanese Journal of Physiology, 39,* 1-19.

Barnes, K.J. (1986). Improving prehension skills of children with cerebral palsy: A clinical study. *Occupational Therapy Journal of Research, 6,* 227-240.

Barnes, K.J. (1989). Relationship of upper extremity weight bearing to hand skills of boys with cerebral palsy. *Occupational Therapy Journal of Research, 9,* 143-154.

Cooper, S. (1960). Muscle spindle and other muscle receptors. In G.H. Bourne (Ed.). *The structure and function of muscle.* New York: Academic Press.

Devandan, M.S., Ghosh, S., & John, K.T. (1983). A quantitative study of muscle spindle and tendon organs in the Bonnet monkey. *The Anatomical Record, 207,* 265-266.

Duffy, F.H., & Burchfiel, J.L. (1971). Somatosensory system: Organizational hierarchy from single units in monkey area 5. *Science, 172,* 273-275.

Gentilucci, M., Fogassi, L., Luppino, G., Matelli, M., Camarda, R., & Rizzolatti, G. (1988). Functional organization of inferior area 6 in the macaque monkey. *Experimental Brain Research, 71,* 475-490.

Heffner, R.S., & Masterton, R.B. (1983). The role of the corticospinal tract in the evolution of human digital dexterity. *Brain Behavior, 23,* 165-183.

Iwamura, Y., Tanaka, M., Sakamoto, M., & Hikosaka, O. (1985). Functional surface integration, submodality convergence, and tactile feature detection in area 2 of the monkey somatosensory cortex. In A.W. Goodwin, & I. Darian-Smith (Eds.). *Hand function and the neocortex.* New York: Springer-Verlag.

Jeannerod, M. (1984). The timing of natural prehension movements. *Journal of Motor Behavior, 16,* 235-254.

Jeannerod, M., Michel, F., & Prablanc, C. (1984). The control of hand movements in a case of hemianaesthesia following a parietal lesion. *Brain, 107,* 899-920.

Jenkins, W.M., Merzenich, M.M., Ochs, M.L., Allard T., & Guic-Robles, E. (1990). Functional reorganization of primary somatosensory cortex in adult owl monkeys after behaviorally controlled tactile stimulation. *Journal of Neurophysiology, 63,* 82-104.

Jones, E.G., & Powell, T.P. (1970). An anatomical study of converging sensory pathways within the cerebral cortex of the monkey, *Brain, 93,* 789-821.

Kuypers, H.G. (1962). Corticospinal connections: Postnatal development in the rhesus monkey. *Science, 138,* 678-680.

Kuypers, H.G. (1981). Anatomy of the descending pathways. In J.M. Brookhart, & V.B. Mountcastle (Eds.). *Handbook of physiology, Section I, Volume II: Motor control, Part 1.* Bethesda, Maryland: American Physiological Society.

Lawrence, D.G., & Hopkins, D.A. (1976). The development of motor control in the rhesus monkey: Evidence concerning the role of corticomotoneuronal connections. *Brain, 99,* 235-254.

Lawrence, D.G., & Kuypers, H.G. (1968a). The functional organization of the motor system in the monkey. I. The effects of bilateral pyramidal lesions. *Brain, 91,* 1-14.

Lawrence, D.G., & Kuypers, H.G. (1968b). The functional organization of the motor system in the monkey. II. The effect of lesions of the descending brain-stem pathways. *Brain, 91,* 15-36.

Lemon, R. (1981). Functional properties of monkey motor cortex neurons receiving afferent input from the hand and fingers. *Journal of Physiology, 31,* 497-519.

Lemon, R. (1990). Contributions to the history of psychology: LXVII. Henricus (Hans) Kuypers F.R.S. 1925-1989. *Perceptual and Motor Skills, 70,* 1283-1288.

Lemon, R., Bennett, K.M., & Werner, W. (1990). The cortico-motor substrate for skilled movements of the primate hand. In J. Requin, & G.E. Stelmack (Eds.). *Tutorials in motor neuroscience.* Boston: Kluwer Academic Press.

Matelli, M., Camarda, R., Glickstein, M., & Rizzolatti, G. (1986). Afferent and efferent projections of the inferior area 6 in the macaque monkey. *The Journal of Comparative Neurology, 251,* 281-289.

Mountcastle, V.B. (1981). Central nervous mechanisms in mechanoreceptive sensibility. In J.M. Brookhart, & V.B. Mountcastle (Eds.). *Handbook of physiology, Section I, Volume III: Motor control, Part 2.* Bethesda, Maryland: American Physiological Society.

Mountcastle, V.B., Lynch, J.C., Georgopoulos, A., Sakata, H., & Acuna, C. (1975). Posterior parietal association cortex of the monkey: Command functions for operations within extrapersonal space. *Journal of Neurophysiology, 38,* 871-908.

Muir, R.B. (1985). Small hand muscles in precision grip: A corticospinal prerogative. In A.W. Goodwin, & I. Darian-Smith (Eds.). *Hand function in the neocortex.* New York: Springer-Verlag.

Muir, R.B., & Lemon, R.N. (1983). Corticospinal neurons with a special role in precision grip. *Brain Research, 261,* 312-316.

Mushiake, H., Inase, M., & Tanji, J. (1991). Neuronal activity in the primate premotor, supplementary, and precentral motor cortex during visually guided and internally determined sequential movements. *Journal of Neurophysiology, 66,* 705-718.

Napier JR. (1962). The evolution of the hand. *Scientific American, 207,* 56–62.

Nudo, R.J., Jenkins, W.M., Merzenich, M.M., Prejean, T., & Grenda, R. (1992). Neurophysiological correlates of hand preference in primary motor cortex of adult squirrel monkeys. *Journal of Neuroscience, 12,* 2918-2947.

Passingham, R., Perry, H., & Wilkinson, F. (1978). Failure to develop a precision grip in monkeys with unilateral neocortical lesions made in infancy. *Brain Research, 145,* 410-414.

Pause, M., Kunesch, E., Binkofski, F., & Freund, H. (1989). Sensorimotor disturbances in patients with lesions of the parietal cortex. *Brain, 112,* 1599-1625.

Recanzone, G.H., Merzenich, M.M., Jenkins, W.M., Grajski, K.A., & Dinse, H.R. (1992). Topographic reorganization of the hand representation in cortical area 3b of owl monkeys trained in a frequency-discrimination task. *Journal of Neurophysiology, 67,* 1031-1056.

Rizzolatti, G., Camarda, R., Fogassi, L., Gentilucci, M., Luppino, G., & Matelli, M. (1988). Functional organization of inferior area 6 in the macaque monkey. II. Area F5 and the control of distal movements. *Experimental Brain Research, 71,* 491-507.

Rizzolatti, G., & Gentilucci, M. (1988). Motor and visual-motor functions of the premotor cortex. In

P. Rakic, & W. Singer (Eds.). *Neurobiology of the neocortex.* London: John Wiley & Sons.

Roland, P.E., Larsen, B., Lassen, N.A., & Skinhoj, E. (1980). Supplementary motor area and other cortical areas in organization of voluntary movements in man. *Journal of Neurophysiology, 43,* 118-136.

Rosen, I., & Asanuma, H. (1972). Peripheral afferent inputs to the forelimb area of the monkey cortex: Input-output relations. *Experimental Brain Research, 14,* 257-273.

Rothwell, J.C., Traub, M.M., Day, B.L., Obeso, J.A., Thomas, P.K., & Marsden, C.D. (1982). Manual motor performance in a deafferented man. *Brain, 105,* 515-542.

Sakamoto, T., Arissian, K., & Asanuma, H. (1989). Functional role of the sensory cortex in learning motor skills in cats. *Brain Research, 503,* 258-264.

Sakamoto, T., Porter, L., & Asanuma, H. (1987). Long-lasting potentiation of synaptic potentials in the motor cortex produced by stimulation of the sensory cortex in the cat: A basis of motor learning. *Brain Research, 413,* 360-364.

Sakata, H., & Iwamura, I. (1978). Cortical processing of tactile information in the first somatosensory and parietal association areas in the monkey. In G. Gordon (Ed.). *Active touch.* New York: Pergamon Press.

Sanes, J.N., Mauritz, K., Dalakas, M.C., & Evarts, E.V. (1985). Motor control in humans with large-fiber sensory neuropathy. *Human Neurobiology, 4,* 101-114.

Scheibel, A., Conrad, T., Perdue, S., Tomiyasu, U., & Wechsler, A. (1990). A quantitative study of dendrite complexity in selected areas of the human cerebral cortex. *Brain and Cognition, 12,* 85-101.

Spinelli, D.N., Jensen, F.E., & DiPrisco, G.V. (1980). Early experience effect on dendritic branching in normally reared kittens, *Experimental Neurology, 68,* 1-11.

Stein, J.F. (1989). Representation of egocentric space in the posterior parietal cortex. *Quarterly Journal of Experimental Physiology, 74,* 583-606.

Taira, M., Mine, S., Georgopoulos, A.P., Murata, A., & Sakata, H. (1990). Parietal cortex neurons of the monkey related to the visual guidance of hand movements. *Experimental Brain Research, 83,* 29-35.

Westling, G., & Johansson, R.S. (1984). Factors influencing the force control during precision grip. *Experimental Brain Research, 53,* 277-284.

2

Anatomy and Kinesiology of the Hand

James W. Strickland

EMBRYONIC DEVELOPMENT

**ANATOMY OF THE FULLY
DEVELOPED HAND**
Osseous Structures
Joints
Muscles and Tendons
Nerve Supply

FUNCTIONAL PATTERNS

One cannot expect to adequately understand the development and function of the hand and arm without a solid working knowledge of the intricate anatomic and kinesiologic relationships of the upper extremity, including the embryonic growth stages through which the extremity progresses. Only through comprehension of the normal formation and anatomy of the human hand can one adequately develop an appreciation for the disturbance in function that accompanies injury, disease, or dysfunction. It is appropriate, therefore, that an early chapter in a book devoted to development of fine motor coordination be concerned with the embryology, anatomy, kinesiology, and biomechanics of the hand. Since it is impossible in this chapter to review in great detail the enormous amount of literature that has been written about these fields of knowledge, readers are directed to the Suggested Readings.

EMBRYONIC DEVELOPMENT

Inspection of a normal newborn's hands never ceases to evoke awe and wonderment. The tiny

nails punctuating the ends of intricately formed fingers and opposable thumbs, each delicately marked with familiar patterns of joint wrinkles, immediately identify the newcomer as human. All of the ingredients that will eventually provide an unbelievably extensive continuum of function from exquisitely fine dexterity to great power are present in the tiny waving arms and hands. However, the normal embryonic process through which the upper extremities develop is both predictable and consistent (Arey, 1980; Bora, 1986; Bunnell, 1944; Moore, 1982).

Upper limb buds are discernible at 4 weeks of gestation. The scapula, humerus, radius, and ulna are apparent at 5 weeks as cartilage, and by 6 weeks upper arm, forearm, and hand divisions are present. Also at 6 weeks the webbed swellings of the three central digits appear and are soon followed by the two border digits. The metacarpals are present as cartilage, as are the proximal phalanges of the index through small fingers. Initially, each extremity is aligned longitudinally with the body trunk, but at 7 weeks the arms rotate outward and forward at the shoulder level to assume a hand-to-face position with the flexor surface of the forearm and hand turned inward toward the body and the extensor surface turned outward. Elbows and wrists are slightly flexed. Innervation of the limbs has already occurred at this point, and vessels extend to the distal extremity. Muscles, muscle groups, joint hollows, and digital cleavages, including thumb differentiation, are also present at 7 to 8 weeks. Webbing between the digits diminishes, and the fingers and thumb are independent of each other by 8 weeks. Carpal bones are cartilaginous, and the os centrale fuses

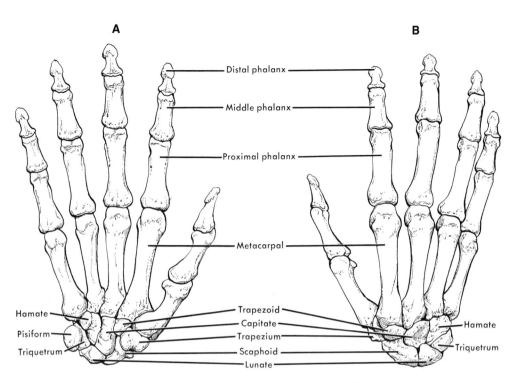

Figure 2-1. Bones of the right hand. **A,** Palmar surface. **B,** Dorsal surface.

(From Fess, E. E., & Phillips, C. A. [1987]. *Hand splinting: Principles and methods.* St. Louis: Mosby.)

to the scaphoid at 8 weeks. For the remainder of gestation after 8 weeks, limb changes primarily involve growth of already present structures.

ANATOMY OF THE FULLY DEVELOPED HAND

The anatomy of the hand must be approached in a systematic fashion with individual consideration of the osseous structures, joints, musculotendinous units, and nerve supply. However, it is obvious that the systems do not function independently, but that the integrated presence of all these structures is required for normal hand function. In presenting this material, we stray into the important mechanical and kinesiologic considerations that result from the unique anatomic arrangement of the hand and briefly try to indicate the problems resulting from various forms of pathologic conditions in certain areas.

Osseous Structures

The unique arrangement and mobility of the bones of the hand (Figure 2-1) provide a structural basis for its enormous functional adaptability. The osseous skeleton consists of eight carpal bones divided into two rows: the proximal row articu-

lates with the distal radius and ulna (with the exception of the pisiform, which lies palmar to and articulates with the triquetrum); the distal four carpal bones in turn articulate with the five metacarpals. Two phalanges complete the first ray, or thumb unit, and three phalanges each comprise the index, long, ring, and small fingers. These 27 bones, together with the intricate arrangement of supportive ligaments and contractile musculotendinous units, are arranged to provide both mobility and stability to the various joints of the hand. Although the exact anatomic configuration of the bones of the hand need not be memorized in detail, it is important to develop a knowledge of the position and names of the carpal bones, metacarpals, and phalanges and an understanding of their kinesiologic patterns to proceed with the management of many hand problems.

The bones of the hand are arranged in three arches (Figure 2-2), two transversely oriented and one that is longitudinal. The proximal transverse arch, the keystone of which is the capitate, lies at the level of the distal part of the carpus and is reasonably fixed, whereas the distal transverse arch passing through the metacarpal heads is more mobile. The two transverse arches are connected by the rigid portion of the longitudinal arch, consisting of the second and third metacarpals, the

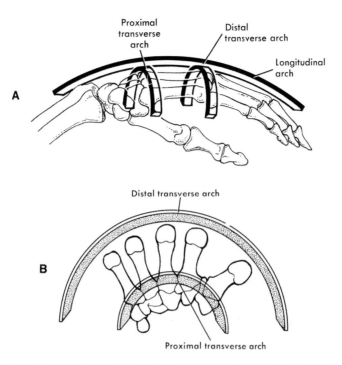

Figure 2-2. A, Skeletal arches of the hand. The proximal transverse arch passes through the distal carpus; the distal transverse arch through the metacarpal heads. The longitudinal arch is made up of the four digital rays and the carpus proximally. **B,** Proximal and distal transverse arches.

(From Fess, E. E., & Phillips, C. A. [1987]. *Hand splinting: Principles and methods.* St. Louis: Mosby.)

index and long fingers distally, and the central carpus proximally. The longitudinal arch is completed by the individual digital rays, and the mobility of the first, fourth, and fifth rays around the second and third allows the palm to flatten or cup itself to accommodate objects of various sizes and shapes.

To a large extent the intrinsic muscles of the hand are responsible for changes in the configuration of the osseous arches, and collapse in the arch system resulting from injury to the osseous skeleton, paralysis, or weakness of the intrinsic muscles can contribute to significant functional problems. Flatt (1972) has pointed out that grasp depends on the integrity of the mobile longitudinal arches and that, when dysfunction at the carpometacarpal joint, metacarpophalangeal joint, or proximal interphalangeal joint interrupts the integrity of these arches, lack of function and even crippling deformity may result.

Joints

The multiple complex articulations between the distal radius and ulna, the eight carpal bones, and the metacarpal bases comprise the wrist joint, whose proximal position makes it the functional

key to the motion at the more distal digital joints of the hand. Functionally the carpus transmits forces through the hand to the forearm. The proximal carpal row consisting of the scaphoid (navicular), lunate, and triquetrum articulates distally with the trapezium, trapezoid, capitate, and hamate; there is a complex motion pattern that relies both on ligamentous and contact surface constraints. The major ligaments of the wrist (Figure 2-3) are the palmar and intracapsular ligaments. There are three strong radial palmar ligaments: the radioscaphocapitate, or sling, ligament, which supports the waist of the scaphoid; the radiolunate ligament, which supports the lunate; and the radioscapholunate ligament, which connects the scapholunate articulation with the palmar portion of the distal radius. This ligament functions as a checkrein for the scaphoid flexion and extension. The ulnolunate ligament arises intraarticularly from the triangular articular meniscus of the wrist joint and inserts on the lunate and, to a lesser extent, the triquetrum. The radial and ulnar collateral ligaments are capsular ligaments, and V-shaped ligaments from the capitate to the triquetrum and scaphoid are known as the deltoid ligaments. Dorsally, the radiocarpal ligament connects the radius to the triquetrum and acts as a dorsal sling for the lunate, maintaining

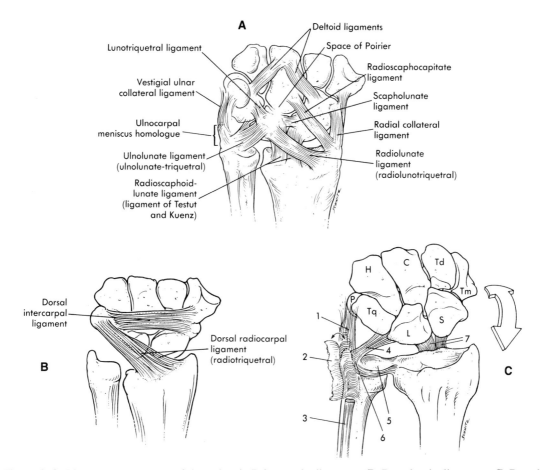

Figure 2-3. Ligamentous anatomy of the wrist. **A,** Palmar wrist ligaments. **B,** Dorsal wrist ligaments. **C,** Dorsal view of the flexed wrist, including the triangular fibrocartilage. *1,* Ulnar collateral ligament; *2,* retinacular sheath; *3,* tendon of extensor carpi ulnaris; *4,* ulnolunate ligament; *5,* triangular fibrocartilage; *6,* ulnocarpal meniscus homologue; *7,* palmar radioscaphoid lunate ligament. *P,* pisiform; *H,* hamate; *C,* capitate; *Td,* trapezoid; *Tm,* trapezium; *Tq,* triquetrum; *L,* lunate; *S,* scaphoid.

(From Fess, E. E., & Phillips, C. A. [1987]. *Hand splinting: Principles and methods.* St. Louis: Mosby.)

the lunate in apposition to the distal radius. Further dorsal carpal support is provided by the dorsal intracarpal ligament. These strong ligaments combine to provide carpal stability while permitting the normal range of wrist motion.

The distal ulna is covered with an articular cartilage (Figure 2-3, *C*) over its most dorsal, palmar, and radial aspects, where it articulates with the sigmoid or ulnar notch of the radius. The triangular fibrocartilage complex describes the ligamentous and cartilaginous structure that suspends the distal radius and ulnar carpus from the distal ulna. Blumfield and Champoux (1984) have indicated that the optimal functional wrist motion to accomplish most activities of daily living is from 10 degrees of flexion to 35 degrees of extension.

Taleisnik (1985) has emphasized the importance of considering the wrist in terms of longitudinal columns (Figure 2-4). The central, or flexion

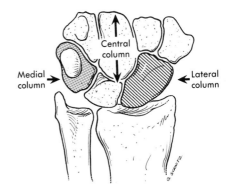

Figure 2-4. Columnar carpus. The scaphoid is the mobile or lateral column. The central, or flexion extension, column comprises the lunate and the entire distal carpal row. The medial, or rotational, column comprises the triquetrum alone.

(From Fess, E. E., & Phillips, C. A. [1987]. *Hand splinting: Principles and methods.* St. Louis: Mosby.)

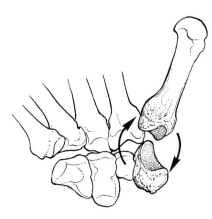

Figure 2-5. Saddle-shaped carpometacarpal joint of the thumb. A wide range of motion *(arrows)* is permitted by the configuration of this joint.

(From Fess, E. E., & Phillips, C. A. [1987]. *Hand splinting: Principles and methods.* St. Louis: Mosby.)

extension, column consists of the lunate and the entire distal carpal row; the lateral, or mobile, column comprises the scaphoid alone; and the medial, or rotation, column is made up of the triquetrum. Wrist motion is produced by the muscles that attach to the metacarpals, and the ligamentous control system provides stability only at the extremes of motion. The distal carpal row of the carpal bones is firmly attached to the hand and moves with it. Therefore during dorsiflexion the distal carpal row dorsiflexes, during palmar flexion it palmar flexes, and during radial and ulnar deviation it deviates radially or ulnarly. As the wrist ranges from radial to ulnar

deviation, the proximal carpal row rotates in a dorsal direction, and a simultaneous translocation of the proximal carpus occurs in a radial direction at the radiocarpal and midcarpal articulations. This combined motion of the carpal rows has been referred to as the rotational shift of the carpus. It was once taught that palmar flexion takes place to a greater extent at the radiocarpal joint and secondarily in the midcarpal joint, but, since dorsiflexion occurs primarily at the midcarpal joint and only secondarily at the radiocarpal articulation, this now appears to be a significant oversimplification. The complex carpal kinematics are beyond the scope of this chapter, and the reader is referred to the works of Weber (1982) and Taleisnik (1976) to gain a thorough understanding of this difficult subject.

The articulation between the base of the first metacarpal and the trapezium (Figure 2-5) is a highly mobile joint with a configuration thought to be similar to that of a saddle. The base of the first metacarpal is concave in the anteroposterior plane and convex in the lateral plane, with a reciprocal concavity in the lateral plane and an anteroposterior convexity on the opposing surface of the trapezium. This arrangement allows for the positioning of the thumb in a wide arc of motion (Figure 2-6), including flexion, extension, abduction, adduction, and opposition. The ligamentous arrangement about this joint, while permitting the wide circumduction, continues to provide stability at the extremes of motion, allowing the thumb to be brought into a variety of positions for pinch and

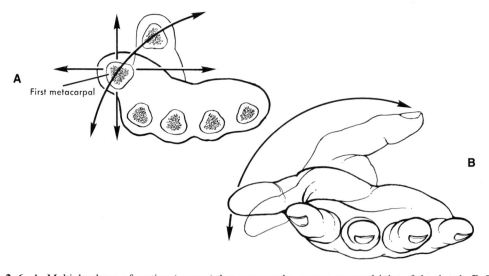

First metacarpal

A

B

Figure 2-6. A, Multiple planes of motion *(arrows)* that occur at the carpometacarpal joint of the thumb. **B,** The thumb moves *(arrow)* from a position of adduction against the second metacarpal to a position of extension abduction away from the hand and fingers and can then be rotated into positions of opposition and flexion.

(From Fess, E. E., & Phillips, C. A. [1987]. *Hand splinting: Principles and methods.* St. Louis: Mosby.)

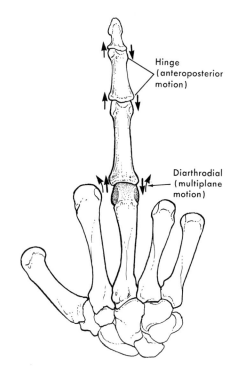

Figure 2-7. Joints of the phalanges. The diarthrodial configuration of the metacarpophalangeal joint permits motion in multiple planes, whereas the biconcave-convex hinge configuration of the interphalangeal joints restricts motion to the anteroposterior plane.

(From Fess, E. E., & Phillips, C. A. [1987]. *Hand splinting: Principles and methods.* St. Louis: Mosby.)

grasp but maintaining its stability during these functions. The articulations formed by the ulnar half of the hamate and the fourth and fifth metacarpal bases allow a modest amount of motion (15 degrees at the fourth carpometacarpal joint and 25 to 30 degrees of flexion and extension at the fifth carpometacarpal

joint). A resulting "palmar descent" of these metacarpals occurs during strong grasp.

The metacarpophalangeal joints of the fingers are diarthrodial joints with motion permitted in three planes and combinations thereof (Figure 2-7). The cartilaginous surfaces of the metacarpal head and the bases of the proximal phalanges are enclosed in a complex apparatus consisting of the joint capsule, collateral ligaments, and the anterior fibrocartilage or palmar plate (Figure 2-8). The capsule extends from the borders of the base of the proximal phalanx proximally to the head of the metacarpals beyond the cartilaginous joint surface. The collateral ligaments, which reinforce the capsule on each side of the metacarpophalangeal joints, run from the dorsolateral side of the metacarpal head to the palmar lateral side of the proximal phalanges. These ligaments form two bundles, the more central of which is referred to as the *cord portion of the collateral ligament* and inserts into the side of the proximal phalanx; the more palmar portion joins the palmar plate and is termed the *accessory collateral ligament*. These collateral ligaments are somewhat loose with the metacarpophalangeal joint in extension, allowing for considerable "play" in the side-to-side motion of the digits (Figure 2-9). With the metacarpophalangeal joints in full flexion, however, the cam configuration of the metacarpal head tightens the collateral ligaments and limits lateral mobility of the digits.

The palmar fibrocartilaginous plate on the palmar side of the metacarpophalangeal joint is firmly attached to the base of the proximal phalanx and loosely attached to the anterior surface of the neck of the metacarpal by means of the joint capsule at the neck of the metacarpal. This arrangement

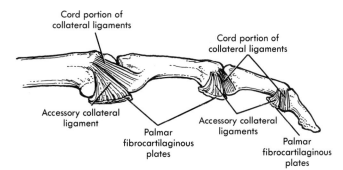

Figure 2-8. Ligamentous structures of the digital joints. The collateral ligaments of the metacarpophalangeal and interdigital joints are composed of a strong cord portion with bony origin and insertion. The more palmarly placed accessory collateral ligaments originate from the proximal bone and insert into the palmar fibrocartilaginous plate. The palmar plates have strong distal attachments to resist extension forces.

(From Fess, E. E., & Phillips, C. A. [1987]. *Hand splinting: Principles and methods.* St. Louis: Mosby.)

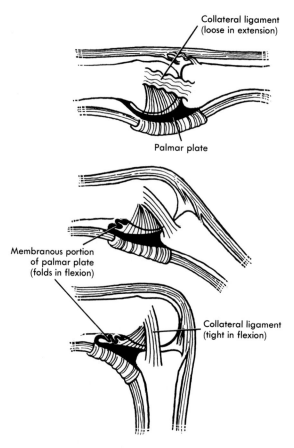

Figure 2-9. At the metacarpophalangeal joint level, the collateral ligaments are loose in extension but become tightened in flexion. The proximal membranous portion of the palmar plate moves proximally to accommodate for flexion.

(Modified from Wynn Parry, C.B., et al. [1973]. *Rehabilitation of the hand.* London: Butterworth.)

allows the palmar plate to slide proximally during metacarpophalangeal joint flexion. The flexor tendons pass along a groove anterior to the plate. The palmar plates are connected by the transverse intermetacarpal ligaments, which connect each plate to its neighbor.

The metacarpophalangeal joint of the thumb differs from the others in that the head of the first metacarpal is flatter, and its cartilaginous surface does not extend as far laterally or posteriorly. Two small sesamoid bones are also adjacent to this joint, and the ligamentous structure differs somewhat. A few degrees of abduction and rotation are permitted by the ligament arrangement of the metacarpophalangeal joint at the thumb, which is of considerable functional importance in delicate precision functions. There is considerable variation in the range of motion present at the thumb metacarpophalangeal joints. The amount of motion varies from as little as 30 degrees to as much as 90 degrees.

The digital interphalangeal joints are hinge joints (see Figure 2-7) and, like the metacarpophalangeal joints, have capsular and ligamentous enclosure. The articular surface of the proximal phalangeal head is convex in the anteroposterior plane with a depression in the middle between the two condyles, which articulates with the phalanx distal to it. The bases of the middle and distal phalanges appear as a concave surface with an elevated ridge dividing two concave depressions. A cord portion of the collateral ligament and an accessory collateral ligament are present, and the collateral ligaments run on each side of the joint from the dorsolateral aspect of the proximal phalanx in a palmar and lateral direction to insert into the distally placed phalanx and its fibrocartilage plate (Figure 2-10). A strong fibrocartilaginous (palmar) plate is also present, and the collateral ligaments of the proximal and distal interphalangeal joints are tightest with the joints in near full extension.

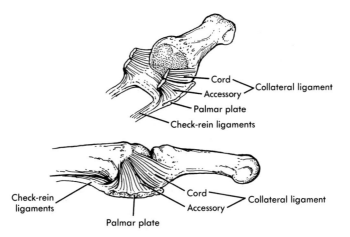

Figure 2-10. Strong, three-sided ligamentous support system of the proximal interphalangeal joint with cord and accessory collateral ligaments and the fibrocartilaginous plate, which is anchored proximally by the check-rein ligamentous attachment.

(Modified from Eaton, R.G., [1971]. *Joint injuries of the hand.* Springfield, Ill.: Charles C. Thomas.)

The stability of the proximal interphalangeal joint is ensured by a three-sided supporting cradle produced by the junction of the palmar plate with the base of the middle phalanx and the accessory collateral ligament structures (Figure 2-10). The confluence of ligaments is strongly anchored by proximal and lateral extensions referred to as the *checkrein ligaments.* This system has been described as a three-dimensional hinge that results in remarkable palmar and lateral restraint.

A wide range of pathologic conditions may result from the interruption or laxity of the supportive ligament system of the intercarpal or digital joints. At the wrist level, interruption or elongation of key radiocarpal or intercarpal ligaments may result in patterns of wrist instability that are often difficult to diagnose and treat. In the digits, disruption or elongation of the collateral ligaments or the fibrocartilaginous palmar plates will produce joint laxity, which is more obvious.

Muscles and Tendons

The muscles acting on the hand can be grouped as extrinsic, when their muscle bellies are in the forearm, or intrinsic, when the muscles originate distal to the wrist joint. It is important to thoroughly understand both systems. Although their contributions to hand function are distinctly different, the integrated function of both systems is important to the satisfactory performance of the hand in a wide variety of tasks. A schematic representation of the origin and insertion of the extrinsic flexor and extensor muscle tendon units

of the hand is provided in Figure 2-11. The important nerve supply to each muscle group is reviewed in this figure and again when discussing the nerve supply to the upper extremity.

Extrinsic Muscles

The extrinsic flexor muscles (Figure 2-11) of the forearm form a prominent mass on the medial side of the upper part of the forearm: the most superficial group comprises the pronator teres, the flexor carpi radialis, the flexor carpi ulnaris, and the palmaris longus; the intermediate group the flexor digitorum superficialis; and the deep extrinsics the flexor digitorum profundus and the flexor pollicis longus. The pronator, palmaris, wrist flexors, and superficialis tendons arise from the area about the medial epicondyle, the ulnar collateral ligament of the elbow, and the medial aspect of the coronoid process. The flexor pollicis longus originates from the entire middle third of the palmar surface of the radius and the adjacent interosseous membrane, and the flexor digitorum profundus originates deep to the other muscles of the forearm from the proximal two thirds of the ulna on the palmar and medial side. The deepest layer of the palmar forearm is completed distally by the pronator quadratus muscle.

The flexor carpi radialis tendon inserts on the base of the second metacarpal, whereas the flexor carpi ulnaris inserts into both the pisiform and fifth metacarpal base. The superficialis tendons lie superficial to the profundus tendons as far as the digital bases, where they bifurcate and wrap around the profundi and rejoin over the distal half

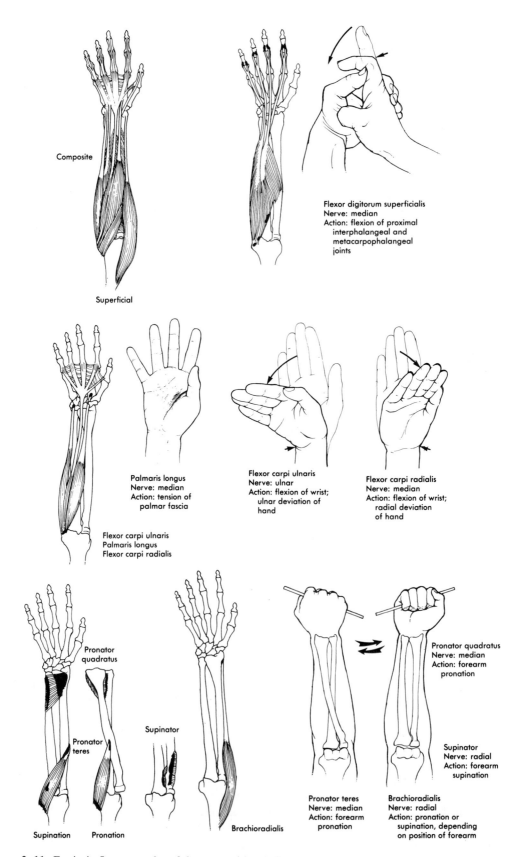

Composite

Superficial

Flexor digitorum superficialis
Nerve: median
Action: flexion of proximal
    interphalangeal and
    metacarpophalangeal
    joints

Palmaris longus
Nerve: median
Action: tension of
    palmar fascia

Flexor carpi ulnaris
Palmaris longus
Flexor carpi radialis

Flexor carpi ulnaris
Nerve: ulnar
Action: flexion of wrist;
    ulnar deviation of
    hand

Flexor carpi radialis
Nerve: median
Action: flexion of wrist;
    radial deviation
    of hand

Pronator
quadratus

Pronator
teres

Supinator

Supination   Pronation

Brachioradialis

Pronator quadratus
Nerve: median
Action: forearm
    pronation

Supinator
Nerve: radial
Action: forearm
    supination

Pronator teres
Nerve: median
Action: forearm
    pronation

Brachioradialis
Nerve: radial
Action: pronation or
    supination, depending
    on position of forearm

Figure 2-11. Extrinsic flexor muscles of the arm and hand. (Dark areas represent origins and insertions of muscles.)

(Modified from Marble, H.C. [1960]. *The hand, a manual and atlas for the general surgeon.* Philadelphia: W.B. Saunders.)   *Continued.*

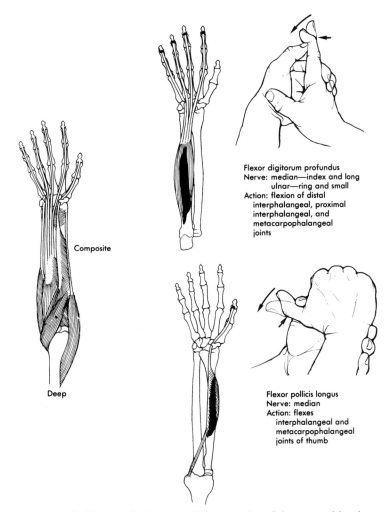

Flexor digitorum profundus
Nerve: median—index and long
        ulnar—ring and small
Action: flexion of distal
    interphalangeal, proximal
    interphalangeal, and
    metacarpophalangeal
    joints

Composite

Deep

Flexor pollicis longus
Nerve: median
Action: flexes
    interphalangeal and
    metacarpophalangeal
    joints of thumb

Figure 2-11, *cont'd.* Extensive flexor muscles of the arm and hand.

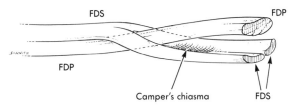

FDS   FDP

FDP

SCHNITZ

FDP

Camper's chiasma   FDS

Figure 2-12. Anatomy of the relationship between the flexor digitorum superficialis *(FDS),* flexor digitorum profundus *(FDP),* and the proximal portion of the flexor tendon sheath. The superficialis tendon divides and passes around the profundus tendon to reunite at Camper's chiasma. The tendon once again divides prior to insertion on the base of the middle phalanx.

(From Fess, E. E., & Phillips, C. A. [1987] *Hand splinting: Principles and methods.* St. Louis: Mosby.)

of the proximal phalanx as Camper's chiasma (see Figure 2-11). The superficialis tendon again splits for a dual insertion on the proximal half of the middle phalanges (Figure 2-12). The profundi continue through the superficialis decussation to insert on the base of the distal phalanx. The flexor pollicis longus inserts on the base of the distal phalanx of the thumb.

At the wrist the nine long flexor tendons enter the carpal tunnel beneath the protective roof of the deep transverse carpal ligament in company with the median nerve. In this canal the common profundus tendon to the long, ring, and small fingers divides into the individual tendons that fan out distally and proceed toward the distal phalanges of these digits (Figure 2-13). At approximately

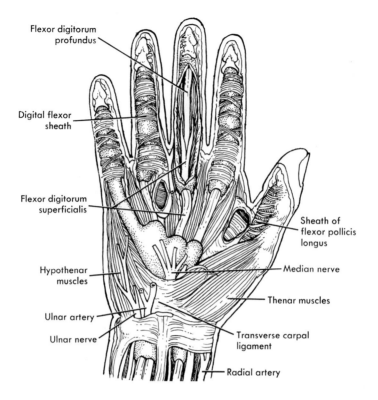

Figure 2-13. Flexor tendons in the palm and digits. Fibroosseous digital sheaths with their pulley arrangement are shown, as is a division of the superficialis tendon about the profundus in the proximal portion of the sheath.

(From Fess, E. E., & Phillips, C. A. [1987]. *Hand splinting: Principles and methods.* St. Louis: Mosby.)

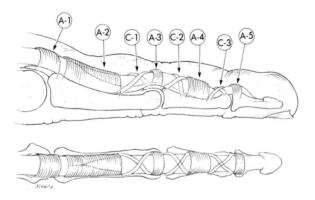

Figure 2-14. Components of the digital flexor sheath. The sturdy annular pulleys *(A)* are important biomechanically in guaranteeing the efficient digital motion by keeping the tendons closely applied to the phalanges. The thin pliable cruciate pulleys *(C)* permit the flexor sheath to be flexible while maintaining its integrity.

(Modified from Doyle, J.R., & Blythe, W. [1975]. In *American Academy of Orthopaedic Surgeons: Symposium on tendon surgery in the hand.* St. Louis: C.V. Mosby.)

the level of the distal palmar crease the paired profundus and superficialis tendons to the index, long, ring, and small fingers and the flexor pollicis longus to the thumb enter the individual flexor sheaths that house them throughout the remainder of their digital course. These sheaths with their predictable annular pulley arrangement (Figure 2-14) not only serve as a protective housing for the flexor tendons but also provide a smooth gliding

surface by virtue of their synovial lining and an efficient mechanism to hold the tendons close to the digital bone and joints. There is an increasing recognition that disruption of this valuable pulley system can produce substantial mechanical alterations in digital function, resulting in imbalance and deformity.

Extension of the wrist and fingers is produced by the extrinsic extensor muscle tendon system, which consists of the two radial wrist extensors, the extensor carpi ulnaris, the extensor digitorum communis, and the extensor digiti quinti proprius (extensor digiti minimi) (Figure 2-15). These muscles originate in common from the lateral epicondyle and the lateral epicondylar ridge and from a small area posterior to the radial notch of the ulna. The brachioradialis originates from the epicondylar line proximal to the lateral epicondyle, and, because it inserts on the distal radius, it does not truly contribute to wrist or digit motion. The extensor carpi radialis longus and brevis insert proximally on the bases of the second and third metacarpals, respectively, and the extensor carpi ulnaris inserts on the base of the fifth metacarpal. The long digital extensors terminate by insertions on the bases of the middle phalanges after receiving and giving fibers to the intrinsic tendons to form the lateral bands that are destined to insert on the bases of the distal phalanx. Digital extension, therefore, results from a combination of the contribution of both the extrinsic and intrinsic extensor systems. The extensor pollicis longus and brevis tendons, together with the abductor pollicis longus, originate from the dorsal forearm and, by virtue of their respective insertions into the distal phalanx, proximal phalanx, and first metacarpal of the thumb, provide extension at all three levels. The extensor pollicis longus approaches the thumb obliquely around a small bony tubercle on the dorsal radius (Lister's tubercle) and therefore functions not only as an extensor but as a strong secondary adductor of the thumb. The extensor indicis proprius also originates more distally than the extensor communis tendons from an area near the origin of the thumb extensor and long abductor. It lies on the ulnar aspect of the communis tendon to the index finger and inserts with it in the dorsal approaches of that digit. The extensor digiti quinti proprius arises near the lateral epicondyle to occupy a superficial position on the dorsum of the forearm with its paired tendons lying on the fifth metacarpal ulnar to the communis tendon to the fifth finger. It inserts into the extensor apparatus of that digit.

At the wrist the extensor tendons are divided into six dorsal compartments (Figure 2-16). The first compartment consists of the tendons of the abductor pollicis longus and extensor pollicis brevis, and the second compartment houses the two radial wrist extensors, the extensor carpi radialis longus and brevis. The third compartment is composed of the tendon of the extensor pollicis longus, and the fourth compartment allows passage of the four communis extensor tendons and the extensor indicis proprius tendon. The extensor digiti quinti proprius travels through the fifth dorsal compartment, and the sixth houses the extensor carpi ulnaris.

Intrinsic Muscles

The important intrinsic musculature of the hand can be divided into muscles comprising the thenar eminence, those comprising the hypothenar eminence, and the remaining muscles between the two groups (Figure 2-17). The muscles of the thenar eminence consist of the abductor pollicis brevis, the flexor pollicis brevis, and the opponens pollicis, which originate in common from the transverse carpal ligament and the scaphoid and trapezium bones. The abductor brevis inserts into the radial side of the proximal phalanx and the radial wing tendon of the thumb, as does the flexor pollicis brevis, whereas the opponens inserts into the whole radial side of the first metacarpal.

The flexor pollicis brevis has a superficial portion that is innervated by the median nerve and a deep portion that arises from the ulnar side of the first metacarpal and is often innervated by the ulnar nerve. The hypothenar eminence in a similar manner is made up of the abductor digiti quinti, the flexor digiti quinti brevis, and the opponens digiti quinti, which originate primarily from the pisiform bone and the pisohamate ligament and insert into the joint capsule of the fifth metacarpophalangeal joint, the ulnar side of the base of the proximal phalanx of the fifth finger, and the ulnar border of the aponeurosis of this digit. The strong thenar musculature is responsible for the ability to position the thumb in opposition so that it may meet the adjacent digits for pinch and grasp functions, whereas the hypothenar group allows a similar but less pronounced rotation of the fifth metacarpal.

Of the seven interosseous muscles (Figure 2-18), four are considered in the dorsal group (Figure 2-18, *B*) and three as palmar interossei (Figure 2-18, *C*). The four dorsal interossei originate from the adjacent sides of the metacarpal bones and, because of their bipinnate nature with two individual muscle bellies, have separate insertions into the tubercle and the lateral aspect of the proximal phalanges and into the extensor expansion. The more palmarly placed three palmar interossei (Figure 2-18, *C*) have similar insertions and origins and are responsible for adducting the digits together, as opposed to the spreading or abducting function of the dorsal interossei. In

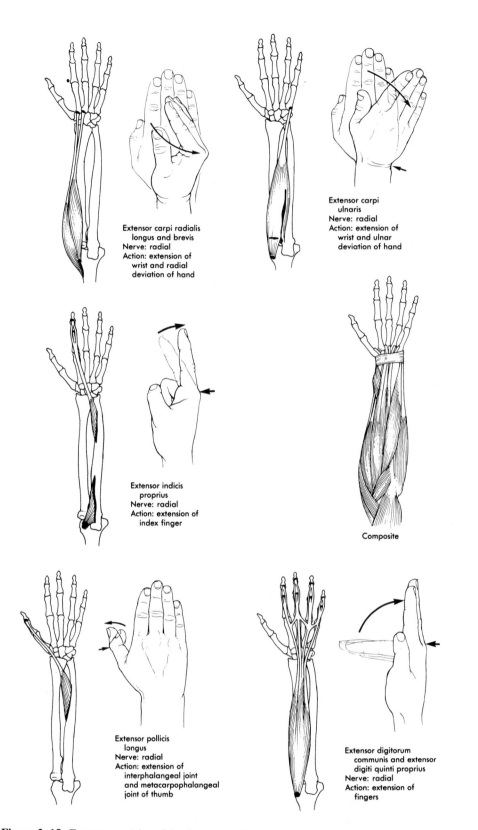

Extensor carpi radialis
longus and brevis
Nerve: radial
Action: extension of
wrist and radial
deviation of hand

Extensor carpi
ulnaris
Nerve: radial
Action: extension of
wrist and ulnar
deviation of hand

Extensor indicis
proprius
Nerve: radial
Action: extension of
index finger

Composite

Extensor pollicis
longus
Nerve: radial
Action: extension of
interphalangeal joint
and metacarpophalangeal
joint of thumb

Extensor digitorum
communis and extensor
digiti quinti proprius
Nerve: radial
Action: extension of
fingers

Figure 2-15. Extensor muscles of the forearm and hand.

(Modified from Marble, H.C. [1960]. *The hand, a manual and atlas for the general surgeon.* Philadelphia: W.B. Saunders.)

Continued.

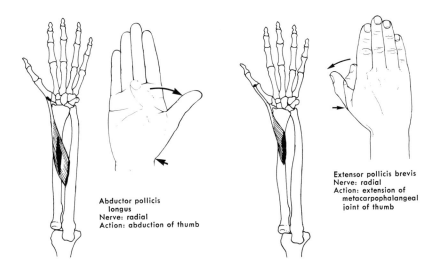

Extensor pollicis brevis
Nerve: radial
Action: extension of
    metacarpophalangeal
    joint of thumb

Abductor pollicis
longus
Nerve: radial
Action: abduction of thumb

Figure 2-15, *cont'd.* Extensor muscles of the forearm and hand.

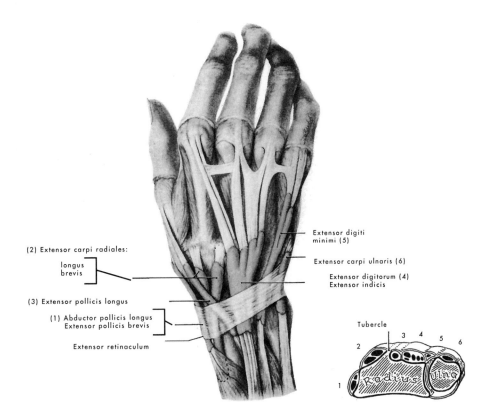

Extensor digiti
minimi (5)

Extensor carpi ulnaris (6)

Extensor digitorum (4)
Extensor indicis

(2) Extensor carpi radiales:

longus
brevis

(3) Extensor pollicis longus

(1) Abductor pollicis longus
Extensor pollicis brevis

Extensor retinaculum

Tubercle

Figure 2-16. Arrangement of the extensor tendons in the compartments of the wrist.

(Modified from Moore, K. L. [1980]. *Clinical human anatomy.* Baltimore: Williams & Wilkins.)

addition, four lumbrical tendons (Figure 2-19, *A*) arising from the radial side of the palmar portion of the flexor digitorum profundus tendons pass through their individual canals on the radial side of the digits to provide an additional contribution to the complex extensor assemblage of the digits. The arrangement of the extensor mechanism, in-cluding the transverse sagittal band fibers at the metacarpophalangeal joint and the components of the extensor hood mechanism that gain fibers from both the extrinsic and intrinsic tendons, can be seen in Figure 2-19, *B* and *C*.

An oversimplification of the function of the intrinsic musculature in the digits would be that

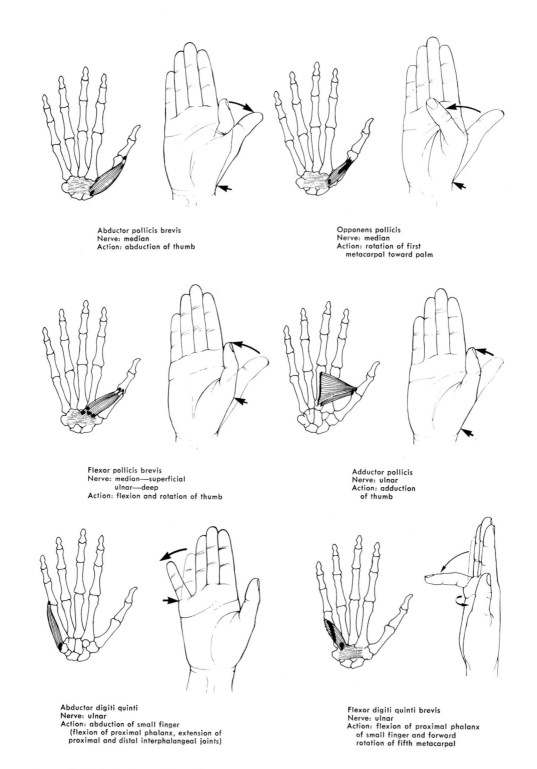

Abductor pollicis brevis
Nerve: median
Action: abduction of thumb

Opponens pollicis
Nerve: median
Action: rotation of first
        metacarpal toward palm

Flexor pollicis brevis
Nerve: median—superficial
        ulnar—deep
Action: flexion and rotation of thumb

Adductor pollicis
Nerve: ulnar
Action: adduction
        of thumb

Abductor digiti quinti
Nerve: ulnar
Action: abduction of small finger
        (flexion of proximal phalanx, extension of
        proximal and distal interphalangeal joints)

Flexor digiti quinti brevis
Nerve: ulnar
Action: flexion of proximal phalanx
        of small finger and forward
        rotation of fifth metacarpal

Figure 2-17. Intrinsic muscles of the hand.

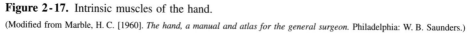

(Modified from Marble, H. C. [1960]. *The hand, a manual and atlas for the general surgeon.* Philadelphia: W. B. Saunders.)

Continued.

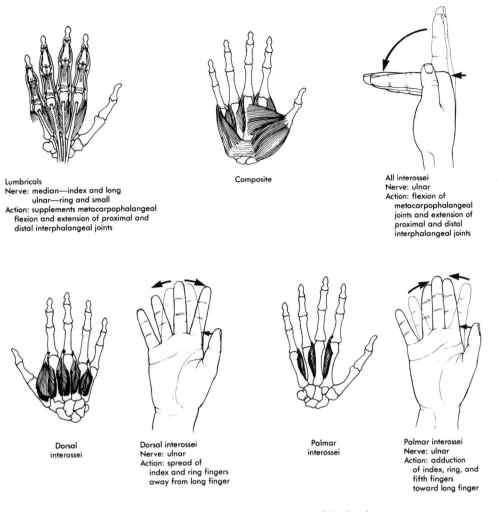

Lumbricals
Nerve: median—index and long
        ulnar—ring and small
Action: supplements metacarpophalangeal
        flexion and extension of proximal and
        distal interphalangeal joints

Composite

All interossei
Nerve: ulnar
Action: flexion of
        metacarpophalangeal
        joints and extension of
        proximal and distal
        interphalangeal joints

Dorsal
interossei

Dorsal interossei
Nerve: ulnar
Action: spread of
        index and ring fingers
        away from long finger

Palmar
interossei

Palmar interossei
Nerve: ulnar
Action: adduction
        of index, ring, and
        fifth fingers
        toward long finger

Figure 2-17, *cont'd.* Intrinsic muscles of the hand.

they provide strong flexion at the metacarpophalangeal joints and extension at the proximal and distal interphalangeal joints. The lumbrical tendons, by virtue of their origin from the flexor profundi and insertion into the digital extensor mechanism, function as a governor between the two systems, resulting in a loosening of the antagonistic profundus tendon during interphalangeal joint extension. The interossei are further responsible for spreading and closing of the fingers and, together with the extrinsic flexor and extensor tendons, are invaluable to digital balance. A composite, well-integrated pattern of digital flexion and extension is reliant on the smooth performance of both systems, and a loss of intrinsic function will result in severe deformity.

Perhaps the most important intrinsic muscle, the adductor pollicis (see Figure 2-18, *A*), originates from the third metacarpal and inserts on the ulnar side of the base of the proximal phalanx of the thumb and into the ulnar wing expansion of the extensor mechanism. This muscle, by virtue of its strong adducting influence on the thumb and its stabilizing effect on the first metacarpophalangeal joint, functions together with the first dorsal interosseous to provide strong pinch. The adductor pollicis, deep head of the flexor pollicis brevis, ulnar two lumbricals, and all interossei, as well as the hypothenar muscle group, are innervated by the ulnar nerve. Ulnar nerve function has a profound influence on hand function.

Muscle Balance and Biomechanical Considerations

When there is normal resting tone in the extrinsic and intrinsic muscle groups of the forearm and hand, the wrist and digital joints will be maintained in a balanced position. With the forearm midway between pronation and supination, the wrist dorsiflexed, and the digits in moderate flexion, the hand is in the optimum position from which to function.

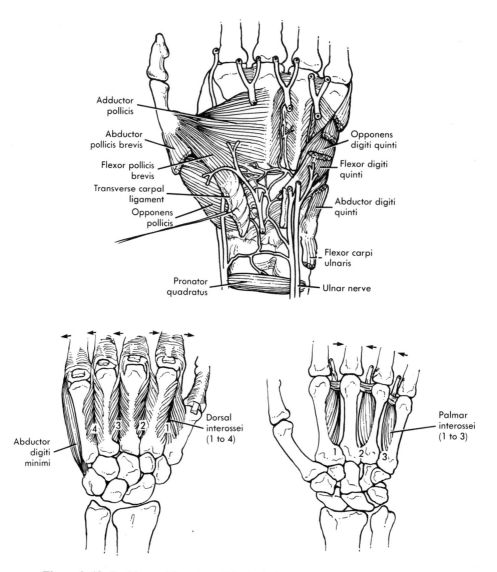

Figure 2-18. Position and function of the intrinsic muscles of the hand.

(Modified from Lampe, E.W. [1969]. In *Clinical Symposia,* New York: CIBA, illustrated by F. H. Netter.)

It may be seen that muscles are usually arranged about joints in pairs so that each musculotendious unit has at least one antagonistic muscle to balance the involved hoint. To a large extent the wrist is the key joint and has a strong influence on the long extrinsic muscle performance at the digital level. Maximal digital flexion strength is facilitated by dorsiflexion of the wrist, which lessens the effective amplitude of the antagonistic extensor tendons while maximizing the contractural force of the digital flexors. Conversely, a posture of wrist flexion will markedly weaken grasping power.

At the digital level, metacarpophalangeal joint flexion is a combination of extrinsic flexor power supplemented by the contribution of the intrinsic muscles, whereas proximal interphalangeal joint extension results from a combination of extrinsic extensor and intrinsic muscle power. At the distal interphalangeal joint the intrinsic muscles provide a majority of the extensor power necessary to balance the antagonistic flexor digitorum profundus tendon.

Nerve Supply

In considering the nerve supply to the forearm, hand, and wrist, it is important to realize that these nerves are a direct continuation of the brachial plexus and that at least a working knowledge of the multiple ramifications of the plexus is necessary if one is to fully appreciate the more distal

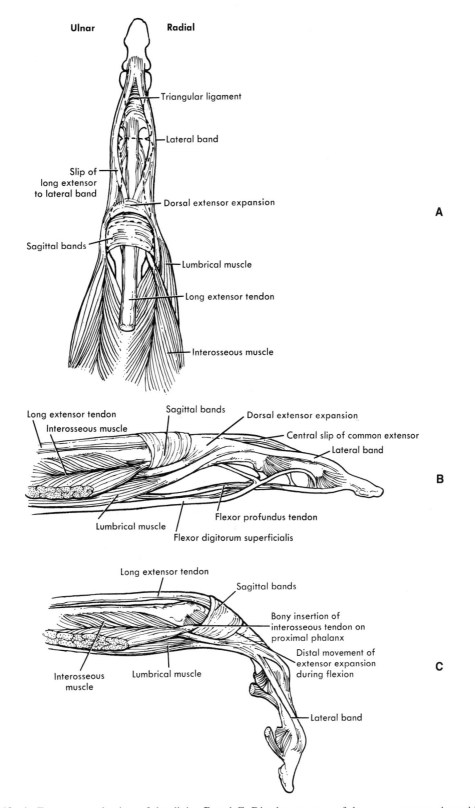

Ulnar   **Radial**

Triangular ligament

Lateral band

Slip of
long extensor
to lateral band

Dorsal extensor expansion

A

Sagittal bands

Lumbrical muscle

Long extensor tendon

Interosseous muscle

Long extensor tendon   Sagittal bands   Dorsal extensor expansion
Interosseous muscle   Central slip of common extensor
                                           Lateral band

B

Lumbrical muscle   Flexor profundus tendon
                 Flexor digitorum superficialis

Long extensor tendon
                        Sagittal bands
                        Bony insertion of
                        interosseous tendon on
                        proximal phalanx
                        Distal movement of
                        extensor expansion
                        during flexion

C

Interosseous   Lumbrical muscle
muscle
                        Lateral band

Figure 2-19. **A,** Extensor mechanism of the digits. **B** and **C,** Distal movement of the extensor expansion with metacarpophalangeal joint flexion is shown.

(Modified from Lampe, E. W. [1969]. In *Clinical Symposia,* New York: CIBA, illustrated by F. H. Netter.)

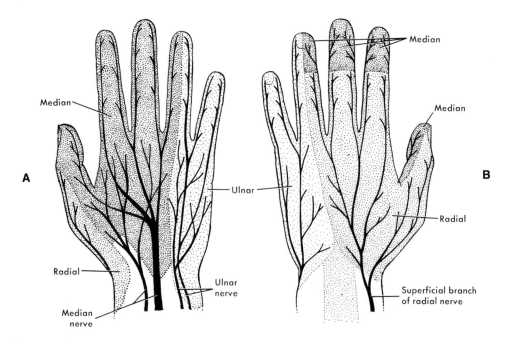

Figure 2-20. Cutaneous distribution of the nerves of the hand. **A,** Palmar surface. **B,** Dorsal surface.

(From Fess, E. E., & Phillips, C. A. [1987]. *Hand splinting: Principles and methods.* St. Louis: Mosby.)

motor and sensory contributions of the nerves of the upper extremity. Injuries at either the spinal cord or plexus level or to the major peripheral nerves in the upper extremity result in a substantial functional impairment.

The median, ulnar, and radial nerves, as well as the terminal course of the musculocutaneous, are responsible for the sensory and motor transmission to the forearm, wrist, and hand. The superficial sensory distribution is shared by the median, radial, and ulnar nerves in a fairly constant pattern (Figure 2-20). This chapter is concerned with the most frequent distribution of these nerves, although it is acknowledged that variations are common.

The palmar side of the hand from the thumb to a line passed longitudinally from the tip of the ring finger to the wrist receives sensory innervation from the median nerve. The remainder of the palm as well as the ulnar half of the ring finger and the entire small finger receive sensory innervation from the ulnar nerve. On the dorsal side the ulnar nerve distribution again includes the ulnar half of the dorsal hand and the ring and small fingers, whereas the radial side is supplied by the superficial branch of the radial nerve. Some innervation to an area distal to the proximal interphalangeal joints is supplied by the palmar digital nerves originating from the median nerve. The area around the dorsum of the thumb over the metacar-

pophalangeal joint is frequently supplied by the end branches of the lateral antebrachial cutaneous nerve.

The extrinsic and intrinsic musculature of the forearm and hand is supplied by the median, ulnar, and radial nerves (Figure 2-21). The long wrist and digital flexors, with the exception of the flexor carpi ulnaris and the profundi to the ring and small fingers, are all supplied by the median nerve. The pronators of the forearm and the muscles of the thenar eminence, with the exception of the deep head of the flexor pollicis brevis and the adductor pollicis, which are innervated by the ulnar nerve, are also supplied by the median nerve. All muscles of the hypothenar eminence, all interossei, the third and fourth lumbrical muscles, the deep head of the flexor pollicis brevis, the adductor pollicis brevis, as well as the flexor carpi ulnaris and the ulnarmost two profundi, are supplied by the ulnar nerve. The radial nerve supplies all long extensors of the hand and wrist as well as the long abductor and short extensor of the thumb and the brachioradialis.

When considering sensibility, one should remember that the hand is an extremely important organ for the detection and transmission to the brain of information relating to the size, weight, texture, and temperature of objects with which it comes in contact. The types of cutaneous sensation have been defined as touch, pain, hot, and cold.

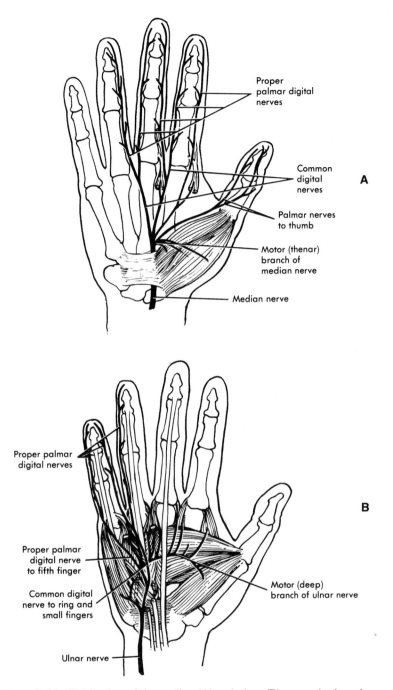

Figure 2-21. Distribution of the median (**A**) and ulnar (**B**) nerves in the palm.
(From Fess, E. E., & Phillips, C. A. [1987]. *Hand splinting: Principles and methods.* St. Louis: Mosby.)

Although most of the nervous tissue in the skin is found in the dermal network, smaller branches course through the subcutaneous tissue following blood vessels. Several types of sensory receptors have been described, and in most areas of the hand there is an interweaving of nerve fibers that allows each area to receive nerve input from several sources. In addition, deep sensibility from nerve

endings in muscles and tendons is important in the recognition of joint position. Moberg (1958) described the hand as being blind when sensation is impaired or absent. Even in the presence of normal motor function, parts of a hand that lack normal sensation are poorly used or avoided entirely in favor of normally innervated segments. Inspection of the skin for dryness and lack of callus formation helps identify potential sensibility problems. Testing with the Semmes-Weinstein monofilaments further defines areas of sensibility pathology (Bell-Krotoski, 1990).

FUNCTIONAL PATTERNS

The prehensile function of the hand depends on the integrity of the kinetic chain of bones and joints extending from the wrist to the distal phalanges. Interruptions of the transverse and longitudinal arch systems formed by these structures will always result in instability, deformity, or functional loss at a more proximal or distal level. Similarly, the balanced synergism-antagonism relationship between the long extrinsic muscles and the intrinsic muscles is a requisite for the composite functions required for both power and precision functions of the hand. It is important to recognize that the hand cannot function well without normal sensory input from all areas.

Many attempts have been made to classify the different patterns of hand function, and various types of grasp and pinch have been described. Perhaps the more simplified analysis of power grasp and precision handling as proposed by Napier (1956) and refined by Flatt (1972) is the easiest to consider.

As generally stated, power grip is a combination of strong thumb flexion and adduction with the powerful flexion of the ring and small fingers on the ulnar side of the hand. The radial half of the hand employing the delicate tripod of pinch between the thumb, index, and long fingers is responsible for more delicate precision function.

An analysis of hand functions requires that one consider the thumb and the remainder of the hand as two separate parts. Rotation of the thumb into an opposing position is a requirement of almost any hand function, whether it be strong grasp or delicate pinch. The wide range of motion permitted at the carpometacarpal joint is extremely important in allowing the thumb to be correctly positioned. Stability at this joint is a requirement of almost all prehensile activities and is ensured by a unique ligamentous arrangement, which allows mobility in the midposition and provides stability at the extremes. As can be seen in Figure 2-22, the thumb moves through a wide arc from the side of the index finger tip to the tip of the small finger, and the adaptation that occurs between the thumb and digits as progressively smaller objects are held occurs primarily at the metacarpophalangeal joints of the digits and the carpometacarpal joint of the thumb.

For power grip the wrist is in an extended position that allows the extrinsic digital flexors to press the object firmly against the palm while the thumb is closed tightly around the object. The thumb, ring, and small fingers are the most important participants in this strong grasp function, and the importance of the ulnar border digits cannot be minimized (Figure 2-23). In a power grip all the extrinsic muscles of the hand are involved along with the muscles of the thenar eminence and the interossei (Long et al., 1970).

In precision grasp, wrist position is less important, and the thumb is opposed to the semiflexed fingers with the intrinsic tendons providing most of the finger movement. Compression force is primarily provided by the extrinsic muscles assisted by the interossei, flexor pollicis brevis, and adductor pollicis. The opponens assists through rotation of the first metacarpal (Long et al., 1970). With soft opposition of the thumb to the fingers, the opponens pollicis is the most active of the thenar muscles and the flexor pollicis brevis the least active (Basmajian, 1980). When a small object is held by the pads of the fingers and the thumb and rotated, the interossei impose the necessary rotation force on the object. If, instead, the held object is moved away from the palm, as in threading a needle, the interossei and the lumbrical are active and provide intrinsic compression, metacarpophalangeal flexion, and interphalanageal extension. If the object is moved back toward the palm, the lumbricals are silent and the interossei provide intrinsic compression and rotation forces (Long et al., 1970).

When the intrinsic muscles are paralyzed, the balance of each finger is markedly disturbed. The metacarpophalangeal joint loses its primary flexors, and the interphalangeal joints lose the intrinsic contribution to extension. A dyskinetic finger flexion results in which the metacarpophalangeal joints lag behind the interphalangeal joints in flexion. When the hand is closed on an object, only the fingertips make contact rather than the uniform contact of the fingers, palm, and thumb that occurs with normal grip (Figure 2-24).

Certain activities may require combinations of power and precision grips, as seen in Figure 2-25. Pinching between the thumb and the combined index and long fingers is a further refinement of precision grip and may be classified as either tip grip, palmar grip, or lateral grip (Figure 2-26), depending on the portions of the phalanges brought to bear on the object being handled. In these functions the strong contracture of the adductor pollicis brings the thumb into contact

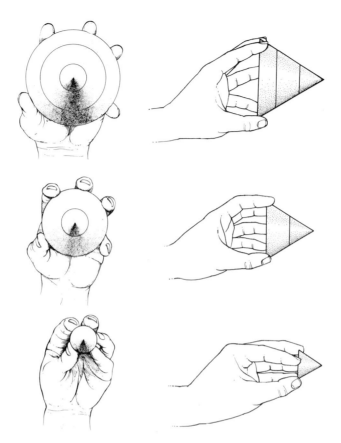

Figure 2-22. Progressive alterations in precision grasp with changes in object size. Adaptation takes place primarily at the carpometacarpal joint of the thumb and the metacarpophalangeal joints of the digits.

(From Fess, E. E., & Phillips, C. A. [1987]. *Hand splinting: Principles and methods.* St. Louis: Mosby.)

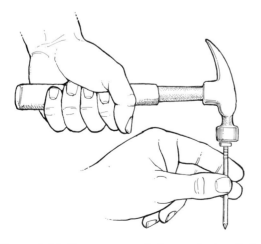

Figure 2-23. Strong power grip imparted primarily by the thumb, ring, and small fingers around the hammer handle with delicate precision tip grip employed to hold the nail.

(From Fess, E. E., & Phillips, C. A. [1987]. *Hand splinting: Principles and methods.* St. Louis: Mosby.)

against the tip or sides of the index or index and long fingers with digital resistance imparted by the first and second dorsal interossei. The size of the object being handled dictates whether large thumb and digital surfaces, as in palmar grip, or smaller surfaces, as in lateral or tip grasp, are utilized.

The patterns of action of the normal hand depend on the mobility of the skeletal arches, and alterations of the configuration of these arches is produced by the balanced function of the extrinsic and intrinsic muscles. Whereas the extrinsic contribution resulting from the large powerful forearm muscle groups is more important to hand strength, the fine precision action imparted by the intrinsic musculature gives the hand an enormous variety of capabilities. Although one need not specifically memorize the various patterns of pinch, grasp, and combined hand functions, it is important to understand the underlying contribution of the various muscle-tendon groups, both extrinsic and intrinsic, to these activities.

Figure 2-24. A, Normal hand grasping a cylinder. Uniform areas of palm and digital contact are shaded. **B,** Intrinsic minus (claw hand grasping the same cylinder). The area of contact is limited to the fingertips and the metacarpal heads.

(From Brand, P. W. [1985]. *Clinical mechanics of the hand.* St. Louis: C. V. Mosby.)

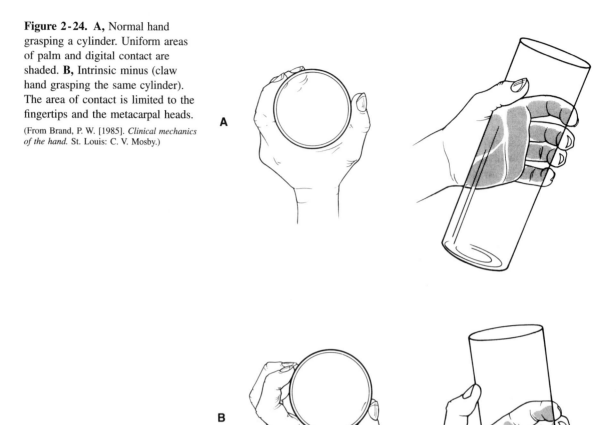

A

B

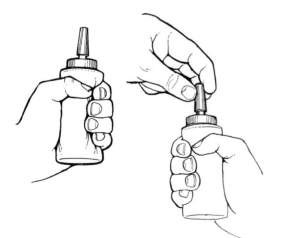

Figure 2-25. Power grip used to hold the squeeze bottle with precision handling of the bottle top by the opposite hand.

(From Fess, E. E., & Phillips, C. A. [1987]. *Hand splinting: Principles and methods.* St. Louis: Mosby.)

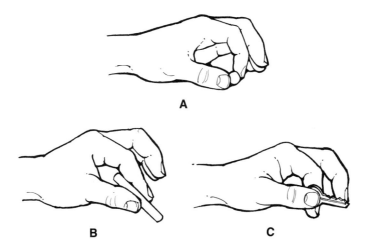

Figure 2-26. Types of precision grip. **A,** Tip grip. **B,** Palmar grip. **C,** Lateral grip.
(Modified from Flatt, A. E. [1974]. *The care of the rheumatoid hand.* St. Louis: C. V. Mosby.)

ACKNOWLEDGEMENTS

I am extremely grateful to Gary W. Schnitz for many of the excellent illustrations used in this chapter.

This chapter has been edited by Elaine Ewing Fess, M.S., O.T.R., F.A.O.T.A., C.H.T., for inclusion in this book. The original unabridged work may be found in Fess, E., & Philips, C. (1987). Hand splinting principles and methods (2nd ed.). St. Louis: Mosby.

REFERENCES

Arey, L. (1980). *Developmental anatomy* (7th ed.). Philadelphia: W.B. Saunders.

Basmajian, J.U. (1980). Electromyography—dynamic gross anatomy: a review. *American Journal of Anatomy, 159,* 245-260.

Bell-Krotoski, J. (1990). Light touch–deep pressure testing using Semmes-Weinstein monofilaments. In J. Hunter, L. Schneider, E. Mackin, & A. Callahan (Eds.). *Rehabilitation of the hand* (3rd ed.). St. Louis: Mosby.

Blumfield, R.H., & Champoux, J.A. [1984]. A biomechanical study of normal functional wrist motion. *Clinical Orthopedics, 187,* 23-25.

Bora, F.W. (1986). *The pediatric upper extremity.* Philadelphia: W.B. Saunders.

Bunnell, S. (1944). *Surgery of the hand.* Philadelphia: J.B. Lippincott.

Flatt, A.E. (1972). Restoration of rheumatoid finger joint function. III. *Journal of Bone & Joint Surgery, 54A,* 1317-1322.

Long C., Conrad, M.S., Hall, E.A., & Furler, M.S. (1970). Intrinsic-extrinsic muscle control of the hand in power grip and precision handling. *Journal of Bone & Joint Surgery, 52A,* 853-867.

Moberg, E. (1958). Objective methods of determining the functional value of sensibility of the hand. *Journal of Bone & Joint Surgery, 40B,* 454-476.

Moore, K.L. (1982). *The developing human: Clinically oriented embryology* (3rd ed.). Philadelphia: W.B. Saunders.

Napier, J.R. (1956). The prehensile movements of the human hand. *Journal of Bone & Joint Surgery, 38B,* 902-913.

Taleisnik, J. (1976). Wrist anatomy, function, and injury. In American Academy of Orthopedic Surgeons. *Instructional lecture course series* (Vol. 27). St. Louis: Mosby.

Taleisnik, J. (1985). *The wrist.* New York: Churchill-Livingstone.

Weber, E.R. (1982). Concepts governing the rotational shift of the intercalated segment of the carpus. *Orthopedic Clinics of North America, 15,* 193-207.

SUGGESTED READINGS

Chase, R.A. (1973). *Atlas of hand surgery.* Philadelphia: W.B. Saunders.

Chase, R.A. (1984). *Atlas of hand surgery* (Vol. 2). Philadelphia: W.B. Saunders.

Clemente, C.D. (Ed.). (1990). *Gray's anatomy of the human body* (14th ed.). Philadelphia: Lea & Febiger.

Hunter, J., Schneider, L., Mackin, E., & Callahan, A. (Eds.). (1990). *Rehabilitation of the hand (3rd ed.).* St. Louis: Mosby.

Kaplan, E.B. (1965). *Functional and surgical anatomy of the hand (2nd ed.).* Philadelphia: J. B. Lippincott.

Landsmere, J. (1976). *Atlas of anatomy of the hand.* Edinburgh: Churchill-Livingstone.

Rasch, P., & Burke, R. (1990). *Kinesiology and applied anatomy (9th ed.).* Philadelphia: Lea & Febiger.

Zancolli, E. (1968). *Structural and dynamic basis of hand surgery.* Philadelphia: J.B. Lippincott.

3

Sensorimotor Integration of Normal and Impaired Development of Precision Movement of the Hand

Ann-Christin Eliasson

The hand is an effective tool used in many different tasks in daily life. Coordination of movements and somatosensory control develop rapidly during the first years of life. The refinement continues for many years, and children do not reach adultlike sensorimotor control until the early teenage years. Cognition, perception, and sensory functions are involved in the motor act. This chapter discusses how sensory information of an object is integrated with the motor processing during development to achieve smooth, coordinated movements of the hand and describes how impairment such as cerebral palsy affects sensorimotor control.

CENTRALLY INITIATED MOVEMENTS

At the beginning of this century, sensory stimuli were thought to be responsible for the generation of movements. This concept was based on studies by Mott and Sherrington (1895) on deafferented monkeys. By transecting the dorsal roots, researchers cut sensory fibers and left the motor fibers intact. The complete sensory loss resulted in permanent abolishment of almost all voluntary movements, especially in the distal segments. A model was proposed in which the movements were generated by chain reflexes, where the sensory information from the first muscle contraction elicited the subsequent spinal reflex.

This reflex origin of movement was disputed by Brown (1911), who studied locomotion in spinal cats. He suggested instead a central origin in which neuronal networks could generate basic locomotor activity in the absence of sensory information (half center model). The task of the afferents was restricted to modifying and compensating for ongoing movements. Recently, there have been several elegant studies that indicate that innate neural networks control rhythmic motor behavior. This has been supported by studies in a variety of species such as locusts, lampreys, and cats (Wilson, 1964; Grillner et al., 1991; Forssberg et al., 1980a,b). Neural networks, referred to as central pattern generators (CPGs), consist of a group of interneurons that interact in an organized manner to produce a motor act. Detailed knowledge of how one CPG operates has been demonstrated in the lamprey, a primitive vertebrate fish. The lamprey is especially suited for such studies because the spinal cord survives in vitro for several days, and neurons involved in the locomotor network for swimming are visible under the microscope, which facilitates microelectrode recording. The swimming can be initiated by stimulation of specific areas in the brainstem, by sensory stimuli if some skin areas are left innervated, and by bath-applied excitatory amino acids. Information about the networks has also been used for computer simulation (Grillner et al., 1991).

The central origin of motor behavior has been further demonstrated in other rhythmic movements such as mastication, swallowing, and respiration (Lund and Olsson, 1983; Miller, 1972; Feldman and Grillner, 1983). Swallowing occurs after the denervation of muscles activated early in the sequence, indicating that the brain sets the motor program for the whole motor act in advance. This, however, does not diminish the importance of afferent signals for modulation and learning of movements. Movements are activated by efferent signals from several higher levels of the central nervous system (CNS), which are modulated by afferent signals from the sensory system and by visual, auditory, somatosensory (that is, vestibular) information.

There are many reasons to believe that the human nervous system is organized in the same way. Spontaneous movements in the human fetus appear from the eighth gestational week, just after the first functional synapses between neurons are developed. The movements seem to be generated by neural networks, and the afferents may not be needed for initiating the movements but are used mainly to adjust and compensate for disturbances (de Vries et al., 1982; Okado, 1980, 1981). Innate motor programs such as breathing, sucking, and swallowing function at birth. The complex pattern of infant stepping is also innate, but this program is immature in the newborn and cannot be used for independent walking until the child has learned to control and adjust the patterns to external conditions. The system develops both through practice and by the process of maturation, where connections with higher central and afferent sensory input continue to be established.

LEARNED MOVEMENTS

Voluntary movements in humans are complex. It is difficult to demonstrate a simple fixed pattern from a CPG although skilled movements appear to depend on a set of motor programs. According to Brooks (1986), "Motor programs are a set of muscle commands that are structured before the motor acts begin and that can be sent to the muscles with the correct timing so that the entire sequence can be carried out in the absence of peripherial feedback" (p. 7), or, in other words, can follow an initial plan. In well-learned, fast movements the trajectory exactly follows this initial plan. The initiation and the termination are planned together, and the movements are almost impossible to stop until completed. This is true, for example, when throwing a ball and in more complex action such as typing. Even continuous movements of moderate speed, such as handling well-known objects, are programmed but allow some amount of sensory feedback. Both kinds of movements are called anticipatory or feed-forward controlled movements, with the characteristic bell-shaped, single-peaked velocity profile (see further discussion).

Slow movements are generally not programmed, allowing time for correction of the ongoing movement by afferent signals, demonstrated by a discontinuous velocity profile (Brooks, 1986). The motor programs are learned by practice when the afferent information adjusts the ongoing movement and updates the motor program for the final movement. The importance of sensory information is demonstrated by birdsong learning in the European chaffinch. Normally the young birds are exposed to singing by their mothers but do not start singing themselves until 10 months of age. If the birds are not exposed to the adult song, they will produce only rudimentary sequences. If the birds are exposed to adult song during the first 4 months of life and then isolated from songs during the month following, they start to sing properly. This indicates that auditory experience is necessary for the motor program to be fully developed. If the birds are deafened after 4 months but before they start to sing, they sing in a very awkward way. Deafening after they start to sing, however, does not affect the song. This indicates that birds also need to compare the initial motor program for singing with the actual song, that is, afferent information is also necessary to be able to learn to use the program of singing. The afferent information corrects the song and updates the program, which could be used without afferent feedback when the song was established (Konishi, 1965; Nottebohm, 1970).

AFFERENT INFORMATION

The importance of afferent information is seen in patients with large sensory fiber neuropathies, in which the large afferent fibers generating proprioceptive and tactile information degenerate. Unless these patients see their limbs, they do not know their position and cannot detect limb motion. When reaching toward a target without seeing the moving hand, they make large errors; if they look at the hand before reaching, the hand comes closer to the target. This indicates that these patients can compensate for the lack of somatosensory information visually and also use vision to program the reaching in advance. Since the patients cannot stop the movement precisely at the desired target, information from various receptors in the skin is essential for precise movements (Ghez et al., 1990).

Proprioception

The proprioceptive system gives information about the stationary position of the limbs (limb position sense) and movements of the limb (kinesthesia). The latter information is mediated from tendon organs and muscle spindles and also from receptors in the skin, sensitive to skin stretch. The tendon organ signals information about the strength of muscle contraction, increased signaling indicating increased tension. Signals from the muscle spindle regulate the length of the muscle fibers. The receptors are rather complicated and, despite intensive research, their function is not fully understood. It has been agreed, however, that the muscle spindle is responsible for small changes in muscle contraction, which may be important for force regulation during the grasping

act. There are muscle spindles in almost all skeletal muscles, and they mediate information mainly through Ia afferents to the spinal cord. The muscle spindle also has efferent innervation to intrafusal muscle fibers, in which the primary and secondary endings set the sensitivity to the afferent signals. The different contractions of intrafusal muscle fibers are probably crucial for the information sent to the central nervous system. Alpha and gamma motor neurons are coactivated by central mechanisms to maintain the sensitivity of the muscle spindles throughout the range of almost all movements. There have been different models for the coactivation of alpha and gamma motor neurons, but it appears that descending commands activate both, as demonstrated by Vallbo (1970) in studies of microneurography. The afferent signals are used to update and correct the motor programs, and the information can be used in a conscious way to give knowledge about the limb movement and position in space.

Touch

The tactile system is used to discriminate between different surfaces and shapes and also provides sensory input to the CNS, which regulates the force of the muscles during grasping and holding of objects. Touch transmits nerve impulses from mechanoreceptors to the CNS via axons with different diameters. Large fibers, with a fast conduction rate, mediate tactile sensation from the skin, whereas thin fibers, with a slow conduction rate, mediate sensation of pain and temperature. The receptors mediating tactile sensation can be classified on the basis of their receptive fields and morphology. Two receptor types, Meissner and Pacini corpuscles, are fast adapting. Meissner corpuscles have small, sharply delineated sensory fields, and Pacini corpuscles have large and diffuse sensory fields. Two other types of receptors that are slow-adapting units are Merkel corpuscles, with small and sharply delineated sensory fields, and Ruffini corpuscles, with large and diffuse fields. Mechanoreceptors with small receptive fields are suitable for fine spatial discrimination since they have a high sensitivity over the entire field, whereas mechanoreceptors with large receptive fields have a central area of high sensitivity and decreased sensitivity in the border of the receptive field. Since there are about 17,000 tactile units in the hand and approximately 70% of them have small receptive fields, it can be postulated that the tactile system of the hand is highly

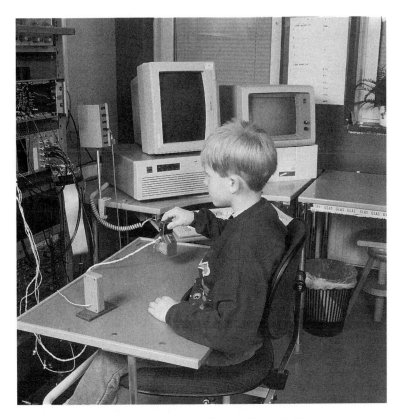

Figure 3-1. Child lifting the experimental object.

developed to detect small movements and discriminate between different surfaces (Johansson and Vallbo, 1983).

We explore the surface of an object by manipulation of the fingers. The difference between exploring known and unknown surfaces is the speed of the finger movements (Roland et al., 1989). A relevant movement for exploring the different surfaces of an object is by touch through digital manipulation, whereas a more adequate way to explore the shape is by rotation of the wrist and bimanual hand activity. The fingertips are very sensitive to tactile information, and tactile discrimination occurs early during development. Children one year old can recognize dissimilar objects, and they are able to use the two different exploratory maneuvers for objects differing in texture or shape (Ruff, 1984). Newborn monkeys can distinguish different textures by choosing the texture that gives milk (Carlson, 1984). These examples indicate that, despite an immature nervous system, there is early interaction between somatosensory signals and motor output.

BASIC COORDINATION OF FORCES DURING GRASPING

During the last decade Johansson and Westling (1984, 1987, 1988, 1990) have been studying grasping movement to understand how somatosensory information is integrated with motor control. In adults, movements of the hand and fingers are precise and the forces of the fingers well controlled. This is not an innate behavior; in fact, these functions develop during early childhood and may be dysfunctional if there is damage in the central nervous system (Forssberg et al., 1991, 1992, unpublished; Gordon et al., 1992; Eliasson et al., 1991, 1992, 1994).

Most grasping acts involve lifting and holding objects, grasping with the fingers and lifting with the arm. The object seen in Figures 3-1 and 3-2 measures grip force from each grip surface (thumb and index finger), a combined vertical load force by strain-gauge transducers, and vertical movement by a photoresistor (Eliasson et al., 1991). With this instrument it has been possible to define different phases of the lift and to understand

Figure 3-2. Experimental instrument where the grip surfaces are exchangeable and the weight can be covaried without any visual changes.

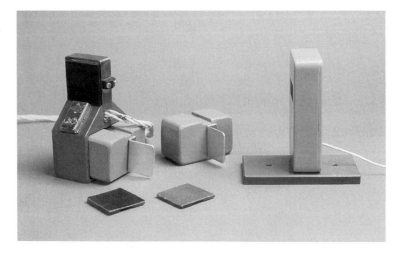

how they are linked to produce smooth movements. When grasping the instrument, there is a short delay before the vertical load force starts to increase. This preload phase is important for establishment of the grasp. During the loading phase the grip force and load force increase in parallel until the instrument starts to move. The rates of grip and load forces have mainly bell-shaped profiles (see later discussion) adjusted to the weight, size, and frictional character of the surface of the object. Following the loading phase there is a transition phase, where the lift reaches the final position and the forces are well adjusted to the current properties of the object. In the final, static, phase the object is held in the air (Figure 3-3).

Tactile information triggers different motor commands and links the different phases together. The different types of receptors respond differently during the lift, which has been demonstrated by microneurography from single tactile units innervating the glabrous skin of the fingers. Fast-adapting receptors send bursts of impulses when first touching an object, at the beginning of the loading phase, and at lift-off but are silent during the static phase. Slow-adapting receptors send impulses continuously during the static phase (Johansson and Vallbo, 1983). This ability makes it possible to handle small fragile objects without crushing them. To investigate how separate components affect the grasping act, the object has a slot where blocks of different weights may be inserted while the visual appearance remains constant; the contact pads can be covered with silk or sandpaper, each having different frictional character, and the size can be adjusted by boxes of

different size attached to the instrument (Figure 3-2).

Development of Manipulatory Forces

During the loading phase, just before the movement starts, the grip and load forces are generated in parallel for coordinated movements. This parallel increment of both grip and load force increases with heavier objects, resulting in prolonged latency until lift-off. If the contact surface changes, the grip force increases more for slippery material compared to rough materials while the load force remains the same. This parallel force generation forms a lifting synergy to simplify movements (Bernstein, 1967). It develops from the second year when the pincer grasp is fully developed. Smaller children cannot generate grip and load forces in parallel; they initiate forces sequentially with prolonged and uncontrolled shift of the phases during the lift. This is clearly seen in Figure 3-4; most of the grip force increases before the onset of load force. The force rate profile is irregular and has several peaks in young children, whereas older children and adults perform mainly a bell-shaped force rate profile, adjusted to the weight of the object at lift-off, indicating anticipatory controlled movements (Figure 3-5) (Forssberg et al., 1991; Brooks. 1986).

Small children also have more variation than adults since they cannot repeatedly produce similar movements. However, children of 1 year can use tactile and proprioceptive information to adjust the forces by sensory feedback during the static phase. All phases are prolonged, and the different

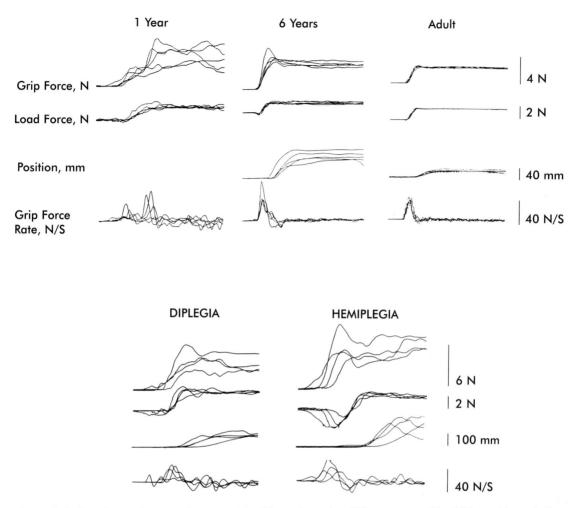

Figure 3-3. Superimposed traces of representative lifts performed at different ages and in children with cerebral palsy. Grip force, load force, position, and grip force rate are shown as functions of time. When lifting the object, the grip force starts to increase; then the grip force and load force increase until the object starts to move. When the forces overcome gravity, the signal measuring position increases, followed by a static phase when the object is held in the air.

(Modified from Forssberg, H., Eliasson, A.C., Kinoshita, H., Johansson, R.S., & Westling, G. [1991]. Development of human precision grip. I. Basic coordination of force. *Experimental Brain Research, 85,* 451-457, and Eliasson, A.C., Gordon, A.M., & Forssberg, H. [1991]. Basic coordination of manipulative forces in children with cerebral palsy. *Developmental Medicine and Child Neurology, 33,* 661-670.)

phases are not triggered elegantly as in adults (Forssberg et al., unpublished). There is increased difference between thumb and finger contact, probably due to an immature ability to adjust the finger toward the object's size (von Hofsten and Rönnquist, 1988). This uncoordinated movement in small children is likely attributable to immature motor output and sensory processing. There is rapid development until age 2. The refined coordination then progressively develops until leveling out at ages 4 to 6 and continues gradually until teenage years, when the lifts are completely adult-like (Forssberg et al., 1991).

DEVELOPMENT OF ANTICIPATORY CONTROL

Anticipatory control of manipulation apparently requires the nervous system to efficiently use sensory information to integrate and store information for internal representation of an object. This internal representation is necessary to produce rapid and well-coordinated transitions between the various movement phases due to a long delay between motor command and sensory feedback. This is true for reaching, grasping, and lifting movements as well as for movement involving the

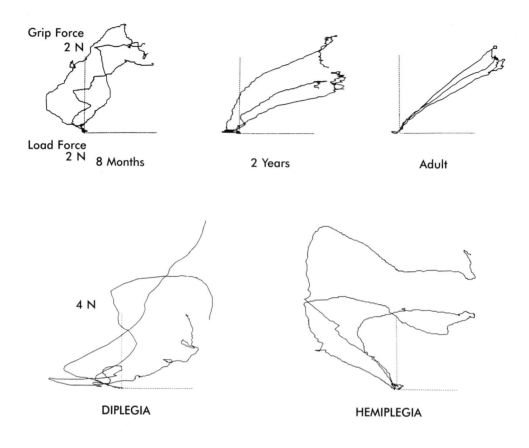

Figure 3-4. Grip force during the preload and the loading phase (before lift-off) is plotted against load force in children of different ages and children with cerebral palsy. Trials are superimposed for each subject.

(Modified from Forssberg, H., Eliasson, A.C., Kinoshita, H., Johansson, R.S., & Westling, G. [1991]. Development of human precision grip. I. Basic coordination of force. *Experimental Brain Research, 85,* 451-457, and Eliasson, A.C., Gordon, A.M., & Forssberg, H. [1991]. Basic coordination of manipulative forces in children with cerebral palsy. *Developmental Medicine and Child Neurology, 33,* 661-670.)

whole body. In the lifting task the motor output is based on internal representation of the object's properties learned by prior experience. Therefore adults and older children base their programming of motor output on internal representation of weight, friction, size, and haptic cues of the object (Johansson and Westling, 1990; Gordon et al., 1991 a,b).

Weight

When the weight of the object is varied but the visual appearance remains constant, adults typically scale the grip and load force rates based on internal representation of the object's weight. This is indicated by higher grip and load force rates for heavier objects. The forces are decreased at lift-off to harmonize with the weight of the object, resulting in similar acceleration independent of the object's weight. The anticipatory mechanism can be further demonstrated when lifting an unexpectedly light object preceded by a heavier object. Lifting the light object results in a faster lift with higher force rates since the event is based on the previous lift and the information of the weight is not available until lift-off. For example, if one lifts an unopened but empty can of soda, the lift will probably be too high since a heavier can is expected. However, this will occur only once for the same can. Somatosensory information adjusts the forces

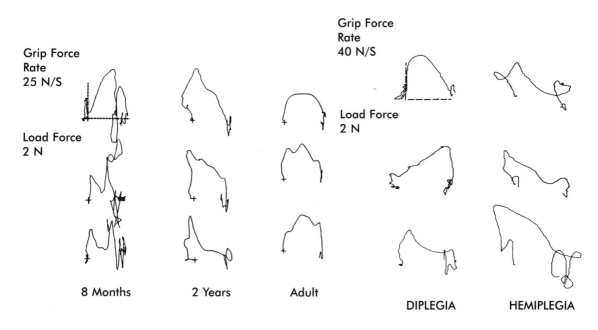

Figure 3-5. Grip force rate as a function of load force in consecutive trials with children of different ages and children with cerebral palsy.

(Modified from Forssberg, H., Eliasson, A.C., Kinoshita, H., Johansson, R.S., & Westling, G. [1991]. Development of human precision grip. I. Basic coordination of force. *Experimental Brain Research, 85,* 451-457, and Eliasson, A.C., Gordon, A.M., & Forssberg, H. [1991]. Basic coordination of manipulative forces in children with cerebral palsy. *Developmental Medicine and Child Neurology, 33,* 661-670.)

to the object's actual weight during the static phase and updates the internal representation of the object for a smooth movement the next time the object is lifted.

Children cannot handle this type of situation as efficiently as adults. However, despite uncoordinated force generation and large variation of grip and load force rates, 2-year-old children start to scale the forces toward different weights. It takes several years until the anticipatory control of weight is fully developed. Children between the ages of 6 and 8 are nearly adultlike although the variation is still larger than in adults (Figure 3-6). This indicates that anticipatory scaling of forces occurs before maturation of coordinated movement (Forssberg et al., 1992).

Size

Anticipatory control is also predicted from visual information about an object's size (Gordon et al., 1991a, b). When the object is kept proportional to the volume, there are appropriately scaled forces toward the expected weight relative to the volume. When only the size of the object is covaried and the weight kept constant, the employed grip force rate is higher for the larger object than for the smaller object. However, adults and older children perceive the small object as heavier. This indicates a dichotomy between the perceptual and motor systems due to the size-weight illusion (Charpentier, 1891). We predict a big object to be heavier than a small one, yet this is not always true. This understanding of the discrepancy between size and weight and a proper scaling of the motor output starts to develop at 3 years. Children younger than 3 are not able to control the motor output according to size but do use higher grip force rate for heavier objects. This suggests that the associative transformation between the object's size and weight involves additional demands of cortical processes, requiring further cognitive development. From 3 to 7 years of age the difference between large and small objects is larger than in adults. Older children seem capable of reducing the effect if it is not purposeful for

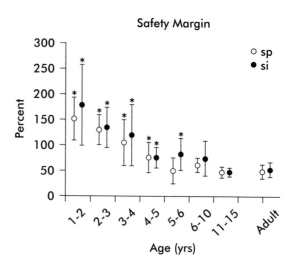

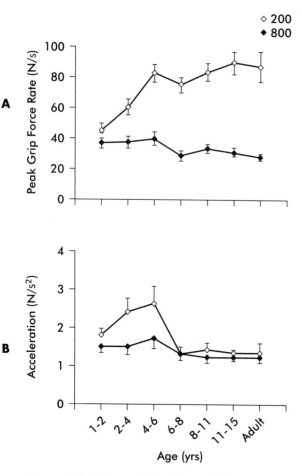

Figure 3-6. Influence of the 200-g and 800-g weight (400 g for 1- to 2-year-old children) in the constant lifting series for peak grip force rate (**A**) and peak acceleration (**B**). The means and SEMs of the individual means for each subject indicate the major changes during development.

(Modified from Forssberg, H., Kinoshita, H., Eliasson, A.C., Johansson, R.S., & Westling, G. [1992]. Development of human precision grip. II. Anticipatory control of isometric forces targeted for object's weight. *Experimental Brain Research, 90,* 393-398).

Figure 3-7. The mean and standard deviation of individual means of the safety margin for lifts with sandpaper and silk plotted for different age groups. The safety margin is expressed in percent of the slip ratio. Significant differences are indicated by * (p <.05).

manipulation, whereas younger children still strongly rely on visual information (Gordon et al., 1992).

Friction

Tactile influence on the force coordination is available on touching an object, contrary to weight influence, which is not available until lift-off. Tactile information from fingertips triggers pre-structured motor commands based on sensorimotor memories and adjusts the force coordination based on the friction of the contact surface. The employed grip forces are different when one holds a slippery bottle than when holding a tool covered with rubber, even if they have the same weight. When contact pads on the test object are altered by exchangeable contact surfaces of silk and sandpaper, the relationship between grip force and load force is changed before lift-off. In adults there is an initial adjustment to the new frictional condition during the first 0.1 second and secondary adjustments during the loading and static phases (Johansson and Westling, 1987). These adjustments are important in establishing an adequate safety margin, which prevents one from dropping the object. The ratio between grip and load force actually used, minus the slip ratio necessary to prevent the object slipping out of the hand, makes up the safety margin.

One-year-old children have a larger safety margin than adults. Gradually, the safety margin decreases in conjunction with increased coordination and less variability during the first 5 years (Figure 3-7). Some children of 18 months can scale the grip force based on tactile information in the beginning of the lift. They have a higher grip force for slippery materials than for rough ones during consecutive lifts with the same friction. Several years are required before children can handle objects with different frictional surfaces in the same elegant way that adults do. Children below 6 years of age, sometimes up to 10 or 12 years, need several lifts and a predictable order to adjust the grip force to the current friction and to form an internal representation before setting the parameters of the programmed motor output. The difference between adaptation to weight and adaptation to friction is that frictional conditions appear directly upon touching the object whereas weight information is likely more crucial for anticipatory control since the weight is not available until lift-off. Grip forces of high amplitude are a useful compensatory strategy to avoid dropping objects (Forssberg et al., unpublished).

IMPAIRED FORCE COORDINATION IN CHILDREN WITH CEREBRAL PALSY

Many children with cerebral palsy (CP) have disturbed hand function because primary or secondary lesions involve the sensorimotor cortex and the corticospinal tract, both of which have great implication for precision grip and independent finger movements (Lawrence and Kuypers, 1968; Muir and Lemon, 1983). Clinically these children are known to be slow and weak with disturbed mobility of finger movements (Ingram, 1966; Brown, 1987). In addition, they have different degrees of spasticity and, especially in children with hemiplegia, disturbed tactile discrimination (Brown, 1987; Uvebrant, 1988). Investigations of locomotion, posture, and isometric force coordination demonstrate deficits in motor control with impaired temporal and spatial coordination (Berger et al., 1982; Nashner et al., 1983; Neilson, 1990). This is in agreement with the studies of manipulatory force coordination in children with hemiplegia and diplegia (Eliasson et al., 1991, 1992, 1993).

Children with CP seem to remain at an early level of development, and sometimes they have exaggerated patterns not seen during normal development. In the lift there is greater delay between the different fingers contacting the object, indicating disturbed coordination of finger mobility and shaping of the fingers toward the size of the object. The parallel grip and load force coordination is rarely seen. Instead, they increase the forces sequentially, with grip force increasing before load force (see Figure 3-4). Consequently they do not produce the force rates in mainly bell-shaped profiles but in stepwise, irregular, and

extremely variable profiles (see Figure 3-5). Also, the phases are prolonged, the grip force is increased and unstable during the lift, and there is large variability between lifts (see Figure 3-3) (Eliasson et al., 1991). However, this slow, sequential initiation of movements is an adequate strategy providing security in a manipulative task where coordination of force generation is not fully functional.

During normal development small children are able to scale the forces in advance, according to weight as well as size and friction of the object, before the parallel force coordination with the mainly bell-shaped force rate profile is developed. Almost none of the children with CP scale the force amplitude for different weights. They increase the forces in steps, permitting sensory feedback, until lift-off. This results in a prolonged loading phase for heavier objects but fairly well-adjusted forces according to the weight of the object during the static phase (Eliasson et al., 1992). The forces are also adjusted to different friction of the contact surfaces during the static phase; however, the grip force increases with large variation resulting in a high safety margin preventing objects from dropping. During the initial part of the lift, most of the children can adjust the forces fairly well after consecutive lifts with the same frictional contact surfaces. Thus processing of tactile information is probably disturbed; they need more than two consecutive lifts with the same frictional conditions for appropriate scaling of the motor output and even for adjustment of the forces in the early static phase. To compensate for this lack of anticipatory control and slow adaptation, they use an increased grip force, not dropping the object (Eliasson et al., 1993).

All children perceive the difference between weight and frictional contact surfaces despite inadequate two-point discrimination for some children with CP, but children with CP seem to have impaired ability to transform sensory information in order to set the motor command. As a result, it appears that sensory processing of proprioceptive and tactile information and the ability to build internal representation and store information are not fully functional. The similar force amplitude for contact pads with different friction and the inability to scale the forces to different weights of the objects even during consecutive presentation of lifts, indicate that this may be the case. In addition, it demonstrates that the perception of different weights and textures requires mechanisms different from those for appropriate force regulation of movement.

ORGANIZATION OF SENSORIMOTOR CONTROL

These studies have enhanced our knowledge of the mechanisms underlying sensorimotor integration and anticipatory control in a grasping task. For this manipulatory act visual, tactile, and proprioceptive information is probably integrated with memories of similar objects from previous manipulative experience in order to update the internal representation. The appropriate muscles are then activated in the proper sequence and timing, resulting in a coordinated grasping and lifting movement. The act may include selection of motor programs that control orientation of the hand and the subsequent limb trajectories. These programs may be stored in a sensorimotor memory and used in an unconscious way, different from declarative memory used in conscious recall of facts, events, and percepts (Squire, 1986). The existence of sensorimotor memory has been demonstrated by disorders in higher brain function. It seems that networks involving cortical function, especially posterior parietal cortex, are important for anticipation. Jeannerod (1986) has described deficit in shaping the fingers toward the size of the object in patients with damage to the parietal area. The ability to construct an internal representation used for anticipatory control of force in grasping-lifting movement is apparently disturbed in children with CP although the damage causing it may have occurred at different stages in development, is located in different areas of the CNS, or may vary in extent. Thus many different areas of the CNS (although varying in extent) are most likely involved in sensorimotor memories.

In conclusion, the maturation of control mechanisms for the grasping movement continues throughout childhood. All measured parameters rapidly develop during the first years. During the second year children start to generate grip and load forces in parallel and scale the forces toward the object's different weight and friction. Tactile and proprioceptive information is used to regulate the forces by sensory feedback in the static phase. In 4-year-old children the motor output is less varied and more coordinated, in conjunction with a decreased safety margin. At that age there is even force scaling to the size of the object. However,

the appropriate anticipatory scaling with acceleration of the lift to harmonize with the weight of the object is not developed until 6 to 8 years of age. Even so, there are still large variations in the ability to properly scale the forces according to frictional demands. It is not until ages 10 to 12 that scaling approaches adult levels.

The maturation processes probably occur at many levels. Both the motor cortex and the corticospinal tract, with monosynaptic connections, are important for precision grip and are highly related to force generation. In monkeys the monosynaptic projections to the spinal cord are not fully developed until the end of the first year (Lawrence and Hopkins, 1976). Myelination of the axons and increased conduction rate of cortical motor neuronal activity develop over several years and probably influence the temporal parameters of the lift (Muller et al., 1991). Since many areas of the brain are apparently involved in the grasping act, its full development obviously depends on establishment of appropriate synaptic connections between the cortex and all other areas associated with the act. These maturation processes are shown by reorganization of reflex responses with more efficient and faster triggering, which continues until adolescence (Issler and Stephens, 1983; Evans et al., 1990; Forssberg et al., 1991). There are cortical networks mediating monosynaptic corticospinal projections to the motor neurons controlling distal muscles (Fetz and Cheney, 1980; Muir and Lemon, 1983), which are active in fine manipulation and force regulation (Smith, 1981; Wannier et al., 1986). There may exist subcortical motor centers and even networks in the spinal cord important for storing certain motor acts; for example, the C3-C4 propriospinal system in cats can be used to mediate and update cortical commands for visually guided reaching (Alstermark et al., 1987). This provides several solutions for a particular movement through a wide range of central and peripheral inputs. During development there may be reorganization of networks in the spinal cord caused by increased descending control on premotor neurons. The descending control may be break up the innate grasp reflex synergy allowing independent finger movement and may form a grip/lift synergy (Forssberg et al., 1991).

Young children and children with CP have difficulty storing and recalling information on an object's physical properties. They require many consecutive lifts to perform a programmed movement. Learning motor activities proceeds by trial and error, and it is not really understood how the information from subsequent lifts is stored in memory to result in efficient programming. It is known that the anterior lobe of the cerebellum is involved in force regulation prior to a lift since the amplitude of the force is correlated with activity in neurons in this region, which have cutaneous and muscle afferent inputs from the hand (Espinoza and Smith, 1990). There are radical changes in synaptic activity, reflected in regional cerebral blood flow, during learning of motor sequence for finger movements. In the initial part of learning there is activation of the cortical areas, the cerebellum, and structures providing information to those areas, namely the anterior language area and the somatosensory association areas. As learning progresses, the activation in the language areas of the cortex disappears, leaving a reduced region in the somatosensory area, whereas different motor structures and the cerebellum show consistent increase in activity. This may mean that motor programs for motor sequence learning of finger movements are established and can be produced in a feed-forward strategy with less sensory information. It appears that memories are not stored in a single cell or in one particular cortical structure (Seitz et al., 1990).

CLINICAL IMPLICATIONS

Functional hand movements during daily life are built up by motor sequences related to sensory, perceptual, and cognitive functions. We have to decode the task and choose strategies before setting the motor commands. Force regulation during a grasping/lifting task is only one parameter involved in manipulation; therefore those results are not directly transferred to manipulatory actions. However, in some aspects it is possible to relate the development of force regulation to the development of skills. The force coordination is poorly developed in 1-year-old children; for example, they will usually crush an ice cream cone, whereas children of 2 years manage quite well. At 4, children have more coordinated and adjusted movements when they carry a kitten, handle fragile objects such as flowers, or efficiently play with building blocks. To produce discrete movements, as in writing with a pen, is still difficult, but this skill develops rapidly during the following years. Efficient control of finger movements continues to develop until adolescence, when children can learn to play musical instruments and develop good handwriting with accurate speed. Obviously, there is parallel processing of cognitive functions and sensorimotor control

during normal development. The qualitative aspect, such as smoothness and coordination or making skills more efficient, is related to force coordination and anticipatory control.

Most children with CP have no functional sensorimotor integration during the grasping task. The force generation is usually unstable with a high safety margin and large variations. This makes the child unsure in handling objects, and it sometimes results in dropping objects. They also feel unsure when carrying the same objects in different environments; they need to focus attention on the task and have to find compensatory strategies for their poorly developed force coordination. They are slow because they have poor anticipatory control and have to use increased grasping forces since they cannot rely on stable force generation or efficient sensory feedback. This compensatory behavior has to be integrated with the child's mental capacity and social life, but it is the knowledge of the sensorimotor mechanisms that should form the basis for treatment.

Sensory information is crucial for precise movements; therefore therapists should investigate how the individual child relies on different kinds of sensory information for motor output. It is important to find tasks for which different sensory information is crucial. Tactile information is important for discrete finger movements, whereas proprioception is more important for reaching in different directions and handling objects of different weight. To button up a shirt, especially without vision, gives information about the child's ability in using tactile information. Vision strongly influences manipulatory actions and could easily be excluded to understand more about the somatosensory systems. Tasks such as opening a door with a key, pulling tape from a holder, and picking raspberries give much information on how children can use proprioceptive and tactile information to modulate the motor act. Observing a child handling objects with different properties gives qualitative information about force regulation and will also illustrate how a child uses sensory information for manipulation.

Sensory information is important in learning movements; the sensory signal corrects and adjusts the movement and updates the motor program for correct execution the next time the program is used. If some kinds of sensory signals are less functional, other sensory signals have to be increased to effect optimal learning. When sensory input or processing is less functional, the anticipation is disturbed and children have a problem in building internal representations and thus in executing precise movements. Although most children are still able to handle objects with different properties, they are often clumsy or immature since they are relying mainly on immediate sensory feedback rather than learned motor programs. Smoothness in the tasks is dependent on anticipatory control that links different movement phases based on previous experience.

Anticipatory control can be investigated by observing the child catching a ball or objects moving at different speeds. Other simple tasks with repetitive movements are making a string of pearls and picking up coins; those kinds of tasks give some clue as to what extent the movements are anticipated. It is probably difficult to learn smoothness when certain control mechanisms are missing or disturbed; children with CP have to rely on sensory feedback, which makes the movement slow due to the delay between sensory feedback and motor commands. In clinical investigations the therapists have to interpret information from different tasks to find trends that may help the child understand how to learn and handle objects in certain situations and to encourage them to find their own compensatory strategy for safe grasping.

We do not know the relationship between maturation of the central nervous system and the practice of different tasks. What we do know is that practice is necessary, and it seems logical that a less efficient nervous system needs more practice than an appropriately functioning one. We also know that improvement in any task strongly depends on motivation. The improvement by motivation is nicely shown in a task measuring pronation and supination of the hand. The children increase their range of movement when hitting a drum compared to just performing the movement (van der Weel, 1991). For the child the game itself is the goal; they are not interested in the specific movement of arms and hands. This is important for the therapist to remember.

In conclusion, intervention by the therapist must help children understand how their own nervous system works and help them find compensatory and reliable strategies despite disturbed sensorimotor control. Second, for success in skills, the therapist should encourage children to find tasks they are motivated to repeat and learn.

REFERENCES

Alstermark, B., Gorska, R., Lundberg, A., Pettersson, L.G., & Walkowska, M. (1987). Effect of different spinal cord lesions on visually guided switching of target-reaching cats. *Neuroscience Research, 5,* 63-67.

Berger, W., Quintern, J., & Dietz, V. (1982) Pathophysiology of gait in children with cerebral palsy. *Electromyography and Clinical Neurophysiology, 53,* 538-548.

Bernstein, N. (1967). *The coordination and regulation of movements.* Oxford: Pergamon.

Brooks, V.B. (1986). *The neural basis of motor control.* New York: Oxford University Press.

Brown, T.G. (1911). The intrinsic factors in the act of progression in the mammal. *Proceedings of the Royal Society of London, 84,* 308-319.

Brown, J.K., van Rensburg, F., Walsh, G., Lakie, M., & Wright, G.W. (1987). A neurological study of hand function of hemiplegic children. *Developmental Medicine and Child Neurology, 29,* 287-304.

Carlson, M. (1984). Development of tactile discrimination capacity in *Macaca Mulatta.* I. Normal infants. *Developmental Brain Research, 16,* 69-82.

Charpentier, A. (1891). Analyse experimental de quelques elements de la sensation de poids. *Archives of Physiology and Normal Pathology, 3,* 122-135.

de Vries, J.I.P., Visser, G.H.A., & Pechtl, H.F.R. (1982). The emergence of fetal behavior. I. Qualitative aspects. *Early Human Development, 7,* 301-322.

Eliasson, A.C., Gordon, A.M., & Forssberg, H. (1991). Basic coordination of manipulative forces in children with cerebral palsy. *Developmental Medicine and Child Neurology, 33,* 661-670.

Eliasson, A.C., Gordon, A.M., & Forssberg, H. (1992). Impaired anticipatory control of isometric forces during grasping by children with cerebral palsy. *Developmental Medicine and Child Neurology, 34,* 216-255.

Eliasson, A.C., Gordon, A.M., & Forssberg H. (In print). Tactile control of isometric finger forces during grasping in children with cerebral palsy. *Developmental Medicine and Child Neurology.*

Evans, A.L., Harrison, L.M., & Stephens, J.A. (1990). Maturation of the cutaneomuscular reflex recorded from the first dorsal interosseous muscle in man. *Journal of Neurophysiology, 428,* 425-440.

Espinoza, E., & Smith, A.M. (1990). Purkinje cell simple spike activity during grasping and lifting objects of different textures and weights. *Journal of Neurophysiology, 64,* 698-714.

Feldman, J.L., & Grillner, S. (1983). Control of vertebrate respiration and locomotion: A brief account. *Physiologist, 26,* 310-316.

Fetz, E.E., & Cheney, P.D. (1980). Post-spike facilitation of forelimb muscle activity by primate corticomotoneural cells. *Journal of Neurophysiology, 44,* 751-772.

Forssberg, H., Eliasson, A.C., Kinoshita, H., Johansson, R.S., & Westling, G. (1991). Development of human precision grip. I. Basic coordination of force. *Experimental Brain Research, 85,* 451-457.

Forssberg, H., Grillner, S., & Halbertsma, J. (1980). The locomotion of the spinal cat. I. Coordination within a hindlimb. *Acta Physiologica Scandinavica, 108,* 269-281.

Forssberg, H., Grillner, S., Halbertsma, J., & Rossignol, S. (1980). The locomotion of the spinal cat. II. Interlimb coordination, *Acta Physiologica Scandinavica, 108,* 283-295.

Forssberg, H., Kinoshita, H., Eliasson, A.C., Johansson, R.S., & Westling, G. (1992). Development of human precision grip. II. Anticipatory control of isometric forces targeted for object's weight. *Experimental Brain Research, 90,* 393-398.

Forssberg, H., Kinoshita, H., Eliasson, A.C., Johansson, R.S., & Westling, G. Development of human precision grip. IV. Tactile adaptation of isometric finger forces to the texture of the contact surface. Unpublished manuscript.

Ghez, C., Gordon, J., Ghilardi, M.F., Christakos, C.N., & Coper, S.E. (1990). Roles of proprioceptive input in the programming of arm trajectories. *Cold Spring Harbor Symposia on Quantitative Biology, 55,* 837-847.

Gordon, A.M., Forssberg, H., Johansson, R.S., & Westling, G. (1991a). The integration of haptically acquired size information in the programming of precision grip. *Experimental Brain Research, 83,* 483-488.

Gordon, A.M., Forssberg, H., Johansson R.S., & Westling, G. (1991b). Visual size cues in the programming of manipulative forces during precision grip. *Experimental Brain Research, 83,* 477-482.

Gordon, A.M., Forssberg, H., Johansson, R.S., Eliasson, A.C., & Westling, G. (1992). Development of human precision grip. III. Integration of visual size cues during the programming of isometric forces. *Experimental Brain Research, 90,* 399-403.

Grillner, S., Wallen, P., & Brodin, L. (1991). Neural network generating locomotor behavior in lamprey: Circuitry, transmittors, membrane properties and simulation. *Annual Review of Neuroscience, 14,* 169-199.

Ingram, T.T.S. (1966). The neurology of cerebral palsy. *Archives of the Diseases of Childhood, 41,* 337-357.

Issler, H., & Stephens, J.A. (1983). The maturation of cutaneous reflexes studied in the upper limb in man. *Journal of Physiology, 335,* 643-654.

Jeannerod, M. (1986). The formation of finger grip during prehension. A cortically mediated visuomotor pattern. *Behavioural Brain Research, 19,* 305-319.

Johansson, R.S., & Vallbo, B. (1983). Tactile sensory coding in the glabrous skin of the human hand. *Trends in Neurosciences, 6,* 27-32.

Johansson, R.S., & Westling, G. (1984). Influence of cutaneous sensory input on the motor coordination during precision manipulation. In C. von Euler, O. Franzen, U. Lindblom, & D. Ottoson (Eds.). *Somatosensory mechanisms.* London: Macmillan Press.

Johansson, R.S., & Westling, G. (1987). Signals in tactile afferents from the fingers eliciting adaptive motor responses during precision grip. *Experimental Brain Research 66,* 141-154.

Johansson, R.S., & Westling, G. (1988). Coordinated isometric muscle commands adequately and erroneously programmed for the weight during lifting task with precision grip. *Experimental Brain Research, 71,* 59-71.

Johansson, R.S., & Westling, G. (1990). Tactile afferent signals in the control of precision grip. In M. Jeannerod (Ed.). *Attention and performance.* Hillsdale, NJ: Erlbaum.

Konishi, M. (1965). The role of auditory feedback in the control of vocalization in the white-crowned sparrow. *Zeitschrift Tierpsychologie, 22,* 770-783.

Lawrence, D.G., & Hopkins, D.A. (1976). The development of motor control in the rhesus monkey: Evidence concerning the role of corticomotoneuronal connections. *Brain 99,* 235-254.

Lawrence, D.G., & Kuypers, H.G.J.M. (1968). The functional organization of the motor system in the monkey. I. The effects of bilateral pyramidal leisions. *Brain, 91,* 1-14.

Lund, J.P., & Olsson, K.A. (1983). The importance of reflexes and their control during jaw movement. *Trends in Neuroscience, 6,* 458-463.

Miller, A.J. (1972). Significance of sensory inflow to swallowing. *Brain Research, 43,* 147-159.

Mott, F.W., & Sherrington, C.S. (1895). Experiments upon the influence of sensory nerves upon movement and nutrition of the limbs. *Proceedings of the Royal Society of London. Series B: Biological Sciences, 57,* 481-488.

Muir, R.B., & Lemon, R.N. (1983). Corticospinal neurons with a special role in precision grip. *Brain Research, 261,* 312-316.

Muller, K., Homberg, V., & Lenard, H.G. (1991). Magnetic stimulation of motor cortex and nerve roots in children. Maturation of corticomotoneural projections. *Electromyography and Clinical Neurophysiology, 81,* 63-70.

Nashner, L.M., Shumway-Cook, A., & Marin, O. (1983). Stance posture control in select groups of children with cerebral palsy: Deficit in sensory organization and muscular coordination. *Experimental Brain Research, 49,* 393-409.

Neilson, P.D., O'Dwyer, N.J., & Nash, J. (1990). Control of isometric muscle activity in cerebral palsy. *Developmental Medicine and Child Neurology, 32,* 778-788.

Nottebohm, F. (1970). Ontogeny of bird song. *Science, 167,* 950-956.

Okado, N. (1980). Development of human cervical spinal cord with reference to synapse formation in the motor nucleus. *Journal of Comparative Neurology, 191,* 495-513.

Okado, N. (1981). Onset of synapse formation in the human spinal cord. *Journal of Comparative Neurology, 201,* 211-220.

Roland, P.E., Ericsson, L., & Widén, L. (1989). *European Journal of Neuroscience, 1,* 3-18.

Ruff, H.A. (1984). Infants' manipulative exploration of objects: Effects of age and object characteristics. *Developmental Psychology, 20,* 9-20.

Seitz, R.J., Roland, P.E., Bohm, C., Greitz, T., & Stone-Elander, S. (1990). Motor learning in man: A positron emission tomographic study. *Neuroreport, 1*(1), 57-66.

Smith, A.M. (1981). The coactivation of antagonist muscles. *Canadian Journal of Physiology and Pharmacology, 59,* 733-747.

Squire, L.R. (1986). Mechanisms of memory. *Science, 232,* 1612-1619.

Uvebrant, P. (1988). Hemiplegic cerebral palsy: aetiology and outcome. *Acta Pediatrica Scandinavica Supplement,* 345.

van der Weel, F.R., van der Meer. A.L.H., & Lee, D.N. (1991). Effect of task on movement control in cerebral palsy: Implications for assessment and therapy. *Developmental Medicine and Child Neurology, 33,* 419-426.

Vallbo, B. (1970). Discharge patterns in human muscle spindle afferents during isometric voluntary contractions. *Acta Physiologica Scandinavica, 80,* 552-566.

von Hofsten, C., & Rönnquist, L. (1988). Preparation for grasping an object: Developmental study. *Journal of Experimental Psychology: Human Perception and Performance, 14*(4), 610-621.

Wannier, T.M.J., Töltl, M., & Hepp-Reymond, M-C. (1986). Neuronal activity in the postcentral cortex related to force regulation during a precision grip. *Brain, 382,* 427-432.

Wilson, D.M. (1964). The origin of the flight-motor command in grasshoppers. In R.F. Qeiss (Ed.). *Neuronal theory and modeling.* Palo Alto: Stanford University Press.

4

Perceptual Functions of the Hand

Janet M. Stilwell   Sharon A. Cermak

The hand has two closely related functions: it is both an executive and a perceptual organ (Hatwell, 1987). As an executive organ it is used for carrying out everyday activities such as tying shoes or buttoning buttons. As a perceptual organ it seeks and processes information such as when searching for a coin in a pocket. The two functions of the hand are closely intertwined. Rochat (1989) emphasized that "from the origin of development, action is under some perceptual or sensorimotor control and the picking up of perceptual information is somehow inherent in any performed act" (p. 871). However, when the hand performs a practical action, its perceptual functioning is regulated by what is needed to achieve this action, whereas when the hand acts primarily as a perceptual system, its motor activity is primarily exploratory and information seeking.

This chapter concerns the hand as a perceptual or information-seeking organ. Focus is on active touch (haptic perception) rather than passive touch. Passive touch involves only the excitation of receptors in the skin and underlying tissue; "active touch involves the concomitant excitation of receptors in the joints and tendons along with new and changing patterns in the skin" (Gibson, 1962, p. 48). Brazelton has suggested that, whereas "passive touch may add to an infant's ability to initiate and maintain control, active touch . . . acts as an alerter and as information. It helps the infant come to a receptive alert state and begin to process information" (Rose, 1990, p. 316). Haptic perception deals with the retrieval, analysis, and interpretation of the tactile properties (such as size, shape, and texture) and identity of objects through manual and in-hand manipulation.

Gibson (1962) considers this process of tactile scanning to be complex and to include the blending of feedback from tactile, kinesthetic, and proprioceptive sensations. The tactile spatial properties of objects are thought to be obtained through the retrieval of information about the relationship of the objects to the body and gravity during active manual exploration.

The study of haptic perception has been closely associated with the study of visual perception. Researchers have attempted to gain insight into how we use our visual and haptic senses to function by comparing the ability of subjects to match objects through the use of vision and through the use of haptic manipulation. These studies typically require the subject to match a standard (test) object to a set of two or more comparison objects. If the subject is asked to do an *intramodal comparison,* both the standard and the comparison objects are analyzed using the same sensory modality (visual or haptic sense). If the subject is asked to do an *intermodal comparison,* the standard object is analyzed using one sense and the comparison objects are analyzed using the other sense. In this chapter research methodology is specified as containing intramodal or intermodal matching while the senses used appear in parentheses (standard-comparison). For example, intermodal (haptic-visual) matching means that the haptic sense was used to analyze the standard or test object and the visual sense was used to select from among the comparison objects. The term *multimodal exploration* refers to the simultaneous use of the visual and haptic senses in object investigation. In this chapter the review of intramodal matching (matching using the same sensory system) is limited to haptic-haptic matching. That is, the subject feels the standard or test object and then feels several comparison objects to find the match.

A goal of the chapter is to provide the reader with an understanding of selected aspects of haptic perception that may influence effective evaluation and treatment of children with suspected and identified CNS impairment. Such children have often been found to have problems in haptic perception (Ayres, 1972b, 1989; Cermak, 1991; Haron and Henderson, 1985; Kinnealey, 1989; Reitan, 1971; Solomons, 1957). The chapter reviews the literature on selected aspects of haptic perception. Topics covered include the development of haptic perception, functions contributing to haptic perception, evaluation of haptic perception in infants and children, and haptic perception in children with disorders. The adult literature has been included to the degree to which it assists in

our understanding of the current status of the pediatric research.

DEVELOPMENT OF HAPTIC PERCEPTION
Haptic Perception in Infants

In the infant the hands and the mouth are both potential sources of haptic information. Ruff (1980) suggests that manipulation may facilitate the learning of an object's characteristics. Results from cross-modal studies show that the mouth can be used to gain information about the shape and the substance of objects (Ruff, 1989). Percheux, Lepecq, and Salzarulo (1988) found evidence suggesting intramodal (haptic-haptic) recognition of shapes inserted into nipples by 2 months of age.

As the infant develops, the hands are a perceptual system that participates in the infant's construction of knowledge (Hatwell, 1987). It is during exploratory play of the first year that infants begin to learn about their environment, their bodies, and how their actions can effect change (Gibson, 1988). During this time the foundations for later symbolic action are laid (Hatwell, 1987). Current research has indicated that haptic abilities are much more efficient in infants than was thought in the past (Hatwell, 1987). Use of the habituation paradigm adapted from vision research has shown that early intramodal (haptic-haptic) manual exploration in infants provides consistent haptic discrimination (Hatwell, 1987; Steri and Pecheux, 1986). In this paradigm infants are given shapes to manually explore with a screen preventing the infants from seeing their hands. The amount of interest the infant devotes to the object is measured by the amount of time the object is grasped. Using two pairs of shapes, Steri and Pecheux (1986) observed a haptic habituation to a familiarized shape and a reaction to novelty when a new shape was presented to 4- and 5-month-old infants. This was noted in infants as young as 2 to 3 months (Steri, 1987). Steri and Pecheux (1986) found that infants required a longer period of time to habituate to tactile stimuli than to visual stimuli. Since information can be obtained more quickly visually than tactually, the authors suggested that this may explain, in part, the differences in habituation time.

Research with infants has also shown that young infants evidence intermodal integration. Rose, Gottfried, and Bridger (1978) concluded that 6-month-old infants can integrate visual and haptic perception as evidenced by their ability to visually recognize a shape after only tactile contact with it.

Another study that supports very early development of visual-haptic integration and haptic object perception is by Steri and Spelke (1988, 1989). Responses of 4- to 5-month-old infants to visual images of objects were assessed following bilateral object handling without opportunity for visual regard of the hands. One object presented was two rings connected by a solid bar; the other object was two rings connected by a string. The infants produced different types of arm movements when holding the different objects. The infants were shown visual displays of two rings either connected or separated, which were moving as they typically did while the infants were holding them. The infants looked longest at the rings that were dissimilar to those which they had held. This was the expected response if the infants perceived the similarities between the rings that they held and moved and those that they saw moving. Steri and Spelke (1988) concluded that "infants evidently perceived connected or separated objects by detecting the patterns of common or independent motion that they themselves produced." They also noted that the infants held the objects for relatively long periods, as much as five times as long as they would have been expected to visually attend to an object. Since these 4-month-old infants were so competent at identifying objects tactually and visually, Steri and Spelke (1988) questioned Piaget's theory that vision and touch become integrated through haptic exploration of objects and suggested that this ability may be present without substantial experience in handling objects.

Haptic Perception in Children

Much of the literature on haptic perception in children deals with the recognition of common objects (e.g., comb, penny) and shapes (e.g., circle, square, diamond). However, the hand is also used to gain information about other object properties, such as texture, hardness, size, weight, and spatial orientation.

Recognition of Common Objects and Shapes

One of the most well-known studies on the development of haptic perception in children is that of Piaget and Inhelder (1948). They presented a series of solid (three-dimensional) common objects and cardboard cutouts of shapes (geometric figures and topologic forms) to a group of 2- to 7-year-old children and asked the children to feel

each figure and then visually select the figure from among a set of figure drawings. The geometric figures used ranged from simple (e.g., circle, ellipse, square) to complex (e.g., star, cross, semicircle). Topologic forms were shapes with irregular surfaces containing one or two holes or having openings or closings on their outer edges. These authors found that the ability of children to identify objects and shapes by touch progressively improved with increased age. Children 2½ to 3½ years of age were able to correctly recognize common objects but were unable to identify shapes. By 3½ to 5 years of age children developed the ability to match topologic forms. Recognition of geometric figures emerged at 4 to 4½ years with the ability to differentiate curvilinear (circle and ellipse) from rectilinear (square and rectangle) shapes. The ability to recognize geometric figures in greater numbers and levels of complexity was shown to progressively improve from 4½ to 7 years of age.

Subsequent research on haptic discrimination of common objects has been infrequent. Benton and Schultz (1949) studied intermodal (haptic-visual) matching of common objects in a group of 156 3- to 5-year-old children. Test performance was found to progressively improve with increasing age. Three-year-old children were typically able to recognize 50% of the items presented (mean 4.0 out of eight items). Four-year-old children performed only slightly better than children in the 3-year-old age group (mean = 4.5). Near perfect performance was typically found by 5 years of age, with most children correctly recognizing at least seven of the eight objects presented.

Hoop (1971a) also studied intermodal (haptic-visual) matching at 3½ to 5½ years. Like Piaget and Inhelder, Hoop found the identification of common objects to be easier than the recognition of topologic forms and geometric figures. There was little variation in the ability of 3½ to 5½-year-old children to match topologic forms (means ranging from 2.3 to 2.6 out of a maximum score of 4). Miller (1971) reported a similar finding. The 3- and 4-year-old children in her study were able to identify less than half of the intermodally (haptic-visual matching) and intramodally (haptic-haptic matching) presented shapes. Like Piaget and Inhelder, Hoop found the recognition of topologic forms through intermodal (haptic-visual) matching to be easier than the identification of geometric figures. However, this has not been a consistent finding.

Research conducted by Lovell (cited in Derevensky, 1979) revealed no difference in the ability of children to recognize topologic forms versus geometric figures. Derevensky (1979) and Derevensky and Petrushka (cited in Derevensky, 1979) used a combination of intramodal and intermodal (visual and haptic) matching test conditions and found topologic forms to be more difficult for children to recognize than geometric figures. These authors suggested that listing shapes as topologic or geometric may be an incorrect method of categorization; they suggested that it may not be whether a shape is topologic or geometric but the nature of the distinctive features that it contains which contributes to task difficulty.

There is general agreement that the ability of children to select geometric figures through intermodal (haptic-visual) matching emerges at about 4 years of age (Abravanel, 1972; Blank and Bridger, 1964; Hoop, 1971a; Micallef and May, 1979; Piaget and Inhelder, 1948). Like the finding of Piaget and Inhelder, all of these studies have noted improvement in accuracy with increasing age.

Another interesting discovery was made by Abravanel (1972), who found that, in a series of intermodal (haptic-visual) matching conditions, it was easier for 6- to 8-year-old children to identify solid (three-dimensional) than flat (two-dimensional) geometric figures. She attributed this finding to possible variation in the usefulness of the manipulation strategies used by the children in shape exploration. This topic is discussed in depth in a later section of this chapter.

Recognition of Texture, Size, and Weight

Haptic discrimination of texture, size, and weight has been shown to improve with increasing age in 4- to 9-year-old children (Gliner, 1967; Miller, 1986; Siegel and Vance, 1970; Solomons, 1957). Gliner further found rough textures to be easier to identify than smooth textures, with third-grade subjects showing a lower threshold (greater sensitivity) to texture stimuli than the kindergarten subjects in her study.

Intermodal (haptic-visual) discrimination of diameter and length has been found to emerge at 4 years and continues to mature into adolescence, with variation in diameter being easier to recognize than variation in length (Abravanel, 1968a, 1968b; Connolly and Jones, 1970; Hulme et al., 1983). When analyzing length, children find tasks requiring intramodal (vision or haptic) discrimination easier than those requiring intermodal (vision and haptic) discrimination for object comparison (Hulme et al., 1982, 1984).

Research comparing children's preference for the use of texture, size, and shape in object recognition suggests that there may be a developmental progression in preferential use of these sensory properties. Preference for the use of texture over shape in object identification during intramodal (haptic-haptic) matching tasks has been found to occur in young children (4 to 5 years of age) but not in older children (Gliner, 1967; Siegel and Barber, 1973; Siegel and Vance, 1970). Size has been shown to be more difficult to discriminate than texture at 4 and 8 years (Miller, 1986). Gliner et al. (1969) further found the preference of kindergartners for texture over shape in object identification in an intramodal (haptic-haptic) matching task to decrease as the textured surfaces became more difficult to identify. Preference for the use of shape over texture and size during intramodal (haptic-haptic) matching of objects was cited by Siegel and Vance (1970) in kindergarten through third-grade children. Miller (1986) further found that variation in shape interfered with accuracy in identification of texture during intramodal (haptic-haptic) matching in 8-year-old children but not in 4-year-old children. She concluded that this may be because 4-year-old children tend to ignore shape cues when texture is available for use in object discrimination. Thus it is possible that, during tasks requiring haptic discrimination, children may choose to use the sensory property that produces the strongest distinctive features. As the ability to recognize shapes improves with age, there may be increased preference for the use of shape over other properties for object identification because shape yields distinctive features that are more useful in object recognition than texture or size. If this hypothesis is correct, then the properties selected for use in object recognition may be age and task dependent. They may vary based on both the degree to which the distinctive features provided by the object are easy to identify and by the developmental level of haptic perception (e.g., texture, shape, size) exhibited by the child being tested.

Recognition of the Spatial Orientation of Objects

Few studies addressed the development of haptic spatial orientation. Perceptual awareness of the constancy of spatial location through the use of vision and haptic exploration has been shown to develop at an early age. Three-year-old blind children were able to identify common objects after 180 degrees of object rotation (Landau,

1991). Hatwell and Sayettat (1991) asked 4- to 7-year-old children to reseat a doll at a table inside a dollhouse after the child, the doll, the table, or the house was rotated. Many of the 4-year-old children were able to successfully reseat the doll in the initial location following rotation using intramodal (visual or haptic) exploration. An age-related increase in accuracy of doll placement occurred between ages 4 and 6 years. The shape of the table had no effect on task performance.

Children of 4½ years in a study by Abravanel (1968a) could visually recognize test objects facing up, down, or rotated but had difficulty when intermodal (haptic-visual) matching was required for task completion. Intermodal recognition of up-down was no better than chance until 5 years of age, and the identification of rotated figures was not possible until 6 years of age. Pick, Klein, and Pick (1966) used intramodal (visual-visual and haptic-haptic) matching tasks to study the ability of children to differentiate the up-down orientation of letterlike forms. They noted that the task could be performed more easily through the use of vision than through the use of touch. No relationship was found between the ability of subjects to perform the task through the use of vision versus touch, leading the authors to conclude that perhaps the method used in coding and discriminating spatial orientation is different for the two sensory modalities. However, it is also possible that the method of CNS processing might not be different for vision and touch; some types of objects might just be better suited for processing through one sensory system than through the other. For example, letterlike forms may represent a type of object that is easily processed through use of the visual system but is not easily analyzed through use of the tactile system.

Sex and Hand Differences in Haptic Recognition and Haptic Accuracy

Several studies have examined whether boys and girls perform differently in the accuracy of haptic perception and whether one hand is more accurate than the other. Research has generally shown that boys and girls 3 to 14 years display equal ability to recognize common objects, shapes, and words through intramodal (haptic-haptic) and intermodal (haptic-visual) matching (Abravanel, 1970; Affleck and Joyce, 1979; Ayres, 1989; Benton et al., 1983; Benton and Schultz, 1949; Cioffi and Kandel, 1979; Cronin, 1977; Etaugh and Levy, 1981; Gliner, 1967; Klein and Rosenfield, 1980;

Kleinman, 1979; Witelson, 1976; Wolff, 1972). Occasionally boys have been identified as exhibiting greater skill than girls in the intramodal (haptic-haptic) matching of objects by texture, size, and shape (Gliner, 1967; Solomons, 1957). In addition, Siegel and Barber (1973) found boys to display a stronger preference than girls for the use of form over texture in the intramodal (haptic-haptic) matching of shapes. Most studies conducted on normal adults have shown there to be no difference in the overall accuracy of haptic perception between men and women (Cronin, 1977; Kleinman, 1979; McGlone, 1980).

Children are often found to display greater left than right hand skill in some forms of haptic perception; however, the strength and age of onset of this difference vary between studies. In a literature review Hahn (1987) concluded that left hand superiority for the recognition of meaningless shapes appears to emerge during childhood, although he cited great variation between studies in the age of onset of this differentiation in hand skill (e.g., Affleck and Joyce, 1979; Etaugh and Levy, 1981; Solomons, 1957).

The finding of greater left than right hand skill on some tasks, particularly those requiring discrimination of meaningless shapes, has been viewed as being related to right hemisphere superiority in the processing of spatial information (e.g., Witelson, 1974, 1976). However, since the age of onset of right-left hand differences varies widely between studies, it is inappropriate to interpret the presence/absence of a hand difference for stereognosis as being related to the maturity of hemispheric specialization for haptic perception in a given child. Consistent evidence of a right-left hand difference for stereognosis does not appear until adolescence.

Summary and Implications for Practice

The ability to distinguish the texture, shape, and substance of objects through the use of intramodal (haptic-haptic) and intermodal (haptic-visual and visual-haptic) exploration develops over a long period. It begins to emerge in early infancy and continues to mature into adolescence.

Infants are amazingly adept at using haptic exploration with the mouth and the hands to learn about objects in their environment. Early haptic discrimination using the mouth is seen at 1 month, and haptic discrimination using the hands appears at 1 to 2 months of age. Intermodal transfer of information between the haptic and visual senses occurs by 4 to 6 months. This means that infants during the second half of the first year of life can explore an object using the hand or the eye and then recognize the same object as being similar or different using the opposite sense.

Haptic perception improves with increasing age. Children find common objects easier to haptically recognize than topologic forms and geometric figures. At 2½ years children can identify many common objects through use of the haptic sense. Haptic recognition of common objects reaches full maturity by about 5 years. Intramodal (haptic) and intermodal (haptic and visual) identification of topologic forms and geometric shapes emerges at 3 to 4 years and continues to develop throughout childhood. With increasing age children are able to match forms/shapes having increasingly complex distinctive features. They are also able to move from recognizing only solid (three-dimensional) shapes to being able to also distinguish flat (two-dimensional) figures.

Like adults, children show greater left than right hand skill in some forms of haptic perception, possibly reflecting specialization of the right hemisphere for the processing of spatial information. Although some authors suggest that haptic perception may be better in boys than in girls, the research on this topic is inconclusive.

The literature contains little information about the development of sensory properties such as texture and weight in childhood. It is known that children find rough textures easier to match than smooth textures. The development of texture discrimination improves between 4 and 9 years, in part because tactile sensitivity increases during this time span (Gliner, 1967). The discrimination of diameter and length begins at about 4 years and continues into adolescence, with variation in diameter being easier to recognize than variation in length. Children as young as 3 to 4 years can recognize the spatial orientation of an object when the child or the object has been rotated, but it is not until 5 to 6 years that children can haptically identify objects as facing up, down, or rotated.

Children's ability to haptically analyze objects having two or more tactile properties is limited. Rather than analyzing several sensory properties simultaneously as adults do, children appear to select one sensory property to use in object analysis. The sensory property selected seems to be the one that is easiest for the child to recognize, perhaps because it exhibits the strongest distinctive features. For example, texture is preferred to shape and size in young children, whereas older children are more likely to match objects by shape than by texture. In addition, the coexistence of several sensory properties in a given object can impair haptic discrimination at some ages. This finding suggests that haptic figure-ground may be an issue in haptic object discrimination, a factor that needs to be considered in the development of tests of haptic perception.

There is much that is still not known about the development of haptic perception in children. We know far more about the development of haptic recognition of common objects and shapes than we do about the development of haptic recognition of properties such as texture, hardness, weight, and temperature. We do not know whether the ability to distinguish objects by shape, size, texture, or weight develops sequentially or simultaneously. Research suggests that children develop the ability to discriminate all of these sensory properties. So it is logical to conclude that we should provide children with ample opportunity to analyze objects having varying sensory properties. When presenting activities designed to promote the development of haptic perception, we need not only to vary objects by one sensory property but also to offer objects with a combination of sensory properties. If the child has the opportunity to sort objects in a variety of ways, he/she is likely to identify or sort objects using the sensory property that has the strongest distinctive features or the one that is most well developed in that child. The sensory properties that the child consistently avoids using may be those which are most delayed and thus most in need of being addressed in treatment. Since little is known about the development of haptic figure-ground perception in children, we do not know if the finding of impaired haptic discrimination in multisensory haptic play activities is normal or a sign of impairment. However, we can be sensitive to the signs of haptic sensory overload in children. It is possible that playing with toys having several sensory properties may be disorganizing for some infants and children. When problems are seen, controlling the variety as well as the quantity of sensory experiences may be necessary to elicit optimum performance during school and play activities.

FUNCTIONS CONTRIBUTING TO HAPTIC PERCEPTION

Most haptic perception tasks are complex. This point is exemplified in a study by Semmes (1965), who found haptic perception to be consistently impaired in adult brain-injured patients with accompanying deficits in somatosensory sensation. Even when the sensory loss was restricted to one hand, bilateral impairment in haptic perception was seen. But she also found deficits in haptic perception among brain-injured patients with normal somatosensory sensation. Research suggests that, in addition to somatosensory processing, manual and in-hand manipulation, along with vision and cognition, contributes to haptic perception.

Role of Somatosensory Sensation in Haptic Perception

Vierck (1976) proposed that sensory feedback processed through the dorsal columns may guide exploratory hand use. Ongoing subcortical and cortical processing of somatosensory sensation has been cited during slow hand movement (Darian-Smith, Sugitani, and Heywood, 1982; Iwamura et al., 1985; Lemon, 1981; Starr and Cohen, 1985). Although the firing of haptic neurons in the sensorimotor cortex is often given credit for guiding exploratory hand use and contributing to the ability to recognize objects by touch, synaptic connections between many CNS structures are involved in the process (Carpenter, 1985; Mountcastle, 1976). Disruption in communication anywhere within this circuit could logically result in loss or impairment in the ability to explore objects with the hands.

A synthesis of information derived from somatosensory receptors provides the hand with a picture of the body and its orientation in space (body scheme) (Gardner, 1988). This internal picture of the body is thought to be used by CNS processes as a framework of the parameters of real world time and space (Brooks, 1986). Upon this framework are scaled motor commands used in motor programing and in executing complex sequenced movements. This internal picture of the body also is thought to serve as a template for interpreting the spatial properties of objects (Gibson, 1962). The precise detail of this internal picture of the body decreases and its spatial complexity increases with progressive afferent processing in the CNS (Brooks, 1986). Research suggests that body scheme may be more important in the performance of complex haptic perception tasks (e.g., stereognosis) than in the performance of tasks requiring less complex haptic discrimination (e.g., discrimination of texture) (Semmes, 1965; Stilwell, 1989).

Not only does somatosensory sensation contribute to the development of body scheme needed for the interpretation of the spatial properties of objects, but it also appears to be necessary for regulating manual and in-hand manipulation during active touch. The sensory control of hand movements is discussed in Chapter 1. At present it seems sufficient to note that, to actively retrieve somatosensory sensation from the environment during active touch, the individual must be able to make rapid and frequent changes in the speed and sequencing of hand movements and regulate force during object manipulation (Hollins and Goble, 1988; Johnson and Hsiao, 1992). These elements of fine motor coordination are thought to be dependent on the processing of tactile, kinesthetic, and proprioceptive sensations for their execution (Brooks, 1986; Johansson and Westling, 1988, 1990).

Role of Manual Manipulation and Exploratory Strategies in Haptic Perception

Interest in the role of in-hand manipulation and other forms of manual exploration in haptic perception appears to have been precipitated by the work of Gibson (1962) on active and passive touch. Using a set of geometric-shaped cookie cutters, adult subjects were either allowed to actively manipulate the cookie cutters or the tactile stimuli were passively presented by the examiner (cookie cutters pressed or pressed and turned in the palm of the subject's hand). The use of active touch contributed to greater accuracy in intermodal (haptic-visual) shape recognition than either of the passive touch conditions although pressing and turning the cookie cutters in the subject's hand (passive pressure with movement) yielded higher scores than the isolated use of passive pressure. Replication of Gibson's study with children yielded similar findings. Haron and Henderson (1985) found children better able to distinguish the cookie cutter shapes through the use of active touch than through the use of passive touch (passive pressure with movement). Cronin (1977) also replicated Gibson's study and obtained slightly different results. She found that shape recognition by school-age children and young adults did not differ between active touch and passive touch (passive pressure with movement) conditions when tactile stimulation was restricted to the palm of the hand in all test conditions; however, she did note that the isolated use of passive pressure (passive pressure without movement) contributed to lower test scores than either of the other two test conditions. In addition, no difference between active touch and passive touch (pressure with movement) was found for the discrimination of texture and tactile maze learning in adults (Lederman, 1981; Richardson, Wuillemin, and MacKintosh, 1981). These findings suggest that it might be movement of the object over the skin surface that produces the tactile feedback needed for object recognition. Although movement of the object in the hand theoretically can be active or passive, it is most commonly produced actively, through the use of manual manipulation and exploratory strategies. This raises the question of how the pattern of tactile feedback generated by variation in the pattern of manual and in-hand manipulation affects the accuracy of object identification. Several researchers in recent years have attempted to answer this question; their findings are discussed in the following section. See Chapter 8 for a discussion of in-hand manipulation. Because most of the research on this topic has been done on adults, this section begins with a summary of the adult research. This is followed by a review of the pediatric literature.

Haptic Manipulation Strategies in Adults

Early research on the influence of manipulation strategies in object recognition was done by Davidson in a series of studies comparing the ability of sighted and congenitally blind subjects to recognize raised curved edges. Davidson (1972) and Davidson and Whitson (1974) found that, when exploring concave, convex, and straight edges, subjects chose to use three manipulation strategies (gripping, pinching the edge, and sweeping the fingers over the top edge). Gripping (grasping the object in the hand) led to fewer errors in identifying the form of the curved edges in both blind and sighted subjects. Gripping was later found to be a useful strategy for obtaining a general understanding of the tactile properties retained by an object (e.g., texture, weight, shape) (Lederman and Klatzky, 1987; Klatzky, Lederman, and Reed, 1987). The method of gripping (referred to as enclosure in some studies) could be modified to aid in differential discrimination of size and shape. Reed and Klatzky (1990) found that subjects preferred to grip with the whole hand when analyzing the size of objects and grip with effort the edges of the object using the fingers and palm when analyzing shape. Although gripping provides subjects with a general classification of object

properties, other strategies are often used when refined analysis is needed.

Contour following (moving the fingers around the edge of the object) was found by Lederman and Klatzky (1987) to be an optimum strategy for use in haptic shape recognition. In a thorough analysis of strategies used in the identification of geometric shapes, Kleinman and Brodzinsky (1978) found that subjects preferred to use a combination of manipulation strategies including an initial scanning of the standard and comparison objects. This was followed by detailed simultaneous comparison of the standard and comparison objects (congruent feature comparison of analogous and mirror-image features and contour following). The initial time spent in scanning the objects was reduced as the shapes became more complex. Locher and Simmons (1978) found the haptic recognition of symmetric shapes to be more difficult than the recognition of asymmetric shapes. Partial trace scanning (contour following along portions of the shape) was common for asymmetric shapes. More complex scanning strategies were used for the identification of symmetric shapes (several repetitions of partial and complete contour following). In a subsequent study Simmons and Locher (1979) found use of the trace scanning strategy (contour following around the complete shape several times using two fingers) to lead to greater accuracy in the identification of asymmetric shapes and the simultaneous apprehension scanning strategy (smooth, continuous movement of thumb and index fingers of both hands over opposite sides of the shape simultaneously) to lead to greater accuracy in the identification of symmetric shapes. The results of these studies suggest that the isolated use of contour following may not always be the most appropriate approach for use in the identification of shapes. It may be necessary to change manipulation strategies to adapt to variation in symmetry of distinctive features and complexity of the objects presented.

Lederman and Klatzky (1987) analyzed manipulation strategies used for the identification of texture, hardness, weight, volume, and temperature. They found that the optimum manipulation strategy (which they termed *exploratory procedures*) for use in object identification differed for each tactile property (Table 4-1). Although contour following was found to be necessary for accurate recognition of shape, several approaches could be used for the identification of most other tactile properties. The most effective strategies were (1)

Table 4-1. Haptic procedures associated with acquiring knowledge about objects

OBJECT DIMENSION	EXPLORATORY PROCEDURES
Substance	
Texture	Lateral motion
Hardness	Pressure
Temperature	Static control
Weight	Unsupported holding
Structure	
Weight	Unsupported holding
Volume	Enclosure; contour following
Global shape	Enclosure
Exact shape	Contour following
Function	
Part motion	Part motion test
Specific function	Function test

Data from Lederman, S. J., & Klatzky, R. L. (1987). Hand movements: A window into haptic object recognition. *Cognitive Psychology, 19,* 342-368.

texture: lateral motion (moving the finger across the surface of the object), (2) hardness: pressure, (3) weight: unsupported holding, (4) volume: enclosure (gripping), and (5) temperature: static contact. Jiggling while holding the object has also been found to aid in the discrimination of weight (Brodle and Ross, 1985).

Preferred manipulation strategies remained unchanged when subjects were asked to determine the gradations of a given tactile property (texture, size, shape, and hardness) and when they needed to simultaneously sort pouches (fabric-covered shapes) by one to three of these tactile properties (Klatzky, Lederman, and Reed, 1989; Lederman and Klatzky, 1987). Enclosure (gripping) was commonly used for all tactile properties, with lateral motion being used primarily for the identification of texture, pressure being primarily used for the identification of hardness, and contour following being used primarily for the identification of shape and size. When pouches needed to be simultaneously sorted by two or three properties, the manipulation strategies were combined, with lateral motion and pressure often being merged into a single finger movement. When the properties of texture and shape needed to be analyzed, adults appeared to search for cues about texture before they searched for cues about the object's shape (Lederman, Brown, and Klatzky, 1988). Subjects showed a preference for the use of manipulation strategies that could be used to simulta-

neously analyze two tactile properties. Exploration time decreased when subjects could use lateral motion and pressure to simultaneously discriminate texture and hardness and when they could use gripping (enclosure) to simultaneously discriminate size and shape (Klatzky, Lederman, and Reed, 1989; Reed and Klatzky, 1990). This finding suggests that subjects may prefer manipulation strategies that can be used to simultaneously explore multiple sensory properties.

Not only do subjects appear to select haptic manipulation strategies based on the tactile properties of objects, they also appear to organize manipulation strategies into a sequence. Lederman and Klatzky (1990) found haptic exploration in adults to consist of a two-stage sequence. The first stage consists of generalized exploration of the object using manipulation strategies such as gripping (enclosure) or unsupported holding (object resting in the palm of the open hand), strategies that provide awareness of the general tactile properties of the object. This is followed by a second stage of refined manipulation, where the subject uses more specialized manipulation strategies (e.g., contour following, lateral motion) to gain specific information about object characteristics. During the second stage the subject often alternates between different manipulation strategies to guide the retrieval of information about the object.

In summary, results of research on haptic manipulation and exploratory strategies provide support for the hypothesis that the pattern of tactile feedback generated by variation in patterns of manual manipulation during active touch contributes to the accuracy of object recognition. Adults select manipulation strategies based on the tactile properties of the object being explored. Furthermore, they combine and sequence the use of these manipulation strategies in situations where conditions require the simultaneous or sequential analysis of several tactile properties. The sophisticated haptic manipulation strategies seen in adults seem to develop throughout childhood.

Haptic Manipulation Strategies in Infants

Haptic exploration begins in early infancy. Neonates and young infants gain much information about objects from action with their mouth. At 2 and 3 months spontaneous interaction with a novel object starts with an oral contact; later, by 4 months, interaction starts with visual inspection (Rochat, 1989). By 4 months, even though vision emerges as the initial modality of exploration, infants continue to frequently bring the object to the mouth. Spontaneous behavior by infants suggests increasing multimodal (visual and haptic) organization of exploration, with vision playing a growing role. According to Rochat (1989), the hands serve both transport and support functions, bringing the object alternately into the oral zone and into the field of view for exploration. According to Ruff (1989), there is a dual role of handling; the hands make information available to the eyes as the object is manipulated at the same time that the hands directly gather haptic information. In the first role the hands are used to manipulate the object and to change the object's location relative to the observer, such as turning the object around to provide different visual perspectives. In the second role the hands gather haptic information about the object, such as by pressing the object to determine its substance or by rubbing the finger across the object to determine its texture or shape.

In conjunction with the early development of multimodal exploration, the characteristics of object manipulation change from 2 to 5 months. At 2 to 3 months the infants' manipulative behaviors are primarily limited to grasping movements, potentially informing the infant about the object's substance. Although slight finger movements are produced at 2 months, by 4 months the occurrence of fingering behavior increases significantly (Rochat, 1989). Before this age, when both hands were involved in contacting an object, it was primarily for transporting the object to the mouth. Rochat (1989) noted that in young infants (2 to 4 months) bimanual coordination is initially linked to the oral system. This observation points to the importance of the mouth in the early manifestation of bimanual action in the context of object manipulation. The hand-mouth coordination seen in the 2- to 4-month-old infant is later combined with vision when behaviors such as fingering emerge.

To more thoroughly assess how infants use object handling skills to gain information for recognition of specific object qualities, Ruff (1984) studied 6-, 9-, and 12-month-old infants and assessed the various manipulation strategies they used, including mouthing, fingering, transferring, banging, and object rotation. With increasing age, fingering increased, particularly with objects that varied in texture. Ruff suggested that this fingering can be crucial for obtaining information about small object details. Hand use for object rotation was also noted to change, with all children using a one-handed rotation pattern, in which the arm or the wrist moves, but only older infants

using two-handed object rotations. Ruff suggested that two-handed rotation can be particularly useful because with rotation the object does not have some parts covered by the hand. She suggested that infants who cannot adjust their handling skills so they can finger objects rather than just hold them, and infants who cannot effectively use two hands together, may be limited in the complexity of information about objects which they can readily gather.

Given that adults use a flexible repertoire of exploratory strategies and that certain actions may be particularly useful for obtaining specific information about objects, the question has also been asked, how, during development, do young infants and children tailor their actions to explore objects (Palmer, 1989)? Whereas earlier work has suggested that infants' actions are not clearly related to object attributes (McCall, 1974), current research has found that exploratory action patterns are indeed influenced by object characteristics and that the actions of the infant are related in functional ways to the structure of the environment (Gibson, 1988).

In a series of studies Ruff (1980, 1984, 1989) examined the effect of object characteristics on infant manipulation strategies. In a study of 9- and 12-month-olds, Ruff (1980) found that infants fingered objects with surface texture more than they fingered smooth blocks. Ruff (1984) investigated 6- to 12-month-old infants' manipulation of a range of objects varying in color, shape, texture, and weight and found that manual exploration was adapted to the visual and the tactual properties of the object. When infants were given objects that varied in shape, they rotated the objects and transferred them from one hand to the other hand; whereas when objects had varying surface textures, infants fingered the objects, often scratching the object's surface. Weight change resulted in less looking and more banging than did other changes in object characteristics. In a more recent study Ruff (1989) found that by 7 to 9 months infants bang hard objects more than soft objects, bang more on hard surfaces than on soft surfaces, and finger textured objects more than smooth objects. In a study of 12-month-old infants' haptic exploration and discrimination, Gibson and Walker (1984) found that infants squeezed, rubbed, and pressed a spongy object more than a rigid object, and that they banged the rigid object more than the spongy object. The results of these studies suggest that infants adjust their manipulative behavior to the characteristics of objects.

Table 4-2. Developmental progression for haptic discrimination of shapes and objects

AGE RANGE	HAPTIC STRATEGY
2½ to 4 years	Children may play with object (e.g., push), but there is no active manual exploration; grasping or touching of object is seen with palm being still when making contact with object; by 3 to 6 years child begins to make discoveries about discriminative features seemingly by chance
4 to 5 years	Exploration often remains passive, with object being grasped between palm and middle fingers; crude manual exploration begins; when manual exploration is seen, it is done in a global haphazard manner, which includes probing for distinctive features
5 to 6 years	Systematic use of both hands (palms and fingers) begins; isolated analysis of distinctive features without studying whole form can be observed
6 to 7 years	Use of systematic method of exploration can be seen; contour following is used

Palmer (1989) also found that infants ages 6, 9, and 12 months tailored their actions to particular object and table characteristics. Palmer recorded the manipulative behavior of infants with 12 different objects of varying rigidity, texture, shape, weight, and sound potential using two different table surfaces (hard wood and foam covered). Research demonstrated that infants made use of both object properties and table surface properties. For example, infants banged more on the wood surface. Age differences in actions were also noted. Palmer suggested that age differences in actions may reflect developing action economy (e.g., waving the bell with a flick of the wrist rather than with the whole arm swing seen in younger infants), new exploratory systems (e.g., changing from mouthing to waving and banging), and increasing fine motor control (e.g., finger individuation).

Recent research suggests that even infants younger than 6 months detect an object's perceptual features that enable particular actions (affordances) for hand and mouth. Rochat (1983, 1987) found that neonates showed differential oral and manual responding to objects varying in substance and texture. In a study of 3-month-old infants, Rochat (1989) noted that the characteristics of manual manipulation and exploration by the infant reflected some relation to the physical properties and affordances of the object.

Steri and Spelke (1988) examined manipulation strategies in 4-month-olds and proposed that longer exploration occurs with two objects than with one object, since the infants tended to handle the rings with a rigid bar for less time than those which were connected by a string and tended to visually attend to the separated rings longer than the connected rings. Thus, even from a very young age, the nature of the object influences the type and extent of haptic exploration.

Haptic Manipulation Strategies in Children

Research with children has been limited primarily to analysis of the role of manipulation strategies in the development of haptic discrimination of shape and size (length). Results of these studies suggest that there is a developmental progression in the acquisition of manipulation strategies, with the accuracy of object identification being related to the level of sophistication of the haptic manipulation strategies used by the children (Abravanel, 1968b; Hoop, 1971b; Jennings, 1974; Kleinman, 1979; Wolff, 1972; Zaporozhets, 1965, 1969). The description of the developmental progression of haptic discrimination of common objects and shapes in Table 4-2 is a summary of the work conducted by Piaget and Inhelder (1948) and Zaporozhets (1965, 1969). Whereas haptic strategies of the 2- to 4-year-old child consist primarily of grasping the object, by age 6 to 7 years systematic exploration with contour following is noted.

Abravanel (1968b) provided a description of the developmental progression in haptic manipulation of size (length) that was strikingly similar to that identified for the analysis of common objects and shapes. She found that the youngest children in her study (3 to 5 years) typically used the palm of the hand, grasping and palpating the objects. By 5 years the children held the ends of the bar used for evaluating length. From 5 through 8 years children used the whole hand (palm with progressively increasing use of the fingers) for manipulation of the bar and displayed a systematic method of determining length. By 9 years, use of the palm was no longer seen; the fingers and fingertips were used for exploration.

Actions Used By Infants in Object Exploration

Grasping	Rubbing
Banging	Pressing
Fingering	Poking
Mouthing	Slapping
Switching (hand to hand)	Scooting
Squeezing	Dropping

Several factors in test design have been found to influence the manipulation strategies used by children. Hoop (1971b) noted that for 5-year-old children common objects required less exploration than topologic forms, and topologic objects required less exploration than geometric figures for their identification. Abravanel (1970) noted that three-dimensional forms can be easily recognized through passive grasping. The 4- and 5-year-old children in her study actively explored three-dimensional geometric shapes but rarely attempted to manipulate similar two-dimensional shapes (2-cm figures cut from hardboard mounted on cardboard) (Abravanel, 1972). This contributed to a large discrepancy in accuracy scores for the two test conditions.

In summary, the results of studies that address analysis of strategies used in the recognition of common objects, shapes, and size (length) suggest that manipulation strategies become more complex with increasing age, a maturational change that seems to contribute to the accuracy of haptic object recognition. Research findings also suggest that structural characteristics of the test materials influence the time spent in haptic exploration, perhaps because they contribute to task difficulty or because they affect the complexity of manipulation strategies needed for object exploration. The effect of object characteristics on the use of manipulation strategies has rarely been addressed in preschool and school-age children although it has been addressed in infants. Infants use a variety of actions in exploring objects (see box above). These actions vary as a function of the object and surface characteristics, that is, they are influenced by the perceptual affordances provided by the environment.

Role of Vision and Cognition in Haptic Perception

Vision

Research suggests that vision plays an important role in the development of haptic perception. Rochat (1989) noted a major link between vision

and fine haptic exploration early in development and suggested that vision may serve as a potential organizer of multimodal exploration and object manipulation in infancy. This is based on research that indicates that fingering starts to manifest itself in coordination with vision. Refined object manipulation is more likely to occur when infants simultaneously look at and manipulate objects. Thus it may be important for infants to see their hands during manual object manipulation. As further support of the role of vision as an organizing factor of object manipulation, Rochat (1989) cites developmental studies of congenitally blind infants who exhibit drastic delays in the use of their hands as exploratory tools (Fraiberg, 1977). Even though congenitally blind toddlers spontaneously develop strategies such as object rotation (Landau, 1988), haptic exploration is primarily oral up to 3 to 4 years of age, much longer than is seen in sighted infants. Thus the use of vision in object exploration may be important for the development of haptic perception.

Hatwell (1990) suggests that even sighted children between the ages of 3 months and 6 years have difficulty using their hands for retrieving haptic information independent of vision. She suggests that the motor functions of young children's hands are primary, with the perceptual capabilities of the hands rarely used except as an adjunct to motor functioning. Hatwell notes that when vision is used, the hands primarily operate under this system of control. Ruff (1989) tempers this view by stating that it may be that the visual system guides exploratory behavior in the haptic system. In this sense, vision would not exclude the contribution from the haptic system as suggested by Hatwell (1987) but would constrain it. Ruff (1989) suggests that there is an "initial tightening of visual control over manipulation around 5 months of age [and] then the loosening of visual control sometime after nine months" (p. 313).

Haptic manipulation is also important in the early learning of object characteristics. Ruff (1980, 1982) points out that infants' manipulation of objects has two potential advantages. First, as infants look at an object they are manipulating, they see the object from different points of view and can learn about its properties. This is critical for the development of object recognition so that the infant can recognize an object in any orientation or in any context. Second, the infant acquires tactile and kinesthetic information about the object through active touch.

Ruff (1980) suggests that movement is particularly important in helping infants to detect the properties of an object that does not vary despite changes in the object's orientations. An important question is what type of movement is necessary. For example, the infant can produce different information about the object through his own movements such as through turning his head to look at the object, by moving his body around the object, or by holding, manipulating, and moving the object.

Alternatively, the infant can get different views of an object when a parent carries the infant around the room, or when the object itself moves as in an infant mobile, or when a parent moves the object, such as in the context of showing a toy to a child. Ruff (1980) suggests that object transformations which occur during movement allow for detection of object characteristics that would not be evident from observing a stationary object. She also suggests that, although both watching object movement and producing object movement are important in learning about objects, producing movement can yield the specific types of information sought and therefore is a more efficient way of learning about objects. The advantage to the individual doing the moving is that infants learn to recognize objects in the context of activity. Ruff (1980) found that 6-month-old infants learned structural differences in objects only when they actually manipulated the objects; viewing object movement did not result in the learning of object characteristics. It should be emphasized that, in the manipulation condition, the infants also visually monitored their movements, thus obtaining both tactile, proprioceptive, and visual information. Ruff suggests that the advantage of object manipulation may be in the simultaneous use of visual and tactile integration in learning about object qualities.

The heavy use of vision in object identification seen in infants may continue into adulthood. Research comparing visual and haptic discrimination has shown visual matching consistently superior to haptic and intermodal (haptic-visual and visual-haptic) matching (Garbin, 1988). This finding has left the impression that vision may be more important than haptic discrimination in object identification. But this may be an incorrect interpretation of the research findings. Klatzky, Lederman, and Metzer (1985) question this conclusion, stating that it may be inappropriate to use objects that can be easily interpreted by the visual system when evaluating function of the tactile system. The superiority of vision diminishes when subjects are given extra time to haptically manipulate objects and when complex three-dimensional objects are

presented for analysis (Butter and Bjorkund, 1973; Davidson, Abbot, and Gershenfeld, 1974; Garbin, 1988).

Rather than vision being superior to haptic manipulation, it would probably be more accurate to say that vision and somatosensory processing both play supportive roles in object identification. Although vision seems to be used by infants and young children to guide exploratory hand use, its purpose may not be to substitute for haptic perception but rather to guide the development of haptic manipulation and make the somatosensory input meaningful. If this is true, then vision would lose its superiority and somatosensory processing would gain in importance with increasing age. Each sensory system would take on increasingly separate roles in object identification with increasing age. Perhaps this is why visual learning is more rapid than haptic learning in young children (Juurmaa and Lehitinen-Railo, 1988). It is not until adolescence that the efficiency of haptic learning approaches that of visual learning.

Cognition

Cognition and vision are closely linked in haptic object identification. Piaget and Inhelder (1968) saw the ability to distinguish objects through the use of touch to be an external reflection of one's capacity to transform tactile properties of objects into visual images (integrate visual and haptic information). This ability to use visual imagery to improve haptic recognition and memory of objects is thought to contribute to children's ability to recognize objects on tests of haptic perception and to reproduce objects through drawing. In fact, research has shown that adults with high spatial ability and skill in mental imagery perform significantly better than their less skilled peers on tests of haptic perception (McCormick and Mouw, 1983).

Verbalization (mental labeling of the haptic properties of objects) also has been found to aid in haptic object identification. Bailes and Lambert (1986) compared the ability of blind and sighted adults to determine if four segments of a stimulus figure matched a completed geometric design. The sighted subjects were faster and more accurate than the blind subjects in their study. Adult subjects who used verbalization had better haptic accuracy scores than subjects who used a mixture of verbalization and mental imagery. Subjects who used solely mental imagery displayed the lowest haptic accuracy scores of the group.

The ability to use cognitive strategies (mental imagery and verbalization) to aid in haptic object recognition appears to develop during childhood. Children 3 to 6 years of age often cannot describe the strategies that they use to aid in haptic object identification (Brink and Bridger, 1964). By the fourth grade some children continue to have no cognitive strategy, several use solely verbalization or mental imagery, whereas most rely on a mixture of verbalization and visual imagery to aid in haptic object identification (Ford, 1973). Adults are evenly mixed in their isolated use of verbalization, isolated use of mental imagery, and combined use of the two cognitive strategies (Bailes and Lambert, 1986).

There has been little research analyzing the development of haptic cognitive strategies in children. But it is logical to assume that such strategies develop over time since they require visual-haptic integration and, in the case of verbalization, the integration of language as well. Thus any factor that impairs attention, memory, or cognitive problem solving could potentially impair test performance.

Summary and Implications for Practice

Several functions contribute to the ability to perform haptic perception tasks. Because an individual performs poorly on tests of haptic perception does not mean that somatosensory processing is impaired. Impairment in somatosensory processing, vision, visual perception, cognition, praxis, and any factor that may alter fine motor coordination has the potential to lower performance on tests of haptic perception. Determining the reason for a child's poor test performance is a necessary prerequisite for effective treatment planning.

In the clinic we may be able to gain some insight into the maturity of the somatosensory system by observing the tendency of infants to mouth and manipulate novel objects. Although infants use vision extensively in object exploration, we should expect to see a combination of visual and oral or manual exploration during play in infancy.

By definition, haptic perception includes oral or manual exploration. Placement of the object in the palm of the hand and movement of the object across the skin's surface improve object recognition. Although optimum performance is seen when manual manipulation is used for object identification, it should be possible to partially assess haptic perception without active manipulation by the patient. This might be accomplished by occluding the patient's vision, having the therapist move the object across the center of the palm, and then asking the patient to identify the object by visual matching or verbal response. For the individual with adequate fine motor skill, analysis of the quality of the haptic manipulation strategies used during test performance might provide useful diagnostic information.

The preferred manual manipulation and exploratory strategies of adults vary for objects with different tactile properties. The manipulation strategy used affects the accuracy of object identification. Research suggests that the development of haptic manual manipulation and exploratory strategies begins early in life, since infants use specific manipulation strategies to explore specific sensory properties. During childhood these manipulation strategies grow in complexity with increasing age. Little is known about how children develop the ability to select manipulation strategies based on the sensory characteristics of the object, or at what age children learn to combine manipulation strategies to improve the speed and efficiency of haptic exploration. We also do not know whether children with problems in haptic perception and fine motor coordination fail to use appropriate manipulation strategies because they have difficulty in the selection or in the execution of haptic manual manipulation and exploratory strategies. However, it is generally recognized that the immature haptic manipulation strategies seen in young children contribute to poor object recognition (Abravanel, 1968b; Derevensky, 1979; Hoop, 1971b; Jennings, 1974; Wolff, 1972; Zaporozhets, 1965, 1969).

Early haptic exploration in infancy is done with the mouth. It is over a year before mouthing is primarily replaced by manual manipulation. We cannot overemphasize the clinical importance of mouthing objects in infancy. Mouthing of objects not only seems to be important for decreasing oral hypersensitivity and facilitating oral-motor development, but it also appears to be important for environmental learning and may contribute to the early development of bilateral hand use. Infants who exhibit little mouthing of objects should be evaluated to determine the cause of the delay. Even older children who exhibit tactile defensiveness and those with problems in haptic discrimination should be encouraged to engage in oral and manual exploration of objects. It takes creativity and close interaction with parents to find socially acceptable ways to encourage mouthing beyond infancy. Children can also show a prolonged need for mouthing of objects. If the behavior is due to oral-tactile defensiveness or poor haptic discrimination, then mouthing should be encouraged. However, if the behavior is due to impaired visual-haptic integration or poor purposeful use of objects, then treatment should be directed toward pairing vision and oral-manual manipulation during purposeful interaction with objects. A bigger challenge is seen in children with multiple handicaps and those who have severe impairment in motor function. We need to help these infants incorporate mouthing of toys into daily play activities and find ways to attach toys to clothing and to positioning equipment so that the toys can easily reach the mouth.

Throughout infancy and early childhood vision is paired with haptic exploration of the mouth and the hands. Vision appears to guide the development of haptic manipulation strategies. It is not until later in life that vision and somatosensory sensations appear to take on separate but supportive roles in object identification and use.

The importance of vision in the development of haptic manipulation is seen in blind infants. Whereas normal infants begin to replace mouthing with manual manipulation at about 4 months, blind infants continue to identify objects orally, with mouthing being the dominant form of exploration until 3 or 4 years of age (Landau, 1988). Because vision appears to be necessary for the development of haptic manual manipulation, the use of haptic exploration with the hands will need to be specifically taught to blind infants; we cannot assume that, since the infant is not using vision, he/she will automatically use the hands for environmental exploration.

An interplay between vision and haptic exploration seems to be needed for environmental learning in infancy and early childhood. Under the age of 5 or 6 years activities should be designed that pair vision and touch rather than emphasize the use of the haptic or visual sense alone. The identification of object features should be integrated in these activities. An exception is seen in children who overuse vision to guide hand use. For these children vision may need to be removed from the play activities to encourage the child to retrieve and use haptic information.

Haptic object identification is made possible by combining vision and cognition. The use of visual imagery and verbalization helps improve haptic memory and discrimination. We cannot assume that children will automatically learn cognitive strategies to aid in haptic task performance. For children with attention deficits, brain injury, and mental retardation, the interpretation and use of haptic information might be enhanced by teaching them to use cognitive strategies such as mental imagery or verbalization techniques during task performance.

EVALUATION OF HAPTIC PERCEPTION IN INFANTS AND CHILDREN

Assessment of haptic perception can be considered from the perspective of standardized vs. nonstandardized assessments and also analyzed according to product/process dimensions. Most of the standardized assessments examine the product—that is, the accuracy of haptic perception, the number of items the child passed. Many of the nonstandardized assessments used primarily for research purposes examine the process, or the way the child approaches a task and the effect of the nature of the task on haptic style or strategy.

There are several standardized assessments to evaluate accuracy of haptic perception. The Miller Assessment for Preschoolers (Miller, 1988) includes a stereognosis item that uses common objects for the younger children (2- to 4-year-olds) and geometric shape matching for older children (3- to 5-year-olds). Although a specific score is not given for this item, percentile equivalents can be determined from the score sheet.

The Sensory Integration and Praxis Tests (SIPT) (Ayres, 1989) are a 17-test battery that assesses aspects of sensory processing (visual, tactile, vestibular) and praxis. They are standardized on children ages 4.0 to 8.11. This battery includes several tests that tap aspects of haptic abilities. The Manual Form Perception (MFP) test, which assesses stereognosis, has two components. The first component is a haptic-visual intermodal matching task. The child feels a geometric shape without the use of vision and must point to its visual counterpart from among a set of choices. The second aspect of the test is a haptic-haptic matching task. The child feels a geometric shape with one hand and with the other hand explores a set of five shapes to find its match. The MFP test is a complex task that, when used in conjunction with the SIPT, can contribute to identification of various problems, including haptic perception, form and space perception deficit across sensory systems, sensory processing inefficiency, problems in visualization, and somatodyspraxia. The haptic-haptic matching component of the test also reflects functional integration of the two sides of the body (Ayres, 1989).

In the Graphesthesia test of the SIPT, the examiner draws a design on the back of the child's hand and the child must reproduce that design with his/her finger. This is not truly a haptic perception task because the tactile input is received passively not through active manipulation. But it is similar to many haptic perception tasks because the child needs to interpret designs received through moving touch applied to the hand and then signify knowledge of the design by a motor response. As with tests of haptic perception, fine motor coordination and motor planning abilities are required for optimal test performance.

Another standardized test that includes aspects of haptic perception is The Luria-Nebraska Neuropsychological Battery: Children's Revision (Golden, 1987), a 149-item test battery designed to assess a broad range of neuropsychologic functions in children ages 8 to 12 years. There are ll different scales, one of which assesses tactile functions. The 16 items on this scale assess tactile localization, tactile discrimination, intensity, tactile spatial discrimination, direction of movement, identification of traced shapes and numbers, and identification of objects. The specific items on the Tactile Function Scale that address aspects of haptic perception include two items that assess stereognosis in which the examiner places an object (quarter, key, paper clip, and eraser) in the child's hand and the child must name the object. If word-finding difficulties are suspected, the examiner can place the four objects in front of the child along with four other objects and ask the child to point to the object he/she just felt. There are also four items which are similar to the Graphesthesia test of the SIPT. In these items the child is required to recognize a cross, triangle, and circle drawn on the back of his/her wrist with a pencil. There are two items in which a number is written on the back of the wrist. In these items the child needs to know only that a number was drawn and does not need to identify the specific number. An overall score is provided for the Tactile Function Scale. Although there is not a specific score for the items assessing haptic perception, the examiner can look at performance on these items. The Luria-Nebraska Scales are usually administered by a neuropsychologist and, like the Sensory Integration and Praxis Tests, require special training. However, the knowledgeable therapist can use results of this test to aid in evaluation.

All the preceding tests examine accuracy of haptic identification. The manipulation strategies used in haptic exploration are not examined. At present there is not a standardized examination of exploratory strategies. However, the work of Zaphorozhets (see Table 4-1) provides guidelines for the therapist wishing to examine this area. If, for example, a therapist notes that a 7-year-old child is using only grasping to examine complex shapes, he/she can infer that this child is using immature and inefficient strategies to gain information about objects. Recently Exner (1992) developed a test to examine in-hand manipulation in children ages 18 months through 6½ years. Although the emphasis of this work is on the hand as a motor instrument used to accomplish specific skilled fine motor tasks with vision present, the process of adjusting objects within the hand after grasp (in-hand manipulation) is critical to enable effective haptic manipulation to gain perceptual information about an object.

There are no standardized assessments to examine haptic identification of object features other than shape such as weight, texture, and length. Research has indicated that adults use different strategies to gain information about these object characteristics. In working with children we need to examine whether they vary the strategy used in exploring different object properties. Although the typical child does not need or receive specific training in how to use the haptic sense, it may be necessary to explicitly teach haptic manipulation strategies in children with disorders.

For therapists wishing to assess haptic abilities in young infants, the best assessments at present are observational rather than standardized testing, although it will be helpful to use a standard protocol to compare infants and to see change in haptic style over time. It has been reported in the literature that from 6 to 12 months there is a decrease in mouthing and an increase in fingering behavior (Ruff, 1980). Thus, if at 12 months an infant is bringing everything to the mouth, one could identify a delay in the use of the hands for manipulation. Similarly, Ruff (1980) noted that 9- and 12-month-old infants adjusted their behavior to the characteristics of objects and more often fingered textured objects with prominent surfaces than smooth objects. Thus one could incorporate giving the infant both smooth blocks and blocks with textures and surfaces and observing his/her response to these different objects.

The information on the role of manipulation in haptic perception also provides guidance for evaluation. Along with noting the frequency of mouthing and the integration of vision and haptic senses in object exploration in infancy and early childhood, it is important to note the manipulation strategy used during performance on tests of haptic perception. Since the identification of common objects matures by 6 years and can be accomplished with little to no haptic manipulation, common objects may be of use only in the assessment of pre–school-age children. Changes in the method of manipulation seen during testing may be a better indication of change in haptic perception than is change in the child's accuracy score. Expanding our assessment beyond the identification of geometric shapes to include the testing of other tactile properties would allow us to look at the maturity and flexibility of manipulation patterns and provide insight into the child's ability to recognize the scope of sensory properties encountered during daily activities.

HAPTIC PERCEPTION IN CHILDREN WITH DISORDERS

Prematurity

The characteristics of touch most fully explored in the infant are those related to social and emotional functioning, and research on the perceptual role of touch often proceeds separately from research on its social role (Rose, 1990). Recently the specific role of tactile stimulation has been examined, and numerous studies have investigated whether the preterm infant will benefit from changes in the quantity, quality, or patterning of stimulation in the environment. The sensory organization and perceptual processing characteristics of the preterm infant have begun to be examined. Rose et al. (1976, 1980) examined the infants' responsivity to (passive) tactile stimulation and their abilities to discriminate different intensities of such stimulation. Infants were assessed at 40 weeks' gestational age, and, while sleeping, they were touched with plastic filaments of different intensities and their cardiac and behavioral responsivity was examined. Results indicated that preterm infants are significantly less responsive to tactile stimulation than are full-term infants.

Rose et al. (1978) also examined differences between preterm and full-term infants at 1 year of age in an active touch multimodal (haptic and visual) task using a habituation paradigm. Preterm infants did not show any evidence of cross-modal transfer, whereas full-term infants showed such transfer. These results indicate that full-term infants are able to gain knowledge about the shape of an object by feeling it and mouthing it and that they are able to make this information available to the visual system. They were able to do this even after only 30 seconds of handling or mouthing of the object. On the other hand, preterm infants did not seem to know that the object that they saw was the same object that they were exploring with their hand or mouth. Overall, preterm infants were limited in acquiring information; they showed evidence of difficulty in perceiving passive touch and in effectively using active touch to explore their world. Interestingly, lower-income full-term infants also showed poorer haptic-visual integration than did full-term middle-income infants. Recognition memory also has been studied in premature infants (Rose, 1983; Rose et al., 1988), who were found to have longer initial exposures and less recovery with novelty, indicating slower and maybe less complete information processing.

Another research paradigm that has been found to discriminate between high-risk infants and their normal peers is manipulative exploration. Early studies of exploratory behavior from a Piagetian perspective documented decreased manipulation in premature infants but interpreted the decreased action to be a reflection of a disordered motor system that provided inadequate or inaccurate information (Kopp, 1974). Kopp examined the performance of clumsy and nonclumsy (based on reach and grasp) premature and full-term 8-month-old infants. The coordinated group of infants showed significantly more exploration of objects, particularly more mouthing. The clumsy infants used more large arm movements and less object manipulation than the nonclumsy infants. Kopp discussed the value of object manipulation in enhancing attention and providing information to infants. However, she also pointed out that infants with poor manipulation skills may give extra attention to motor actions, leaving less attention available for sensory/perceptual processing.

More recent studies have focused on the attentional and organizational differences between preterm and full-term infants. Preterm infants exhibit shorter duration of action and less directed information-seeking action. High-risk infants have also been found to have less organized action and attentional strategies in exploratory manipulation of objects (Ruff, 1986; Ruff et al., 1984). It is not clear whether this disorganization is a purely motor phenomenon or relates to the ability to perceive environmental affordances and act on them.

Mental Retardation

An association between cognition and haptic perception has been identified in normal children. Finlayson and Reitan (1976) compared tactile discrimination to cognitive abilities in a group of younger children (6 to 11 years) and a group of older children (12 to 14 years). Four tests of tactile discrimination (including one test of haptic shape recognition) and three tests of cognitive ability were administered. Verbal IQ scores (Wechsler Intelligence Scale for Children [WISC]) were higher for the children in both age groups who displayed good tactile discrimination (based on combined performance on the four test measures) than for the children who displayed poor tactile discrimination. Good tactile discrimination was also found to be associated with better reading skill and cognitive problem-solving ability in the older age group. This finding was interpreted to suggest that the association between tactile perception and higher-level cognitive processing may become stronger with age. This conclusion gains support from an earlier study conducted by Reed (1967), who found a similar age-related increase in association between performance on tests of finger agnosia and tests of cognitive ability (verbal IQ scores on the WISC and reading skill) in elementary school–age children.

Research conducted with subjects who are mentally retarded provides insight into the relationship between haptic perception and cognitive ability. Much of the research examining the relationship between cognitive abilities and motor skill has been done with children with Down syndrome (e.g., Moss and Hogg, 1981; Sugden and Keogh, 1990). These studies generally found that children with Down syndrome did not show as effective accommodation of their hands to objects after grasp and did not use haptic manipulation and exploratory strategies as readily as typical children. However, it is difficult to directly attribute these results to the child's cognitive abilities since many of these findings can be attributed to the motor problems or other aspects of Down syndrome (Exner, 1991). It is likely that, regardless of the cause of the delay, impairment in the ability to efficiently explore objects will interfere with learning about key object properties (Exner, 1991).

Jones and Robinson (1973) compared the performance of a group of children with mental retardation (mean IQ = 47) to an age-matched group of children with normal intelligence. The accuracy of intramodal (haptic-haptic) and inter-modal (haptic-visual) discrimination of meaningless shapes was found to be poorer for the children with mental retardation than for the children with normal intelligence. When children with mental retardation and typical children were matched for mental age, the between-group difference in accuracy of haptic recognition disappeared (Derevensky, 1976, cited in Derevensky, 1979; Jones and Robinson, 1973; Medinnus and Johnson, 1966). However, two studies were cited that identified subjects with mental retardation as performing better than normal mental age–matched controls in the intramodal (haptic-haptic) and in the inter-modal (haptic-visual) matching of Russian and Greek letters (Hermelin and O'Connor, 1961; Mackay and Macmillan, 1968).

Since matching subjects for mental age often served to eliminate variation in haptic accuracy scores between children with mental retardation and typical children, it can be concluded that some aspect of higher cognitive processing is most likely required for task completion. Two factors apart from verbal intelligence have been found to impact test performance of individuals with mental retardation. Jones and Robinson (1973) noted that typical children tend to perform better on intermodal (visual-haptic and haptic-visual) matching than on intramodal (haptic-haptic) matching of shapes. The addition of visual cues did not seem to help improve the test performance of children with mental retardation. This finding suggests that some factor related to visual perception or neural integration of visual-haptic integration may be impaired in individuals with mental retardation. Subjects with mental retardation have been known to display immature manipulation strategies during tests of haptic perception. The sophistication of haptic manipulation strategies has been shown to be closely related to cognitive ability since manipulation strategies tended not to differ between typical children and children with mental retardation when subjects were matched for mental age (Davidson, 1985; Davidson, Pine, and Wiles-Kettenmann, 1980). An increase in sophistication of manipulation strategies has been shown to occur in close association with an increase in mental age within the population with mental retardation (Davidson, Pine, and Wiles-Kettenmann, 1980). Evidence from research on blind and sighted children with mental retardation and age-matched controls suggests that experience may contribute to improved manipulation and thus accuracy of intramodal (haptic-haptic) matching in individuals with mental retardation, but experience alone cannot fully compensate for the effects of reduced cognitive ability (Davidson, Appelle, and Pezzmenti, 1981). These findings suggest that training can help improve the sophistication of manipulation strategies in individuals with mental retardation, but such improvement in hand function is only partially effective in improving performance on tests of haptic perception.

Brain Injury

Impairment in tactile perception has commonly been seen in children with diagnoses reflecting known brain injury (e.g., cerebral palsy) (Bolanos et al., 1989; Boll and Reitan, 1972; Reitan, 1971; Solomons, 1957; Tachdjian and Minear, 1958). Poor stereognosis (haptic identification of shapes or common objects) was often cited among the tactile functions showing deficit in these studies (Bolanos et al., 1989; Reitan, 1971; Solomons, 1957; Tachdjian and Minear, 1958). Intermodal (visual-haptic) matching of shapes also has been shown to be impaired (Birch and Lefford, 1964). Solomons (1957) also found children with brain injury to be impaired in the haptic discrimination of size and texture. The children with brain injury and the normal children in her study did not differ in their ability to haptically match objects by weight. Although Boll and Reitan (1972) cited no problems in haptic shape recognition, they did note that the children with brain injury in their study performed poorly on a complex tactile performance task that required shape recognition for task completion. Rudel and Teuber (1971) compared the ability of typical children and children with brain injury to discriminate three-dimensional shapes through the use of intramodal (haptic and visual) and intermodal (visual-haptic) matching. Reduced performance in the group with brain injury was seen only in the visual-visual and visual-haptic matching conditions. These authors noted that, unlike the normal controls, who tended to perform better on the test conditions that included the use of vision than on the one requiring solely the use of touch, the addition of visual cues did not seem to assist the subjects with brain injury to improve their test performance. This finding suggests that children with brain injury may have a problem in visual perception or visual-haptic integration. However, this conclusion should be interpreted with caution since the mental ages of the subjects in the group with brain injury were 1½ to 2 years above that of the normal control group. It is possible that, if the subjects

were more equally matched for mental age, greater impairment in haptic perception might have been found within the group with brain injury.

The studies reviewed frequently used children with a mixture of diagnoses (cerebral palsy, encephalitis, traumatic head injury). Thus it was not surprising to find research that cited deficits in manual dexterity (e.g., finger tapping, grip strength, motor coordination) along with dysfunction in tactile perception in the children with brain injury studied (Boll and Reitan, 1972; Reitan, 1971). Solomons (1957) compared the ability of children with brain injury with and without fine motor impairment to perform tests of haptic perception. The children with brain injury with intact hand function were able to more accurately match objects by shape, texture, and size than the children with brain injury with fine motor impairment. The accuracy of haptic discrimination of weight did not differ between the two groups. Deficits in tactile perception (including stereognosis) have been closely associated with poor hand function in children with cerebral palsy (Tachdjian and Minear, 1958). Stereognosis has also been identified as a good predictor of upper-extremity surgical outcome within the cerebral palsied population (Goldner and Ferlic, 1966).

Learning Disabilities and Related Disorders

Impairment in tactile perception has also been cited in children who display learning disabilities and related disorders, conditions where clearly identifiable brain damage has not been found. Poor tactile and kinesthetic perception has been found in children with learning disabilities, language disorders, dyspraxia, and developmental Gerstmann syndrome (Ayres, 1965; Haron and Henderson, 1985; Johnson et al., 1981; Kinnealey, 1989; Kinsbourne and Warrington, 1963; Lord and Hulme, 1987; Spellacy and Barbara, 1978). Stereognosis was among the tactile tests used in some of these studies (Ayres, 1965; Haron and Henderson, 1985; Kinnealey, 1989). Children with learning disabilities were found to be less accurate in the haptic discrimination of shapes and letters than normal age-matched controls (Ayres, 1965; Hughes, 1976; Kinnealey, 1989). Studies comparing the performance of normal and dyspraxic children on tests of haptic discrimination of shapes yielded similar findings. The children with dyspraxia in these studies had lower accuracy scores than the typical children tested (Haron and

Henderson, 1985; Modero, 1970). Research comparing children who were clumsy and typical children on the haptic discrimination of length yielded mixed findings (Hulme et al., 1982, 1984).

Impairment in motor coordination has often been found to accompany poor tactile perception in children with learning disabilities and related disorders. Johnson, Stark, Mellits, and Tallal (1981) found children with language disorders to perform more poorly than a group of normal children matched for age, IQ, and socioeconomic status on tests of tactile perception (simultagnosis, graphesthesia, and finger identification) and motor coordination (hopping, finger opposition, diadochokinesis, and putting coins in a box). Reports of children with developmental Gerstmann syndrome have commonly cited a pairing of impairment in finger identification and constructional praxis (including poor handwriting and difficulty drawing geometric shapes) (Benton and Geschwind, 1970; Kinsbourne and Warrington, 1963; PeBenito, 1987; Spellacy and Barbara, 1978). Several authors have also linked deficits in somatosensory processing (including poor haptic perception) to problems in motor planning (praxis) (Ayres, 1965, 1969, 1971, 1972a, 1977; Ayres, Mailloux, and Wendler, 1987; Gubbay, 1975; Hulme et al., 1982; Walton and Court, 1965; Walton, Ellis, amd Court, 1962).

Research designed to identify factors that may be contributing to impaired haptic perception in children with dyspraxia has been a rare finding. Like typical children, children with dyspraxia have been shown to have greater difficulty matching geometric shapes through the use of passive touch than through the use of active touch (Haron and Henderson, 1985). Haron and Henderson found there to be less difference between the passive touch and active touch accuracy scores of the children with dyspraxia than of the typical children in their study. These authors attributed this finding to the possible presence of attention deficits in the dyspraxic children studied. But this finding could also be partially due to variation between the two groups in the level of sophistication of the manipulation strategies used during the active touch test condition. The contribution of manipulation strategies to the accuracy of haptic perception test scores in children with dyspraxia was conducted by Modero (1970). Children with dyspraxia displayed both lower accuracy scores for intramodal (haptic-haptic) matching of geometric and topologic shapes and less mature manipulation strategies than the normal controls.

There was no relationship found between the haptic accuracy scores and the haptic manipulation scores of either the typical children or children with dyspraxia in this study. Since comparison of intramodal (haptic-haptic) and intermodal (haptic-visual) matching accuracy scores has not been done using dyspraxic children, the extent to which impairment in the use of visual processing may have contributed to reduced haptic-visual matching ability found in these children is unclear. The common finding of a coexistence of deficits in tactile perception and visual perception in children with dyspraxia suggests that impaired visual processing may be a contributing factor to reduced test performance in some children (Ayres, 1969, 1971, 1977; Ayres, Mailloux, and Wendler, 1987; Murray, Cermak, and O'Brien, 1990).

Summary and Implications for Practice

This section provides documented evidence of the existence of problems in haptic perception in children born prematurely and those with a variety of disorders associated with brain injury and learning disabilities. Like much of the literature on haptic perception in children previously discussed, most of the research on haptic perception in children with disorders has been limited to the study of haptic discrimination of shape. The presence of problems in haptic discrimination of shapes does not mean that a child also has equal impairment in haptic discrimination of objects containing other sensory properties (such as texture and weight). Thus we cannot assume that because a child has problems discriminating shapes he/she has global impairment in haptic perception. Future research on disordered children needs to be directed toward the analysis of haptic recognition of objects having a variety of sensory properties. Factors contributing to test performance (such as in-hand manipulation and attention) also need to be addressed if we are to gain the information needed for effective intervention.

The striking similarity in factors contributing to poor haptic perception across the diagnoses was surprising. It was interesting to note that reduced sophistication of manual and in-hand manipulation strategies, problems in visual perception, and visual-haptic integration were cited as possible contributing factors to poor haptic perception in all the conditions reviewed. Although reduced cognitive ability was considered only as a contributing factor to poor haptic perception in children with mental retardation, attention deficits or related cognitive processing problems were cited as possible contributing factors to impairment in haptic discrimination in premature infants and in children with developmental dyspraxia.

CONCLUSIONS

Haptic perception in infants and children has been reviewed in depth in the previous pages of this chapter. It was our intent to provide an overview of the literature on the topic, with emphasis on material relevant to the evaluation and treatment of disorders in haptic perception in children with suspected and identified CNS dysfunction. The literature reviewed provides insight into the development of haptic perception and into the identification of factors that may be contributing to impairment in haptic perception in some children.

Haptic perception emerges in early infancy and continues to mature into adolescence. The infant initially uses oral exploration to learn about objects. The hands first transport objects to the mouth and later become a primary tool for haptic object exploration. Manual manipulation of objects begins with grasping and is later replaced by more specific manipulation patterns (e.g., fingering, banging) that are tailored to the physical properties of the object. Manual manipulation gradually replaces mouthing as the preferred method of object exploration. This is followed by a long period of development where the accuracy of haptic object recognition improves and the complexity of manual manipulation and exploratory strategies increases.

The accuracy of haptic object recognition is related to the choice of haptic manual manipulation and exploratory strategies. Vision appears to guide the development of manual manipulation and helps to bring meaning to the haptic information being retrieved by the hands. It is not until 6 years of age that children can easily explore objects with the hands without the assistance of vision. With time the hands develop the ability to retrieve information from the environment without the aid of vision, making it possible for vision and haptic sensory processing to take on separate supportive roles in daily function. But visual imagery continues to be used by many people to aid in haptic object recognition.

Research suggests that the ability to use cognitive strategies such as visual imagery and verbalization in the cognitive processing of haptic information develops with age. It appears to be related to intelligence, since there is an association between mental age and the accuracy of haptic object recognition.

Review of the literature on haptic perception in children with disorders suggests that impairment in somatosensory processing, manual and in-hand manipulation, vision, visual perception, or cognition can contribute to deficits in haptic perception.

Most of the tests currently used to assess haptic perception measure the product—the number of objects identified correctly. Yet process might be as important as, or even more important than, product when using the results of testing to guide treatment. Assessing the process means considering the quality of manual manipulation and exploratory strategies, along with the degree to which vision and cognitive strategies are being used in task performance.

Therapists need to realize that the tests available to measure haptic perception in children assess only a segment of this function. Because a child shows impairment in shape recognition on a test of stereognosis does not mean that the same child will display problems in haptic discrimination of other sensory properties (e.g., weight, texture). We need to consider developing tests of haptic perception that assess the breadth of haptic sensory properties found in objects. We also need to develop tests that measure the process as well as the product of task performance. We need to test haptic discrimination of several sensory properties to determine the extent of dysfunction, and we need to analyze the process of task performance to determine the reason for low test scores. We also need to know the extent of sensory properties showing deficit and the processes (e.g., vision, manual manipulation) showing impairment to develop treatment strategies that will translate into improvement in the use of haptic perception in daily function.

REFERENCES

Abravanel, E. (1968a). Intersensory integration of spatial position during early childhood. *Perceptual and Motor Skills, 26,* 251-256.

Abravanel, E. (1968b). The development of intersensory patterning with regard to selected spatial dimensions. *Monographs of the Society for Research in Child Development, 33*(2), 1-53.

Abravanel, E. (1970). Choice for shape vs. textural matching by young children. *Perceptual and Motor Skills, 31,* 527-533.

Abravanel, E. (1972). How children combine vision and touch when perceiving the shape of objects. *Perception and Psychophysics, 12*(2A), 171-175.

Affleck, G., & Joyce, P. (1979). Sex differences in the association of cerebral hemispheric specialization of spatial function with conservation task performance. *Journal of Genetic Psychology, 134,* 271-280.

Ayres, A.J. (1965). Patterns of perceptual motor dysfunction in children: A factor analytic study. *Perceptual and Motor Skills, 20,* 335-358.

Ayres, A.J. (1969). Deficits in sensory integration in educationally handicapped children. *Journal of Learning Disabilities, 26,* 13-18.

Ayres, A.J. (1971). Characteristics of types of sensory integrative dysfunction. *American Journal of Occupational Therapy, 26,* 329-334.

Ayres, A.J. (1972a). Types of sensory integrative dysfunction among disabled learners. *American Journal of Occupational Therapy, 26,* 13-18.

Ayres, A.J. (1972b). *Sensory integration and learning disorders.* Los Angeles: Western Psychological Services.

Ayres, A.J. (1977). Cluster analyses of measures of sensory integration. *American Journal of Occupational Therapy, 31,* 362-366.

Ayres, A.J. (1989). *Sensory integration and praxis tests.* Los Angeles: Western Psychological Services.

Ayres, A.J., Mailloux, Z.K., & Wendler, C.L.W. (1987). Developmental dyspraxia: Is it a unitary function? *Occupational Therapy Journal of Research, 7,* 93-110.

Bailes, S.M., & Lambert, R.M. (1986). Cognitive aspects of haptic form recognition by blind and sighted subjects. *British Journal of Psychology, 77,* 451-458.

Benton, A.L., Mamsher, K., Varney, N., & Spreen, O. (1983). *Contributions to neuropsychological assessment.* New York: Oxford University Press.

Benton, A.L., & Schultz, L.M. (1949). Observations on tactual form perception (stereognosis) in preschool children. *Journal of Clinical Psychology, 5,* 359-364.

Benton, D.F., & Geschwind, N. (1970). Developmental Gerstmann syndrome. *Neurology, 20,* 293-298.

Birch, H.G., & Lefford, A. (1964). Two strategies for studying perception in "brain-damaged" children. In H.G. Birch (Ed.). *Brain damage in children.* Baltimore: Williams & Wilkins.

Blank, M., & Bridger, W.H. (1964). Cross-modal transfer in nursery-school children. *Journal of Comparative and Physiological Psychology, 58,* 277-282.

Bolanos, A.A., Bleck, E.E., Firestone, P., & Young, L. (1989). Comparison of stereognosis and two-point discrimination testing of the hands of children with cerebral palsy. *Developmental Medicine and Child Neurology, 31,* 371-376.

Boll, T.J., & Reitan, R.M. (1972). Motor and tactile-perceptual deficits in brain-damaged children. *Perceptual and Motor Skills, 34,* 343-350.

Brodie, E.E., & Ross, H.E. (1985). Jiggling a lifted weight does aid discrimination. *American Journal of Psychology, 98,* 469-471.

Brooks, V.B. (1986). *The neural basis of motor control.* New York: Oxford University Press.

Butter, E.J., & Bjorklund, D.F. (1973). Investigating information gathering capabilities of visual and haptic modalities. *Perceptual and Motor Skills, 37,* 787-793.

Carpenter, M.B. (1985). *Core text of neuroanatomy* (3rd ed.). Baltimore: Williams & Wilkins.

Cermak, S. (1991). Somatosensory dyspraxia. In A. Fisher, E. Murray, & A. Bundy (Eds.). *Sensory integration: Theory and practice.* Philadelphia: F. A. Davis.

Cioffi, J., & Kandel, G.L. (1979). Laterality of stereognostic accuracy of children for words, shapes, and bigrams: A sex difference for bigrams. *Science, 204,* 1432-1434.

Connolly, K., & Jones, B. (1970). A developmental study of afferent-reafferent integration. *British Journal of Psychology, 61,* 259-266.

Cronin, V. (1977). Active and passive touch of four age levels. *Developmental Psychology, 13,* 253-256.

Darian-Smith, I., Sugitani, M., & Heywood, J. (1982). Touching textured surfaces: Cells in somatosensory cortex respond both to finger movements and surface texture. *Science, 218,* 906-909.

Davidson, P.W. (1972). Haptic judgments of curvature by blind and sighted humans. *Journal of Experimental Psychology, 93,* 43-55.

Davidson, P.W. (1985). Functions of haptic perceptual activity in persons with visual and developmental disabilities. *Applied Research in Mental Retardation, 6,* 349-360.

Davidson, P.W., Abbott, S., & Gershenfeld, J. (1974). Influence of exploration time on haptic and visual matching of complex shape. *Perception and Psychophysics, 15,* 539-543.

Davidson, P.W., Appelle, S., & Pezzmenti, F. (1981). Haptic equivalence matching of curvature by nonretarded and mentally retarded blind and sighted persons. *American Journal of Mental Deficiency, 86,* 295-299.

Davidson, P.W., Pine, R, & Wiles-Kettenmann, M. (1980). Haptic-visual shape matching by mentally retarded children: Exploratory activity and complexity effects. *American Journal of Mental Deficiency, 84,* 526-533.

Davidson, P.W., & Whitson, T.T. (1974). Haptic equivalence matching for curvature by blind and sighted humans. *Journal of Experimental Psychology, 102,* 687-690.

Derevensky, J.L. (1979). Relative contributions of active and passive touch to a child's knowledge of physical objects. *Perceptual and Motor Skills, 48,* 1331-1346.

Etaugh, C., & Levy, R.B. (1981). Hemispheric specialization for tactile-spatial processing in preschool children. *Perceptual and Motor Skills, 53*, 621-622.

Exner, C.E. (1991). *The relationship between the development and use of motor and perceptual-cognitive skills.* Unpublished manuscript.

Exner, C.E. (1992). In-hand manipulation skills. In J. Case-Smith, & C. Pehoski (Eds.). *Development of hand skills in the child.* Rockville, MD: The American Occupational Therapy Association.

Finlayson, M.A.J., & Reitan, R.M. (1976). Tactile-perceptual functioning in relation to intellectual, cognitive, and reading skills in younger and older normal children. *Developmental Medicine and Child Neurology, 18*, 442-446.

Ford, M.P. (1973). Imagery and verbalization as mediators in tactual-visual information processing. *Perceptual and Motor Skills, 36*, 815-822.

Friberg, S. (1977). *Insights from the blind.* New York: Basic Books.

Garbin, C.P. (1988). Visual-haptic perceptual nonequivalence for shape information and its impact upon cross-modal performance. *Journal of Experimental Psychology: Human Perception and Performance, 14*, 547-553.

Gardner, E.P. (1988). Somatosensory cortical mechanisms of feature detection in tactile and kinesthetic discrimination. *Canadian Journal of Physiology and Pharmacology, 66*, 439-454.

Gibson, E.J. (1988). Exploratory behavior in the development of perceiving, acting, and the acquiring of knowledge. *Annual Review of Psychology, 39*, 1-41.

Gibson, E.J., & Walker, A.S. (1984). Development of knowledge of visual-tactual affordances of substance. *Child Development, 55*, 453-460.

Gibson, J.J. (1962). Observations on active touch. *Psychological Review, 69*, 477-491.

Gliner, C.R. (1967). Tactual discrimination thresholds for shape and texture in young children. *Journal of Experimental Child Psychology, 5*, 536-547.

Gliner, C.R., Pick, A.D., Pick, H.L., & Hales, J.J. (1969). A developmental investigation of visual and haptic preferences for shape and texture. *Monographs of the Society for Research in Child Development, 34*(6), 1-40.

Golden, C.J. (1987). *Luria-Nebraska neuropsychological battery: Children's revision.* Los Angeles: Western Psychological Services.

Goldner, J.L., & Ferlic, D.C. (1966). Sensory status of the hand as related to reconstructive surgery of the upper extremity in cerebral palsy. *Clinical Orthopedics and Related Research, 46*, 87-92.

Gubbay, S.S. (1975). *The clumsy child.* Philadelphia: W. B. Saunders.

Gubbay, S.S., Ellis, J.N., Walton, J.N., & Court, S. D.M. (1965). Clumsy children: A study of apraxic and agnosic defects in 21 children. *Brain, 88*, 295-312.

Hahn, W.K. (1967). Cerebral lateralization of function: From infancy through childhood. *Psychological Bulletin, 101*, 376-392.

Haron, M., & Henderson A. (1985). Active and passive touch in developmentally dyspraxic and normal boys. *Occupational Therapy Journal of Research, 5*, 101-112.

Hatwell, Y. (1987). Motor and cognitive functions of the hand in infancy and childhood. *International Journal of Behavioral Development, 10*(4), 509-526.

Hatwell, Y. (1990). Spatial perception by eyes and hand: Comparison and cross-modal integration. In C. Bard, M. Fleury, & L. Hay (Eds.). *The development of eye-hand coordination across the life span.* Columbia: University of South Carolina Press.

Hatwell, Y., & Sayettat, G. (1991). Visual and haptic spatial coding in young children. *British Journal of Developmental Psychology, 9*, 445-470.

Hermelin, B., & O'Connor N. (1961). Recognition of shapes by normal and subnormal children. *British Journal of Psychology, 52*, 281-284.

Hollins, M., & Goble, A.K. (1988). Perception of length of voluntary movements. *Somatosensory Research, 5*, 335-348.

Hoop, N.H. (1971a). Haptic perception in preschool children. Part I. Object recognition. *American Journal of Occupational Therapy, 25*, 340-344.

Hoop, N.H. (1971b). Haptic perception in preschool children. Part II. Object manipulation. *American Journal of Occupational Therapy, 25*, 415-419.

Hughes, B.J. (1976). Pressure levels of active touch in normal and learning disabled children. *Dissertation Abstracts International, 37*, 4281A. (University Microfilms No. 76-30, 401).

Hulme, C., Biggerstaff, A., Moran, G., & McKinlay, I. (1982). Visual, kinesthetic, and cross-modal judgments of length by normal and clumsy children. *Developmental Medicine and Child Neurology, 24*, 461-471.

Hulme, C., Smart, A., Moran, G., & McKinlay, I. (1984). Visual, kinesthetic, and cross-modal judgments of length by clumsy children: A comparison with young normal children. *Child Care, Health and Development, 10*, 117-125.

Hulme, C., Smart, A., Moran, G., & Raine, A. (1983). Visual, kinesthetic, and cross-modal development: Relationships to motor skill development. *Perception, 12*, 477-483.

Iwamura, W., Tanaka, M., Skaramoto, M., Hikosaka, M., & Hikosaka, O. (1985). Functional surface integration, submodality convergence, and tactile feature detection in area 2 of the monkey somatosensory cortex. *Experimental Brain Research Supplementum, 10*, 44-58.

Jennings, P.A. (1974). Haptic perception and form reproduction by kindergarten children. *American Journal of Occupational Therapy, 28*, 274-280.

Johansson, R.S., & Westling, G. (1988). Coordinated isometric muscle commands adequately and erroneously programmed for the weight during lifting task with precision grip. *Experimental Brain Research, 71*, 59-71.

Johansson, R.S., & Westling, G. (1990). Tactile afferent signals in the control of precision grip. In M. Jeannerod (Ed.). *Attention and performance. XIII: Motor representation and control.* Hillsdale: Lawrence Erlbaum Associates.

Johnson, K.O., & Hsiao, S.S. (1992). Neural mechanisms of tactile form and texture perception. *Annual Review of Neuroscience, 15*, 227-250.

Johnson, R.B., Stark, R.E., Mellits, D., & Tallal, P. (1981). Neurological status of language impaired and normal children. *Annals of Neurology, 10*, 159-163.

Jones, B., & Robinson, T. (1973). Sensory integration in normal and retarded children. *Developmental Psychology, 9*, 178-182.

Juurmaa, J., & Lehitinen-Railo, S. (1988). Cross-modal transfer of forms between vision and touch. *Scandinavian Journal of Psychology, 29*, 95-110.

Kinnealey, M. (1989). Tactile functions in learning-disabled and normal children: Reliability and validity considerations. *Occupational Therapy Journal of Research, 9*, 3-15.

Kinsbourne, M., & Warrington, E.K. (1983). The developmental Gerstmann syndrome. *Archives of Neurology, 85*, 490-501.

Klatzky, R.L., Lederman, S.J., & Metzger, V.A. (1985). Identifying objects by touch: An "expert system." *Perception and Psychophysics, 37*, 299-302.

Klatzky, R.L., Lederman, S., & Reed, C. (1987). There's more to touch than meets the eye: The salience of object attributes for haptics with and without vision. *Journal of Experimental Psychology: General, 116*, 356-369.

Klatzky, R.L., Lederman, S., & Reed, C. (1989). Haptic integration of objects' properties: Texture, hardness, and planar contour. *Journal of Experimental Psychology: Human Perception and Performance, 15*, 45-57.

Klein, S.P., & Rosenfield, W.D. (1980). The hemispheric specialization for linguistic and non-linguistic tactile stimuli in third-grade children. *Cortex, 16*, 205-212.

Kleinman, J.J. (1979). Developmental changes in haptic exploration and matching accuracy. *Developmental Psychology, 15*, 480-481.

Kleinman, J.M., & Brodzinsky, D.M. (1978). Haptic exploration in young, middle-aged, and elderly adults. *Journal of Gerontology, 33*, 521-527.

Kopp, C.B. (1974). Fine motor abilities of infants. *Developmental Medicine and Child Neurology, 16*, 629-636.

Landau, B. (1991). Spatial representation of objects in young blind children. *Cognition, 38*, 145-178.

Lederman, S.J. (1981). The perception of surface roughness by active and passive touch. *Bulletin of the Psychonomic Society, 18*, 253-255.

Lederman, S.J., Brown, R.A., & Klatzky, R.L. (1988). Haptic processing of spatially distributed information. *Perception and Psychophysics, 44*, 222-232.

Lederman, S.J., & Klatzky, R.L. (1987). Hand movements: A window into haptic object recognition. *Cognitive Psychology, 19*, 342-368.

Lederman, S.J., & Klatzky, R.L. (1990). Haptic classification of common objects: Knowledge-driven exploration. *Cognitive Psychology, 22*, 421-459.

Lemon, R.N. (1981). Functional properties of monkey motor cortex neurons receiving afferent input from the hand and fingers. *Journal of Physiology, 311*. 497-519.

Locher, P.J., & Simmons, R.W. (1978). Influence of stimulus symmetry and complexity upon haptic scanning strategies during detection, learning, and recognition tasks. *Perception and Psychophysics, 23*, 110-116.

Lord, R., & Hulme, C. (1987). Kinaesthetic sensitivity of normal and clumsy children. *Developmental Medicine and Child Neurology, 29*, 720-725.

Mackay, C.K., & Macmillan, J. (1968). A comparison of stereognostic recognition in normal children and severely subnormal adults. *British Journal of Psychology, 59*, 443-447.

McCall, R.B. (1974). Exploratory manipulation and play in the human infant. *Monographs of the Society for Research in Child Development, 39* (2, Serial No. 155).

McCormick, R.V., & Mouw, J.T. (1983). Subject-object and subsystem interactions in problem solving. *Alberta Journal of Educational Research, 29*, 196-205.

McGlone, J. (1980). Sex differences in human brain asymmetry: A critical survey. *Behavioral and Brain Sciences, 3*, 215-263.

Medinnus, G.R., & Johnson, D. (1966). Tactual recognition of shapes by normal and retarded children. *Perceptual and Motor Skills, 22*, 406.

Micallef, C., & May, R.B. (1979). Visual dimensional dominance and haptic form recognition. *Bulletin of the Psychonomic Society, 7*, 21-24.

Miller, L.J. (1982). *Miller assessment for preschoolers.* Littleton, CO: The Foundation for Knowledge in Development.

Miller, S. (1971). Visual and haptic cue utilization by preschool children: The recognition of visual and haptic stimuli presented separately and together. *Journal of Experimental Child Psychology, 12*, 88-94.

Miller, S. (1986). Aspects of size, shape and texture in touch: Redundancy and interference in children's discrimination of raised dot patterns. *Journal of Child Psychology and Psychiatry, 27,* 367-381.

Modero, M.G. (1970). *Manual manipulation and identification in apraxic and normal eight- and nine-year-old children.* Unpublished masters thesis, Boston University, Boston.

Moss, S.C., & Hogg, J. (1981). The development of hand function in mentally handicapped and non-handicapped preschool children. In P. Mittler (Ed.), *Frontiers of knowledge in mental retardation.* Baltimore: University Park Press.

Mountcastle, V.B. (1976). The world around us: Neural command functions for selective attention. *Neurosciences Research Program, 14,* 1-47.

Murray, E., Cermak, S., & O'Brien, V. (1990). The relationship between form and space perception, constructional abilities and clumsiness in children. *American Journal of Occupational Therapy, 44,* 623-645.

Palmer, C.F. (1989). The discriminating nature of infants: Exploratory actions. *Developmental Psychology, 25,* 885-893.

PeBenito, R. (1987). Developmental Gerstmann syndrome: Case report and review of the literature. *Developmental and Behavioral Pediatrics, 8,* 299-232.

Pecheux, M., Lepecq, J., & Salzarulo, P. (1980). Oral activity and exploration in 1- to 7-month-old infants. *British Journal of Developmental Psychology, 6,* 245-256.

Piaget, J., & Inhelder, B. (1948). *The child's conception of space.* New York: Norton.

Pick, H.L., Klein, R.E., & Pick, A.D. (1966). Visual and tactual identification of form orientation. *Journal of Experimental Child Psychology, 4,* 391-397.

Reed, J.C. (1967). Lateralized finger agnosia and reading achievement at ages 6 and 10. *Child Development, 38,* 213-220.

Reed, J.C., & Klatzky, R.L. (1990). Haptic integration of planar size with hardness, texture, and plantar contour. *Canadian Journal of Psychology, 44,* 522-545.

Reitan, R.M. (1971). Sensorimotor functions in brain-damaged and normal children of early school age. *Perceptual and Motor Skills, 33,* 655-664.

Richardson, B.L, Wuillemin, D.B., & MacKintosh, G.J. (1981). Can passive touch be better than active touch? A comparison of active and passive tactile maze learning. *British Journal of Psychology, 72,* 353-362.

Rochat, P. (1983). Oral touch in young infants: Responses to variation of nipple characteristics in the first months of life. *International Journal of Behavioral Development, 6,* 123-133.

Rochat, P. (1987). Mouthing and grasping in neonates: Evidence for the early detection of what hard or

soft substances afford for action. *Infant Behavior and Development, 10,* 435-449.

Rochat, P. (1989). Object manipulation and exploration in 2- to 5-month-old infants. *Developmental Psychology, 25,* 871-874.

Rose, S.A. (1983). Differential rates of visual information processing in full-term and preterm infants. *Child Development, 54,* 1189-1198.

Rose, S.A. (1990). Perception and cognition in preterm infants: The sense of touch. In K. Barnard & T.B. Brazelton (Eds.). *Touch: The foundation of experience.* Madison CT: International Universities Press.

Rose, S., Gottfried, A., & Bridger, W. (1978). Cross-modal transfer in infants: Relationship to prematurity and socioeconomic background. *Developmental Psychology, 14,* 643-652.

Rose, S.A., Schmidt, K., & Bridger, W.H. (1976). Cardiac and behavioral responsivity to tactile stimulation in premature and full-term infants. *Developmental Psychology, 12,* 311-320.

Rose, S.A., Schmidt, K., Riese, M.L., & Bridger, W. H. (1980). Effects of prematurity and early intervention on responsivity to tactile stimuli: A comparison of preterm and full-term infants. *Child Development, 51,* 416-425.

Rudel, R.G., & Teuber, H.L. (1971). Pattern recognition within and across sensory modalities in normal and brain-injured children. *Neuropsychologia, 9,* 389-399.

Ruff, H.A. (1980). The development of perception and recognition of objects. *Child Development, 51,* 981-992.

Ruff, H.A. (1982). Role of manipulation in infants' responses to invariant properties of objects. *Developmental Psychology, 18,* 682-691.

Ruff, H.A. (1986). Components of attention during infants' manipulative exploration. *Child Development, 57,* 105-114.

Ruff, H.A. (1989). The infant's use of visual and haptic information in the perception and recognition of objects. *Canadian Journal of Psychology, 43,* 302-319.

Ruff, H.A., McCarton, C., Kurtzberg, D., & Vaughan, H.G., Jr. (1984). Preterm infants' manipulative exploration of objects. *Developmental Psychology, 55,* 1166-1173.

Semmes, J. (1965). A non-tactual factor in astereognosis. *Neuropsychologia, 3,* 295-315.

Siegel, A.W., & Barber, J.C. (1973). Visual and haptic dimensional preference for planometric stimuli. *Perceptual and Motor Skills, 36,* 383-390.

Siegel, A.W., & Vance, B.J. (1970). Visual and haptic dimensional performance: A developmental study. *Developmental Psychology, 3,* 264-266.

Simmons, R.W., & Locher, P.J. (1979). Role of extended perceptual experience upon haptic perception of nonrepresentational shapes. *Perceptual and Motor Skills, 40,* 987-991.

Solomons, H.C. (1957). *A developmental study of tactual perception in normal and brain injured children*. Unpublished doctoral dissertation, Boston University, Boston, MA.

Spellacy, F., & Barbara, P. (1978). Dyscalculia and elements of the developmental Gerstmann syndrome in school children. *Cortex, 14*, 197-206.

Starr, A., & Cohen, L.G. (1985). "Gating" of somatosensory-evoked potentials begins before the onset of voluntary movement in man. *Brain Research, 54*, 23-32.

Stilwell, J.M. (1989). *Relationship between tactile perception and motor coordination*. Unpublished manuscript. Boston University, Sargent College of Allied Health Professions, Boston, MA.

Streri, A.F. (1987). Tactile discrimination of shape and intermodel transfer in 2- to 3-month-old infants. *British Journal of Developmental Psychology, 5*(3), 213-220.

Streri, A., & Pecheux, M. (1986). Tactual habituation and discrimination of form in infancy: A comparison with vision. *Child Development, 57*, 100-104.

Streri, A., & Spelke, E.S. (1988). Haptic perception of objects in infancy. *Cognitive Psychology, 20*, 1-23.

Streri, A., & Spelke, E.S. (1989). Effects of motion and figural goodness on haptic object perception in infancy. *Child Development, 60*, 1111-1125.

Tachdjian, M.O., & Minear, W.L. (1958). Sensory disturbances in the hands of children with cerebral palsy. *Journal of Bone and Joint Surgery, 40A*, 85-90.

Vierck, D.J. (1978). Interpretations of the sensory and motor consequences of dorsal column lesions. In G. Gordon (Ed.). *Active touch*. New York: Pergamon Press.

Walton, J.N., Ellis, E., & Court, S.D.M. (1962). Clumsy children: Developmental apraxia and agnosia. *Brain, 85*, 603-612.

Witelson, S.F. (1974). Hemispheric specialization for linguistic and nonlinguistic tactual perception using a dichotomous stimulation technique. *Cortex, 10*, 3-17.

Witelson, S.F. (1976). Sex and the single hemisphere: Specialization of the right hemisphere for spatial processing. *Science, 193*, 425-427.

Wolff, P. (1972). The role of stimulus-correlated activity in children's recognition of nonsense forms. *Journal of Experimental Child Psychology, 14*, 427-441.

Zaporozhets, A.V. (1965). The development of perception in the preschool child. *Monographs of the Society for Research in Child Development, 30*(2), 82-101.

Zaporozhets, A.V. (1969). Some of the psychological problems of sensory training in early childhood and the preschool period. In A.N. Leont'ev, A.R. Luria, & A.A. Smirnov (Eds.). *A Handbook of contemporary Soviet psychology*. New York: Basic Books.

5

Reaching and Eye-Hand Coordination

Birgit Rösblad

MATURE REACHING MOVEMENTS
  Movement Speed
  Transport and Grasp Phase
  Role of Vision
  Role of Proprioception
  Integration of Sensory Information

**DEVELOPMENT OF REACHING
  DURING INFANCY**
  Beginning to Master the Reach
  Preparing the Hand for the Grasp
  Anticipatory vs. Feedback Control
  Perceiving Positions and Movements of
    One's Own Body
  Postural Control and Reaching

**REACHING IN CHILDREN WITH
  MOTOR IMPAIRMENTS**

Our hands are extremely important tools for us in our everyday lives, and we are able to use them with grace and skill. To do so we have to be able to bring them to the right place at the right time. This can be illustrated with the example of catching a ball. To catch the ball successfully the hand has to be at the calculated meeting point at exactly the right time. Moreover, it must be prepared for the catch, with the fingers closing around the ball before the moment of contact, or we will fail to catch it. In other types of goal-directed arm movements the arm trajectory as such can be the goal, as when painting or drawing, but in a reaching movement the goal is to transport the hand to the target, with precision in both time and space.

This chapter is organized in three parts: the first deals with the mature reaching movement, the second with the development of reaching in infancy, and the third provides some examples of how the reaching movement can be disturbed in children with motor impairments.

MATURE REACHING MOVEMENTS

Reaching for an object means getting the hand from a starting position to the goal, the object. In doing this, the hand will describe a trajectory. The word *trajectory* can be used in different ways, but here refers to the path taken by the hand as it moves toward a target and the speed as it moves along the path (Abend et al., 1982). The reaching trajectory has several characteristics.

Movement Speed

If the velocity of the hand during a reaching movement is plotted vs. time, as in Figure 5-1, one can see that the tangential velocity curve is bell shaped. The reaching movement is continuous with one single peak of velocity. In the last part of the reaching movement, when the hand is close to the target, the velocity is slow. This typical bell-shaped velocity curve is seen when the reach is carried on with, as well as without, visual feedback (Jeannerod, 1984; Morosso, 1981.) This indicates that the reaching movement to a high degree is programmed in advance of movement onset.

If one considers the reaching movement in terms of accelerations and decelerations, it can be divided into movement units. One phase of acceleration followed by a deceleration can then be said to constitute a movement unit (Brooks, 1976; von Hofsten, 1979). The movement paths within these movement units are relatively straight, and movement direction is changed in between units (Morosso, 1981; von Hofsten, 1991). The number of movement units comprising a movement can be viewed as an index of its degree of programming. A movement consisting of only one movement unit, such as that depicted in Figure 5-1, can then be viewed as being entirely programmed before movement onset. However, if the movement is composed of many movement units, one can assume that it has been programmed several times during execution. A reaching movement, aimed at a stationary object, generally consists of one or two movement units, with the first covering the main part of movement duration.

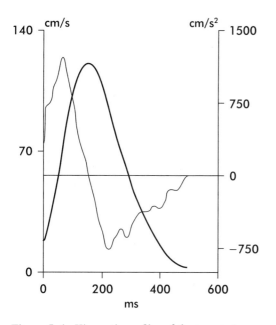

Figure 5-1. Kinematic profiles of the transport component of a reaching movement. The heavy line depicts the velocity of the wrist (*cm/s*) as a function of time. This curve describes a single continuous movement with a single peak of velocity. The two peaks connected by the thin line depict the acceleration of the wrist (*cm/s²*) as a function of time. The positive peak constitutes one phase of acceleration and the negative peak one phase of deceleration, together forming one movement unit.

(From Jeannerod, M., et al. [1992]. Parallel visuomotor processing in human prehension movements. In R. Caminiti, P. B. Johnson, & Y. Burnod [Eds.]. *Control of arm movement in space.* New York: Springer-Verlag.)

Transport and Grasp Phase

Yet another way of viewing the reaching movement is to look for its functional components. Two distinct and coordinated movement components can then be identified (Jeannerod, 1984). The first component is a transportation phase, which brings the hand to the target. In this part of the movement mainly the proximal muscles and joints are involved. The second component is a grasp phase in which the hand is shaped in anticipation of contact with the object. This phase involves mainly the distal joints and muscles. One can also divide the visual information needed to successfully grasp an object into two categories. For the transport phase of the movement knowledge of the position of the object in the room is needed (the object's extrinsic properties). With this information we can program the direction and extent of the movement. For the grasp phase, perception of size and the shape of the object is needed (the object's intrinsic properties). There is evidence for independent neural coding of the two reaching phases (see Jeannerod, 1992, for a review).

Although the grasp and transportation phase of the reach are separately controlled, these two components are coordinated so that the grasp phase starts during the transportation phase. To accomplish a smooth and coordinated grasp, the fingers must initiate the grasp well before encountering the object. Closing the hand too early or too late will prevent capturing or make the grasp impossible or awkward. During the transportation phase the fingers open to a maximum grip aperture. After this maximum opening the fingers start to close in anticipation of contact with the object (Jeannerod, 1981). A small object requires longer reaching time than a larger object. The first part of the movement trajectory seems to be unaffected by object size, but for smaller objects extra movement time is spent in the last part of the movement, after peak acceleration. Moreover, the more precision required, the earlier the hand anticipates the physical characteristics of the object (Marteniuk et al., 1990). The hand will open more fully during the reach when reaching for a larger object and always more than required (von Hofsten and Rönnquist, 1988). If the reach has to be carried out with high speed, the grip aperture will be larger. When we increase the speed of a movement, the accuracy will decrease. Opening the hand more fully during a fast reach could be seen as a way to make sure that the object will be succesfully grasped despite the decreased movement accuracy (Wing et al., 1986).

Role of Vision

It is obvious that vision plays a very important role in our ability to reach out for objects. One need only imagine what it would be like to be blind to realize the importance of vision to reaching. Vision is the sense that provides us with information about the layout of the environment, and when reaching for an object, vision will define both the position and shape of the object. Seeing the environment gives us an opportunity to anticipate upcoming events and therefore plan our movements in an anticipatory fashion. One example of this would be the way we shape our hand prior to contact with an object. A blind person reaching for an object does not have this ability but will have to touch the object first and then, guided by haptic information, shape the hand for grasp. If we can't foresee upcoming events and plan our movements ahead of time, our movements will of necessity be uncoordinated (von Hofsten, 1993).

As early as 1899 Woodworth studied the role of visual information for goal-directed arm movements, and many of the concepts he developed are still valid today. He found that slow movements were performed with more accuracy, compared with fast movements. Another important finding was that visual feedback during the ongoing movement improved movement accuracy, but only for slow movements. Woodworth stated that the bad effect that speed had on movement accuracy was due to an inability to control movements visually when their duration was shorter than a critical value. Several studies carried out since then have proved that movement correction based on visual feedback is a relatively slow process. In 1968 Keele and Posner stated that it takes about 200 msec for visual feedback to influence an ongoing movement. However, there is now considerable evidence that visual feedback might be as fast as 100 msec (Alstermark et al., 1990; Martin and Prablanc, 1992; Paulignan et al., 1991a, b).

As discussed earlier in this chapter, the movement of the hand slows down toward the end of the reaching trajectory, and much of the entire movement time is spent close to the target. One could assume that the slowing down at the end of the movement serves the purpose of guiding the hand with sensory feedback toward the target. This is probably the case. Many experiments have shown that visual feedback is necessary for endpoint accuracy. Buyakas et al. (1980) placed subjects in a completely dark room and asked them to point at a point of light. They found that this was an impossible task. The subjects started out with a rather precise movement that ended close to the target but not on the target. Without vision of the hand and the target, endpoint accuracy is poor (Tillary et al., 1991; von Hofsten and Rösblad, 1988).

However, even if the movement is carried out without visual feedback, the main features of the reaching trajectory remain. One will still see the bell-shaped velocity curve as well as the coordination between movement speed and anticipatory hand shaping (Jeannerod, 1981); that is, if the subject is first allowed to see the spatial position and size of the object, but vision is excluded during the movement itself, the main features of the reach can still be observed. This indicates that to a high degree the reaching movement is programmed in advance of movement onset but can be modified during execution, when necessary, that is, when endpoint accuracy is needed or if we reach for a target that moves in an unpredictable way.

Role of Proprioception

In our muscles, tendons, joints, and skin we have receptors that provide us with information about the positions and movements of our body parts. This is here termed *proprioception,* after Sherrington (1906). Although it is relatively easy to find out how we can move without vision or with degraded vision, proprioceptive information can't be manipulated as easily. Instead, the research on the role of proprioception has focused on animal experiments and patients with sensory loss due to diseases.

One line of research has used deafferented monkeys. When their dorsal spinal roots are sectioned, the monkeys are deprived of sensation from the upper limbs but the motor nerves are unaffected. This technique was used in early experiments by Mott and Sherrington (1895). They reported that the monkeys' limbs became useless after such operations and that the animals would use their upper limbs only if forced to and then in an awkward way. They concluded that afferent information from the limbs was necessary for both movement initiation and control. Similar results were also reported by Lassek (1953). However, later experiments with deafferented monkeys reported different results. Taub and Berman (1968) reported a clear improvement in motor function after the initial disability resulting from the section of the nerves. The animals were able to reach for and grasp objects with a primitive pincer grip a few months after surgery. Recovery of function has also been reported by Knapp et al. (1963). Bossom and Ommanya (1968) have pointed out that motor pathways can easily be damaged during a rhizotomy and that this could be why the degree of recovery of function varied between studies.

Despite the previous diversity in results, there are also similarities. Several investigators have found that, when forced to, the animals are able to use their deafferented limb. Animals that had both forelimbs deafferented regained function to a higher degree than those with only one deafferented forelimb, who could choose to use the normal hand. This latter effect has been called learned nonuse by Taub and Berman (1968) and was explained in terms of an inhibition of the deafferented limb. However, if the animals who had one limb deafferented were forced to use it because the normal limb was restrained, they recovered function to the same degree as the bilaterally deafferented animals (Bossom, 1974; Knapp et al., 1963).

Yet another similarity between the reports is that the deafferented monkeys were capable of both initiating and carrying out motor acts, however uncoordinated. Studies of humans with sensory deficits seem to confirm this. Gordon and Ghez (1992) described patients with large-fiber sensory neuropathy in the following way: "These patients, although able to initiate and carry out complex movement sequences, were severely impaired in most functional activities. For example, none could drink water from a cup without spilling."

The experiments by Ghez et al. (1990) provide us with important information about the role of proprioception in reaching movements. They studied the reaching movement in patients with sensory loss due to large-fiber neuropathy. Without visual feedback the patients would make large directional errors from movement onset and were also unstable at movement endpoint. When allowed to monitor the movement visually, they were able to substitute for the loss of proprioceptive information to some degree, and performance improved. But Ghez et al. (1990) also studied the effect on movement accuracy when the patients were able to look at the limb before movement onset but not during the ongoing movement and found that this also improved function. This indicates that proprioception is not only important for feedback during the ongoing movement but also plays an important role for programming of move-

ments by providing the nervous system with information about the current state of the body parts.

Integration of Sensory Information

A coordinated reaching movement involves processing of both visual and proprioceptive information. This means that the visual and proprioceptive systems have to be in correspondence with each other. One example of when they are not integrated involves wearing a pair of displacing prisms. If we then reach for an object, we perceive the object at a location displaced from its virtual position, and the reach is directed to this erroneous position. However, reaching actively toward the object several times rapidly reintegrates the visual and proprioceptive systems, and within a few minutes adaptation has occurred (Harris, 1965). This can also be experienced when one puts on a pair of new glasses. The distance to the ground seems to be changed, and it takes some minutes of walking before the visual system again is in agreement with the proprioceptive system.

That active movements are important for integrating the visual and proprioceptive systems was also demonstrated in a classic study by Held and Hein (1963). They used an experimental setup in which one kitten was riding in a gondola that was pulled by another kitten. During this gondola ride both kittens received the same visual information about the surroundings. At all other times the kittens were kept in a dark room. On being tested after the experiment, the kitten that had been pulling the gondola proved to have normal visually guided behavior, but the kitten who had been passively riding did not.

DEVELOPMENT OF REACHING DURING INFANCY
Beginning to Master the Reach

Observing a newborn baby's arm movements, one might perceive them as random, performed without meaning. However, even at birth the infant is capable of movements that require some degree of sensory motor integration. Von Hofsten (1982) placed 5-day-old infants in a semireclining seat that gave good support to the trunk and head but allowed free movement of the arms. (When studying infant behavior it is crucial that the infant is in an optimal state, not fuzzy or sleepy. The semireclining position was found to be optimal in maintaining alertness.) The infants were presented with a colorful tuft that moved irregularly and slowly in front of them. The infants' arm movements were recorded with two video cameras, making it possible to calculate the arm trajectory in three-dimensional space. All infants noticed the tuft and were able to follow it with eye and head movements for varying periods. The infants' forward extended arm movements as well as looking behavior were analyzed. When the infants were fixating the tuft, they aimed their reaching movements closer to it than when looking in another direction or closing their eyes. Thus a child only a few days old already has a rudimentary visual control of arm movements. Moreover, when initiating an aimed movement toward a visually fixated target, the infant must "know" where its arm is. Since the neonate is fixating the target, the starting position of the hand must be defined proprioceptively. This indicates that the visual and proprioceptive space are to some degree already connected in the newborn infant. But even though the infants aimed their reaching movements closer to the object while fixating on it, most of the time they did not touch it. Also, at this early age, even if they did touch the object, they were not capable of grasping it. To do so successfully they would have to extend the arm and at the same time flex the fingers around the object, but the arm and hand moved synergetically. When the infants extended the arm, the fingers were also extended, and when flexing the arm the fingers were flexed. Before voluntary grasping of an object is possible, this synergy between arm and hand has to break down. Von Hofsten (1984) reported an emerging ability in infants around 3 months of age to control arm and hand movements independently, and at the same age they increased their reaching attempts.

As discussed earlier in this chapter, the reaching movement can be analyzed in terms of acceleration and deceleration. A phase of acceleration followed by a phase of deceleration then constitutes a movement unit. When around 4 months of age the infants first start to reach and grasp for objects, the movement path is awkward and crooked, and the trajectory consists of many movement units (Fetters and Todd, 1987; von Hofsten, 1979). This changes rapidly within a few months. The movement path straightens out and the number of movement units decreases. At around 6 months of age the reaching movement often consists of just two movement units, with the first covering the main part of the trajectory (von Hofsten, 1979, 1991).

Von Hofsten and Lindhagen (1979) found that at the age children start to reach successfully for stationary objects, they can also catch fast-moving ones. To be able to do this the child has to predict the trajectory of the moving object and reach for the meeting point. Eighteen-week-old infants were found to be able to catch objects that moved at 30 cm/sec. Most of the reaches were aimed at the meeting point from movement onset. This demonstrates an early emerging capacity for anticipatory control of reaching movements. That is, the infant does not reach toward where he/she first sees the object, but rather appears to be anticipating the point where the hand and the object will meet (Figure 5-2).

Preparing the Hand for the Grasp

An adult reaching for an object will shape the hand to fit the properties of the object in anticipation of contacting it. How does this ability emerge in infants? Von Hofsten and Fazel-Zandy (1984) found that infants at the age of 4½ months orient their hand crudely to match a horizontal or vertical rod before contact. Von Hofsten and Rönnquist (1988) studied the coordination between the transport and the grasp phase in infants at 5 to 6, 9, and 13 months of age. The 5- to 6-month-old children were able to control the closing of the hand visually and started to close the hand before making contact with the object. But both they and the 9-month-old children initiated hand closure later during the reaching movement than did the 13-month-olds and adults. The 5- to 6-month-old infants did not adjust their grip aperture to match the object size as did the two older age groups (Figure 5-3). Infants at the age of 10 months have also been found to shape their hand to fit different shapes of objects prior to contact (Pieraut-Le Bonniec, 1990).

Anticipatory vs. Feedback Control

As discussed earlier in this chapter, aimed reaching movements are accomplished by both programming and corrections made during the ongoing movement. Very early in development the child has an emerging capacity for anticipatory control. The low number of movement units during the reach, the ability to catch moving objects, and the shaping of the hand prior to object contact are all evidence of this. There is also evidence that very early the child starts to use visual information to correct ongoing movements. McDonnell (1975)

05:58:51

05:58:31

05:58:11

05:57:91

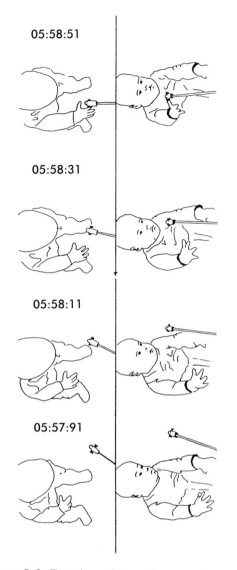

Figure 5-2. Two views of the performance of a well-aimed reach by an infant, 21 weeks of age. The frame on the bottom is the start of the reach. The interval between frames is 0.2 sec (*digital clock reading in the upper portion of each frame*). The child is directing the reach ahead of the object to the point where the object will be at the end of the reaching movement.

(From von Hofsten, C. [1980]. Predictive reaching for moving objects by human infants. *Journal of Experimental Child Psychology, 30,* 369-382.)

to be integrated in a flexible way, and this is not fully matured until adolescence.

Perceiving Positions and Movements of One's Own Body

To reach or point with precision, visual feedback of the hand is necessary. When sewing on a button or doing embroidery, we are reminded of this: since the sewing hand is not visible, we find it difficult to direct the needle accurately. However, we are to a great extent able to replace the missing visual information with proprioceptive and tactual information. How does the ability to direct the hand to a goal, without visual information about the moving hand, develop in children? Von Hofsten and Rösblad (1988) tested children between 4 and 12 years of age. The task was to place pins underneath a tabletop at the locations of four dots placed on the upper side of the table. The pointing hand was always hidden underneath the tabletop while the perceptual information about the target was varied. In the visual condition the child could see the dot but not the pointing hand. In the proprioceptive condition the child placed the index finger of the other hand on the dot to be pointed at, closed his/her eyes, and placed the drawing pin underneath the dot. One finding was that performance was superior when visual information about the target was provided. This was true for all age groups. Another finding was that there was a marked increase in the ability to direct the hand to a goal, without visual information about the moving hand, up to the age of 7 years. In Figure 5-4 the performance of the children ages 5 to 12 years is depicted.

Postural Control and Reaching

If we are perturbed by an external event so that we lose balance, the postural muscles will be activated in a specific way to maintain balance. However, balance is also perturbed by our own voluntary movements. When we reach out with our hands for an object, this creates a shift in the body's center of gravity, but we do not lose our balance. Before the voluntary act takes place we have already prepared ourselves for the perturbation by anticipatory postural adjustments. This has been shown in several experiments, one of which was carried out by Cordo and Nashner (1982). They made standing subjects pull or push a handle. When doing this the postural muscles in the legs were activated before the muscles of the

found that, while wearing displacing prisms during reaching, infants of 4 months of age were able to utilize visual feedback for movement control to some degree. However, the anticipatory and the feedback methods of controlling movements have

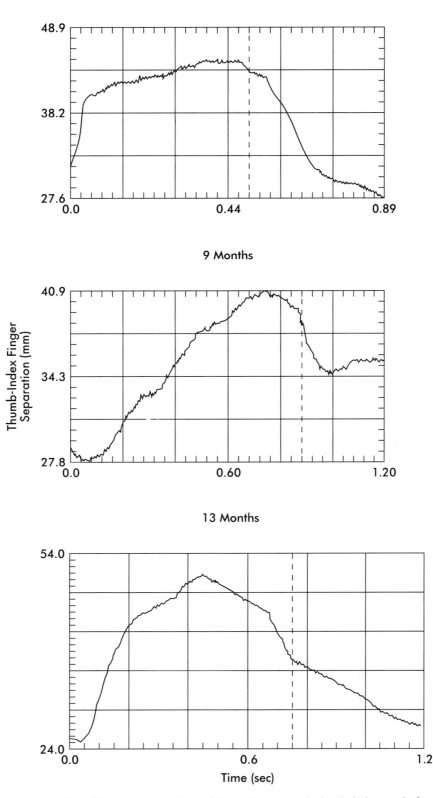

Figure 5-3. Examples of how infants at ages 5, 9, and 13 months prepare the hand, during reach, for grasping an object. The opening of the hand, measured as the distance between the thumb and the index finger, increases and then decreases as the hand nears the object. The *dotted line* represents the moment when the hand first touches the object.

(From von Hofsten, C., & Rönnquist, L. [1988]. Preparation for grasping an object: A developmental study. *Journal of Experimental Psychology: Human Perception and Performance, 14,* 610-621.)

Figure 5-4. The mean error at each age level from 5 to 12 years of age with a child pointing to a target with the pointing hand hidden. Visually, the child is looking at the target but pointing with the hidden hand. In the proprioceptive condition neither hand is seen; the pointing hand reaches toward the felt position of the other hand.

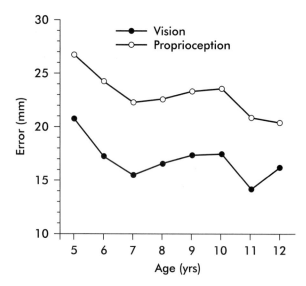

arm. These anticipatory postural adjustments in the legs are also present in children at the age of 4 years, though in a less proficient form (Haas et al., 1989). There is also some evidence that this anticipatory mode of counteracting upcoming forces on the body starts to operate much earlier. Von Hofsten and Woollacott (unpublished manuscript) showed that at 10 months of age children activated the muscles of the trunk prior to voluntary arm movements. This integration between posture and voluntary control is an important prerequisite for coordinated arm and hand movements. Little is known of how children with motor impairments can integrate voluntary movements and posture, but it is possible that this is one contributory factor in these children's fine motor disturbances.

Another study indicating that the development of posture and reaching are linked to each other was carried out by Rochat (1992). When infants started to reach for objects, they tended to use both hands and later in development acquired one-handed reach. A successful object-oriented reach of a young infant is symmetric and synergistic with the hands meeting in midline. Older infants often display an asymmetric one-hand reach. This transition from two-handed to one-handed reach was studied in relation to the development of postural control. The infants, 5 to 8 months of age, were divided into two groups according to whether they were able to sit independently. The study revealed a trend toward more one-hand reaches in the group of independently sitting infants compared to the nonsitting infants. Clinical observations made by Grenier (1981) also indicate that postural control is important for coordinated arm

movements. Infants started to reach successfully for objects at 3 to 4 months of age, but if supported appropriately at the neck and trunk they could perform coordinated arm movements much earlier.

REACHING IN CHILDREN WITH MOTOR IMPAIRMENTS

We still have very limited knowledge concerning the development and coordination of reaching in children with motor impairments. However, the knowledge we have from research carried out on normally developed children and adults can be utilized when asking questions about children with motor impairments. This section reviews some examples of this line of research.

Kluzik et al. (1990) used what is known about reaching trajectories in normally developed children when studying children with motor impairments. They were interested in the short-term effects of neurodevelopmental treatment (NDT) in children with cerebral palsy. The question they asked was whether the reaching movement skills of children with cerebral palsy are amenable to change following one session of NDT. Hand position in three-dimensional space was recorded during a reaching movement, before and after treatment. The authors found that movement time was longer in the children with cerebral palsy and that one reaching movement consisted of an increased number of movement units, compared to normal children. After treatment the number of movement units decreased and the movements become less jerky. The total movement time also decreased significantly. However, the authors did not study the long-term effects of the therapy.

Another example of applying what is known about reaching trajectories in normally developed children is a study by Forsström and von Hofsten (1982), who investigated visually directed reaching in children diagnosed as having minimal brain dysfunction (MBD). The task was to catch a moving object that passed in front of the child. The movement parameters evaluated—speed, number of movement units, and length of movement—revealed a less efficient motor performance in the children with MBD compared to a control group of normally developed children. When reaching for a moving object, a successful strategy is to reach for the meeting point with the object; this was also the strategy adopted by both groups of children participating in this study. The two groups of children mainly differed in that the children diagnosed as having MBD aimed their movements at a point further ahead of the target than did the normally developed children. This gave the children diagnosed as MBD more time and compensated for their less efficient movement. It seemed that these children took their less efficient capacity into account when planning the movement. However, this strategy restricts these children's ability to catch fast-moving objects, since it can be successful only up to a certain speed. That clumsy children have to slow down movement speed to achieve movement accuracy has been proved in several studies (Henderson et al., 1992; van der Meulen et al., 1991a, b). This is of course an important factor to consider when assessing motor performance in these children. The children are most likely to reveal their movement difficulties when they are tested on tasks carried out under a time constraint.

As discussed earlier in this chapter, the ability to perceive the external world as well as our own body is crucial for well-coordinated reaching movements. If a child has an impaired capacity to perceive the layout of the world or an impaired capacity to perceive the positions and movements of his/her own body, this will affect the ability to perform goal-directed arm movements. One line of research has focused on how deficits in the processing of perceptual information may affect motor performance in children with motor impairments. Rösblad and von Hofsten (1992) studied the ability of motor-impaired children to perform goal-directed arm movement when deprived of visual information about the arm and hand. The task was the same as in the study by von Hofsten and Rösblad described above, that is, to place pins underneath a tabletop at positions seen or felt on the tabletop. The test was administered to children with three different medical diagnoses: cerebral palsy, spina bifida, and developmental coordination disorders (DCD). (The essential feature of DCD is a marked impairment in the development of motor coordination, which is not a function of mental retardation and is not due to a known physical disorder.) The reason for choosing children with these medical diagnoses was that they are likely to have disturbed coordination of arm and hand function as well as perceptual problems. The children with motor impairments exhibited large variability in pointing accuracy compared to normally developed children, but as can be seen in Figure 5-5, there is to some extent an overlapping in the performance of the children with motor impairments and the normally developed children. However, some of the children with motor impairments demonstrated marked problems in directing their hand when they could not visually monitor it. A main finding in von Hofsten and Rösblad (1988) was a superior pointing performance with visually defined targets. This effect was found to be even larger in the study of motor-impaired children. If the children with motor impairments could not see the target during the pointing action, the impairment was more obvious.

To perform a coordinated reaching movement, the visual and proprioceptive spaces have to be in correspondence with each other. With a task similar to the one described above, Lee et al. (1990) wanted to see if a noncorrespondence between the two systems would be a problem for children with hemiparetic cerebral palsy. They found that different forms of disorders might be expected. Some children exhibited an impaired capacity to align the unseen hand to a seen target, that is, a disturbed correspondence between the proprioceptive and visual systems. Others revealed an impaired capacity to align the two hands without visual information, that is, a noncorrespondence between the proprioceptive information from the two hands.

When discussing results from studies of children with motor impairments, it is important to point out that the variation within one specific diagnostic group is large. The movement problems within one diagnostic group could of course not be explained by one specific factor. But the knowledge obtained from studies carried out on both normally developed children and children with motor impairments can provide us with knowledge of what processes might be disturbed and what to look for when assessing the children.

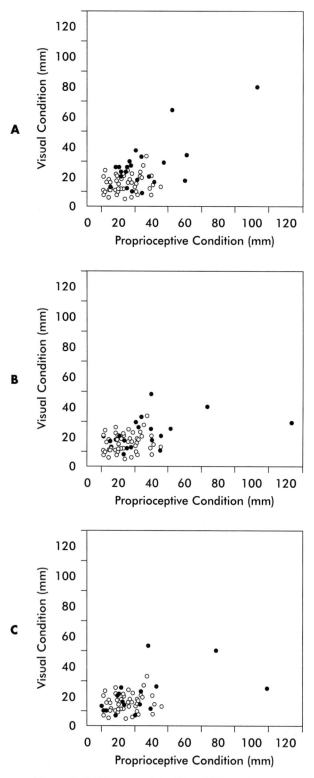

Figure 5-5. The mean error when children are pointing to a target without seeing the pointing hand. *Unfilled circles* denote normally developed 7-year-olds plotted as a frame of reference. *Filled circles* denote children with developmental coordination disorders (**A**), children with spina bifida (**B**), and children with cerebral palsy (**C**).

(Replotted from data presented in von Hofsten, C., & Rösblad, B. [1988]. The integration of sensory information in the development of precise manual pointing. *Neuropsychologia, 26*[6], 805-821.)

ACKNOWLEDGMENT

I am grateful to Claes von Hofsten for valuable comments on an earlier version of the manuscript. This chapter was prepared under support by a grant from the Swedish Council for Social Research (Project No. 92-0113:1C).

REFERENCES

Abend, W., Bizzi, E., & Morasso, P. (1982). Human arm trajectory formation. *Brain, 105,* 331-348.

Alstermark, B., Górska, T., Lundberg, A., & Petterson, L–G. (1990). Integration in descending motor pathways controlling the forelimb in the cat. 16. Visually guided switching of target-reaching. *Experimental Brain Research, 80,* 1-11.

Bossom, J. (1974). Movement without proprioception. *Brain Research, 45,* 285–296.

Bossom, J., & Ommaya, A.K. (1968). Visuomotor adaptation to prismatic transformation of the retinal image in monkeys with bilateral dorsal rhizotomy. *Brain, 91,* 161-72.

Brooks, V.B. (1976). Some examples of programmed limb movements. *Brain Research, 71,* 38-47.

Buyakas, T.M., Vardanyan, G., & Gippenreiter Y. B. (1980). On the mechanisms of precise hand movements (in Russian). *Psichologitsheskij Journal, 1,* 93-103.

Cordo, P.J., & Nashner, L.M. (1982). Properties of postural adjustments associated with rapid arm movements. *Journal of Neurophysiology, 47,* 287-302.

Fetters, L., & Todd, J. (1987). Quantitative assessment of infant reaching movements. *Journal of Motor Behavior, 19*(2), 147-166.

Forsström, A., & von Hofsten, C. (1982). Visually directed reaching of children with motor impairments. *Developmental Medicine and Child Neurology, 24,* 653-661.

Ghez, C., Gordon, J., Ghilardi, M.F., Christakos, C.N., & Cooper, S.E. (1990). Roles of proprioceptive input in the programming of arm trajectories. *Cold Spring Harbor Symposia on Quantitative Biology, 55,* 837-847.

Gordon, J., & Ghez, C. (1992). Roles of proprioceptive input in control of reaching movement. In H. Forsberg, & H. Hirschfeldt (Eds.). *Movement disorders in children. Medicine and Sport Science, Vol. 36.* Basel: Karger.

Grenier, A. (1981). "Motoricité libélrée"par fixation manuelle de la nuque au cours de prémières semaines de la vie. *Archives Francaises de Pediatrie, 38,* 557-561.

Haas, G., Diener, H.C., Rapp, H., & Dichgans, J. (1989). Development of feedback and feedforward control of upright stance. *Developmental Medicine and Child Neurology, 31,* 481-488.

Harris, C.S. (1965). Perceptual adaptation to inverted, reversed and displaced vision. *Psychological Review, 72,* 419-444.

Held, R., & Hein, A. (1963). Movement-produced stimulation in the development of visually guided behavior. *Journal of Comparative and Physiological Psychology, 56*(5), 872-876.

Henderson, L., Rose, P., & Henderson, S. (1992). Reaction time and movement time in children with a developmental coordination disorder. *Journal of Child Psychology and Psychiatry, 33*(5), 895-905.

Jeannerod, M. (1981). Intersegmental coordination during reaching at natural visual objects. In J. Long, & A. Baddeley (Eds.). *Attention and performance.* IX. Hillsdale: Earlbaum.

Jeannerod, M. (1984). The timing of natural prehension movements. *Journal of Motor Behavior, 16*(3):235-254.

Jeannerod, M. (1992). Coordination mechanisms in prehension movements. In G.E. Stelmach & J. Requin (Eds.). *Tutorials in motor behavior.* II, XXX. Amsterdam: Elsevier.

Keele, S.W., & Posner, M.I. (1968). Processing visual feedback in rapid movement. *Journal of Experimental Psychology, 77,* 155-158.

Kluzik, J.A., Fetters, L., & Coryell, J. (1990). Quantification of control: A preliminary study of effects of neurodevelopmental treatment on reaching in children with spastic cerebral palsy. *Physical Therapy, 70*(2), 65-76.

Knapp, H.D., Taub, E., & Berman, A.J. (1963). Movements in monkeys with deafferented forelimbs. *Experimental Neurology, 7,* 303-315.

Lassek, A.M. (1953). Inactivation of voluntary motor function following rhizotomy. *Journal of Neuropathology and Experimental Neurology, 16,* 83-7.

Lassek, A.M., & Moyer, E.K. (1953). An ontogenetic study of motor deficits following dorsal brachial rhizotomy. *Journal of Neurophysiology, 16,* 247-251.

Lee, D.N., Daniel, B.M., Turnball, J., & Cook, M.L. (1990). Basic perceptuo-motor dysfunction in cerebral palsy. In M. Jeannerod (Ed.). *Attention and performance. XIII. Motor representation and control.* New York: Lawrence Erlbaum.

Marteniuk, R.G., MacKenzie, C.L., & Athenes, S. (1990). Functional relationships between grasp and transport components in a prehension task. *Human Movement Science, 9,* 149-176.

Martin, O., & Prablanc, C. (1992). Online control of hand reaching at undetected target displacements. In G.E. Stelmach & J. Requin (Eds.). *Tutorials in motor behavior.* II, XXX. Amsterdam: Elsevier.

McDonnell, P.M. (1975). The development of visually directed reaching. *Perception and Psychophysics, 18,* 181-185.

Morosso, P. (1981). Spatial control of arm movements. *Experimental Brain Research, 42,* 223-227.

Mott, F.W., & Sherrington, C.S. (1895). Experiments upon the influence of sensory nerves upon movement and nutrition of the limbs. *Proceedings of the Royal Society, B57,* 481-488.

Paulignan, Y., MacKenzie, C., Marteniuk, R., & Jeannerod, M. (1991a). Selective perturbation of visual input during prehension movements. 1. The effect of changing object position. *Experimental Brain Research, 83,* 502-512.

Paulignan, Y., Jeannerod, M., MacKenzie, C., & Marteniuk, R. (1991b). Selective perturbation of visual input during prehension movements. 2. The effect of changing object size. *Experimental Brain Research, 87,* 407-420.

Pieraut–Le Bonniec G. (1990). Reaching and hand adjusting to target properties. In H. Bloch & Bertenthal B.I. (Eds.). *Sensory-motor organization and development in infancy and early childhood.* Netherlands: Kluwer Academic Publishers.

Rochat, P. (1992). Self-sitting and reaching in 5- to 8-month-old infants: The impact of posture and its development on eye-hand coordination. *Journal of Motor Behavior, 24*(2), 210-220.

Rösblad, B., & von Hofsten, C. (1992). Perceptual control of manual pointing in children with motor impairments. *Physiotherapy Theory and Practice, 8,* 223-233.

Sherrington, C.S. (1906). *The integrative action of the nervous system.* New Haven: Yale University Press.

Soechting, J.F., & Flanders, M. (1992). Moving in three-dimensional space: Frames of reference, vectors, and coordinate systems. *Annual Review of Neuroscience, 15,* 167-91.

Taub, E., & Berman, A.J. (1968). Movement and learning in the absence of sensory feedback. In S.J. Freedman (Ed.). *The neurophysiology of spatially oriented behaviour.* Homewood: Dorsey Press.

Tillary, M.I., Flanders, M., & Soechting, J.F. (1991). A coordinated system for the synthesis of visual and kinesthetic information. *Journal of Neuroscience, 11*(3), 770-778.

van der Meulen, J.H.P., Denier, J.J., van der Gon, J.J., Gielen, C.C.A.M., Gooskens, R.H.J.M., & Willemse, J. (1991a). Visuomotor performance of normal and clumsy children. I. Fast goal-directed arm movements with and without visual feedback. *Developmental Medicine and Child Neurology, 33,* 40-54.

van der Meulen, J.H.P., Denier, J.J., van der Gon, J.J., Gielen, C.C.A.M., Gooskens, R.H.J.M., & Willemse, J. (1991b). Visuomotor performance of normal and clumsy children. II. Arm-tracking with and without visual feedback. *Developmental Medicine and Child Neurology, 33,* 118-129.

von Hofsten, C. (1979). Development of visually directed reaching: The approach phase. *Journal of Human Movement Science, 5,* 160-178.

von Hofsten, C. (1982). Eye-hand coordination in the newborn. *Developmental Psychology, 18*(3), 450-461.

von Hofsten, C. (1984). Developmental changes in the organization of prereaching movements. *Developmental Psychology, 20*(3), 378-388.

von Hofsten, C. (1991). Structuring of early reaching movements: A longitudinal study. *Journal of Motor Behavior, 23*(4), 280-292.

von Hofsten, C. (1993). Prospective control: A basic aspect of action development. *Human Development. 36,* 253-270.

von Hofsten, C., & Fazel-Zandy, S. (1984). Development of visually guided hand orientation in reaching. *Journal of Experimental Child Psychology, 38,* 208-219.

von Hofsten, C., & Lindhagen, K. (1979). Observations on the development of reaching for moving objects. *Journal of Experimental Child Psychology, 28,* 158-173.

von Hofsten, C., & Rönnquist, L. (1988). Preparation for grasping an object: A developmental study. *Journal of Experimental Psychology: Human Perception and Performance, 14,* 610-621.

von Hofsten, C., & Rösblad, B. (1988). The integration of sensory information in the development of precise manual pointing. *Neuropsychologia, 26*(6), 805-821.

von Hofsten, C., & Woollacott, H.M. (1990). *Postural preparations for reaching in 9-month-old infants.* Unpublished manuscript.

Wing, A.M., Turton, A., & Fraser. C. (1986). Grasp size and accuracy of approach in reaching. *Journal of Motor Behavior, 18,* 245-261.

Woodworth, R.S. (1899). The accuracy of voluntary movement. *Psychological Review Monograph Supplements, 3*(3).

6

Cognition and Motor Skill

Charlotte E. Exner   Anne Henderson

Of all motor skills, manipulative tasks require the greatest interaction of cognitive and motor abilities, and limitations in one of these areas may influence the development of the other. Motor skills and cognitive skills are often addressed together either directly or indirectly in the literature, but the focus of research is usually on cognitive development. In developmental evaluation, motor task performance is used as a method of inferring cognitive functions. The inferences made from the observation of task proficiency may be erroneous because limited task performance may reflect either impairment in motor skills, or impairment in cognitive functioning, or both. For example, block building requires both cognitive and motor skill. However, building a six-block tower requires a higher level of motor skill than building a three-block train, whereas the perceptual-cognitive demands for building the train are greater than for building a block tower. It is through the analysis of tasks such as these that therapists differentiate between subtle motor and cognitive problems. However, with many tasks it is difficult to determine the primary factor in a child's difficulty in the performance of hand activities.

This chapter presents an introduction to the cognitive abilities that are clearly related to the development and execution of fine motor skills. We begin with our working definition of cognition.

Cognition is broadly defined as the capacity by which the individual acquires, organizes, and uses knowledge (Lidz, 1987). This broad definition has been interpreted differently by various authors over the years because the term encompasses multiple mental processes, and the identification of these processes has often differed (Flavell, 1985). In the past, one way of viewing cognition was to limit its definition to very high-level processes such as imagining, solving problems, creating, planning, categorizing information, using symbols, and conceptual thinking. In the viewpoint of other authors, perception, imagery, memory, attention, learning, and, in the case of infants, organized motor movements should be included (Flavell, 1985).

The cognitive constructs an author includes have typically depended on the theory being used to explain the cognitive processes. For example, in the information-processing approach a computer model has been used to explain the reception, coding, storage, retrieval, and use of information (Flavell, 1985). Piaget and Inhelder focused more on the process of "knowing" at varying levels of complexity; the concepts of perception, symbol use, imagery, categorization of information, and problem solving were included in their theory of cognitive development (Gallagher and Reid, 1981). Today cognition is considered to be a global term encompassing multiple classes of mental capacities. Cognitive psychology includes the study of perception, attention, memory, reasoning, problem solving, and language (Glass and Holyoak, 1986). Cognition is a basic and universal human trait that underlies virtually every human activity (Flavell, 1985; Katz, 1992). It then follows that some degree of cognition is necessary to the learning and execution of all motor skills.

Cognitive psychology is a large field of study, and each of the processes introduced here has its separate and extensive body of research. Only a few of the cognitive processes are discussed, and those only briefly for the purpose of illustrating the role of cognition in the execution and development of motor skills. In this chapter we first define and discuss the characteristics of motor skill, then introduce the basic, interrelated processes of attention, perception, and memory, and then discuss thinking (categorizing, reasoning, and problem solving and planning) and learning. A second section of the chapter reviews the theory and research addressing the role of motor function in cognitive development.

COGNITION IN THE ACQUISITION AND EXECUTION OF MOTOR SKILL
Definition and Characteristics of Motor Skill

We define motor skill as precisely executed and organized movement sequences used to accomplish a specific goal. This definition highlights three fundamental characteristics of skilled motor performance: goal direction, proficiency, and organization. The goal-directed nature of the act differentiates skilled movement from other movements. Sugden and Keogh (1990) describe motor skills as being "movements that are intentional, goal directed, organized, and adaptive. . . . Intentionality

indicates a purposefulness that is goal directed in an effort to achieve a desired outcome" (p. 1). Gilfoyle, Grady, and Moore (1981) and Connolly (1973) also describe movement skill in relation to the activity being performed—the fact that the movement must be goal oriented. These definitions imply that not all movements are skillful; those movements that do not involve attempts at goal accomplishment (are not purposeful) do not involve skill. For example, a movement that is simply a change in position in space (Levine, 1987) or a reflex response such as scratching is not a skill. Movements may be possible that do not directly involve cognition, but "movement skill . . . involves knowing and doing" (Sugden and Keogh, 1990, p. 102). Goal orientation requires at the very least the cognitive elements of memory and planning.

The second fundamental characteristic that distinguishes motor skill is the quality and accuracy of the movement (Fitts and Posner, 1967; Paillard, 1960). Paillard defines skilled motor activity as:

. . . a particular category of finely coordinated voluntary movements generally engaging certain privileged parts of the musculature in the performance of various technical acts which have as common characteristics the delicacy of adjustment, the economy of their execution and the accuracy of their achievement (1960, p. 1679).

Finely coordinated voluntary movement requires continuous feedback from those sensory systems that provide continuous spatial and temporal information while a movement is progressing. To be considered skillful, movements must be appropriate in relation to the space and time requirements for the activity. Attention and perception are key processes in the use of feedback in the development and execution of motor skill (Elliott and Connolly, 1974). The ability to adjust movements as they are occurring also depends heavily on the use of perception and cognition (Sugden and Keogh, 1990).

The third fundamental characteristic of motor skill is that "skilled performance always involves an organized sequence of activities" (Fitts and Posner, 1967, p. 1). Almost every daily activity, such as dressing, eating, and typing, is a sequence of actions that is appropriate to the task. Task performance is skillful if sequences of actions are carried out efficiently, rapidly, and with minimal effort (Connolly, 1973; Glass and Holyoak, 1986). Strategy acquisition, learning, problem solving, and planning are important for sequential, organized movements.

There are additional characteristics important to competency in motor skills. A second type of feedback, that of the knowledge of the results of actions, is also critical. Cognitive skills are needed to understand such feedback and to recognize how this feedback will affect future performance. Preparation for subsequent movements based on feedback is also necessary; such preparation involves planning.

For movement to be skillful, there must be competence in accommodating movements to the situational needs (Sugden and Keogh, 1990); skill must also include rules for managing a variety of objects in different situations (Elliott and Connolly, 1974). Both situational planning and the use of rules are cognitive functions.

Tool use is an aspect of motor skill that seems to have a close relationship with cognition. The ability to use tools is very important for almost all types of work performed by adults. Connolly (1973) notes that "the manner in which an adult handles a tool reflects not only his knowledge of the tool and the plan of action which he employs but also the 'reliability' of the sub-routines available to him" (p. 361).

Finally, all motor skills are learned (Glass and Holyoak, 1986). This is most apparent in skills that involve complex sequences of movements, but even the simple action of grasping is practiced over and over by the infant. All motor learning draws on attention and memory, and complex motor learning requires planning and problem solving as well.

In summary, several aspects of cognition are specifically involved in motor skill. These cognitive components include attention, use of sensation and perception to guide the movement, organization/sequencing of movements, learning movement sequences, and modification of these movement sequences in response to situational demands.

Motor Skill and Praxis

Praxis is a detailed and complex area of study and is mentioned here only briefly for its relationship to motor skill. The concept of praxis has been derived from studies of adults and children with central nervous system dysfunction, whereas motor skill has been studied in normal adults and children. The definitions of praxis are varied, but all refer to one or more aspects of motor learning or performance; when the multiple uses of the term are viewed together, a description of praxis is very much like the description of motor skill just presented. The qualifying labels for apraxia and dyspraxia have been derived from differing symptoms observed in association with motor dysfunction or clumsiness. The major categories are (1) ideational apraxia, referring to the loss of the concept of an action; (2) ideomotor apraxia, the inability to plan sequences of actions when the goal is understood; (3) limb-kinetic apraxia, the loss of memory of movements; and (4) somatosensory dyspraxia, identifying the association of poor motor function with diminished tactile and kinesthetic perception. Each of these categories identifies a characteristic of motor skill. It may be that in time the research areas of praxis and motor skill will be combined. For now, however, the reader is referred to Roy (1985) for a comprehensive review of apraxia.

Basic Cognitive Processes in Motor Skill

The characteristics of skilled movement each place a demand on one or more cognitive processes at either a simple or complex level. Attention, perception, and memory enter into all skilled behavior, from the simple action of repetitive reaching to the complex action of tying one's shoe. Thinking enters when behavior requires choice.

Attention

Attention is basic to all cognitive activity, including perception, memory, and action. Attention is selective. Our environment is full of sounds, sights, tastes, and smells. Our minds are full of thoughts and memories. We are aware of only a few of these at any given instant because our attention system has a limited capacity for processing information (Glass and Holyoak, 1986). Conscious attention is voluntary. We choose to focus our attention on something we see or hear, inwardly on a thought or memory, or on something we are doing. The process of attention is a process of selection.

Attention, perception, and memory are closely intertwined. When we consciously attend to something we perceive, our perception is matched to information in our memory. Our awareness of something we see in the environment is determined both by the thing we see and by our memory of what we have seen before. And the "ability to maintain a representation in consciousness is at the center of your ability to control your actions independently of the environment" (Glass and Holyoak, 1986, p. 80).

In his discussion of the role of attention in movement, Klein (1976) noted that the acquisition of most new motor skills occurs only when attention is focused on the skill, but with increasing competence in performing the skill, attention is decreased. Both simple and complex motor skills require the regulation of attention for their development and use, and deciding not to move also requires attention. Attention is important in stimuli selection and in the use of the mental processes that allow for the acquisition and use of motor skills.

Klein (1976) further proposed that attention is limited and that this limitation affects how attention is allocated. When a particular task receives an individual's attention, other tasks are less likely to receive attention. Attention seems to be used most at movement initiation regardless of the type of movement, but attention for termination varies, based on whether an external object will be used to stop the movement or whether the control for stopping needs to be internal. Attention during the movement tends to be minimal. Movements to small targets require much more attention than movements to large targets. This information discussed by Klein seems to pertain primarily to short-duration movements in which the individual is initiating movement for the purpose of contacting an object. It does not seem to apply to sustained movement that would be used in object exploration or handling.

Attention in infant movements. Attention is critical for the development of both motor control and cognitive skills. Attention and perception provide the stimulus for motor activity, and motor activity enhances attention and perception (Corbetta and Mounoud, 1990). Object manipulation and cognitive development in infancy are closely interrelated.

A measure of attention used in the study of infants is their habituation to stimuli, that is, their decrease in response to familiar stimuli. Habituation is often determined by visual fixation but can also be inferred from hand activity (Lecuyer, 1989). In a habituation study Hutt (1967) found that the infant's object manipulation decreased as a 30-minute session progressed, and that with increasing familiarization with a particular object the infant increased banging and dropping behaviors. Object manipulation skills were all accompanied by visual inspection, whereas the behaviors that occurred with habituation were without visual inspection.

Infants' examining behaviors, which include visual inspection, finger movement over the object surface, and rotation of the object, are all indica-

tive of the infants' focused visual attention (Ruff, 1986). Ruff found that the amount of time spent in examining behavior decreases as the infant becomes familiar with a novel object and suggests that the time taken to initiate object examination may "be affected by the arousal properties of the object as well as by the time required for organizing a response; or organization may be faster under conditions of optimal arousal" (p. 110). The kind of motor activity (turning objects, dropping objects) as well as the time spent on a particular motor activity is determined by the infant's attention and interest in the properties of objects. An aspect of manipulation not addressed by Ruff is the extent to which response orientation might be influenced by the differences in the motor control development of individual infants.

A finding of interest in Ruff's studies is that sustained attention may be a stable trait in children. A follow-up study at age 3½ years of the children who were seen at 9 months of age, used the number of times children got out of their seats as an indicator of sustained attention. The measures at 3½ were moderately correlated with variables at 9 months. Both the period of examining at 9 months and the ability of the child to stay in the seat later are indicative of the child's ability to maintain behaviors that allow learning to occur (Ruff, 1986).

Perception

Perception is the process of acquiring information about objects, places, and events (Gibson and Spelke, 1983). Perception is not entirely separable from sensation, attention, memory, or knowledge. We perceive what is specified through our senses as patterns of phenomena such as light and sounds. We selectively attend to particular perceptions. Mental representations of our perceptions are stored in our memory, and perceptions form the basis for our knowledge about our environment.

There is a continuity between perception and cognition, and, although there are different approaches to research and theory, they are interrelated. Gibson and Spelke (1983) wrote that "from our view, there is no firm line to be drawn between perception and cognition" (p. 58). There is a similar continuity between sensation and perception. Therefore, in discussing the aspects of perception essential for skilled hand use, it is sometimes useful to differentiate between perceptual-motor and perceptual-conceptual functions. We identify as perceptual-motor the often unthinking monitoring of movement in environmental space, such as the use of the kinesthetic and visual senses. Perceptual-conceptual activity involves the use of perception and perceptual knowledge in decision making, such as deciding what to do or whether to move. These aspects of perception are not entirely separable, but they do represent different levels of function.

Perceptual-motor function. A general principle of motor control is that "the motor system is tuned to perception" (Rosenbaum, 1991, p. 387). Perceptual-motor skill is the modeling of actions to the physical characteristics of objects, places, and events, such as the shaping of the hand to fit the size and orientation of an object, reaching the required distance and direction for grasp, or timing a reach to grasp a moving object. The use of perceptual feedback in the attainment of movement precision is a perceptual-motor function. Perception is used in the visual and proprioceptive guidance or monitoring of every movement. Spatial perception, object perception, and timing are essential to motor skill.

We are seldom conscious of the constant monitoring of skilled movements by our perceptual systems. The visual system is constructed to directly extract information from the environment. Objects are perceived as separate wholes from their backgrounds. Visual mechanisms provide information about distances between objects and places. Movement of objects or self is directly apprehended; that is, as we reach for a pencil, we are not aware of the movement adjustments we base on the sight of the pencil and our hand. We don't think "move more to the right" or "move further," we simply reach. Our actions usually reach consciousness only if we misreach since, although perceptual-motor control is largely unconscious, it is always available to consciousness with a shift in attention. The perceptual control of movement is discussed in Chapters 3 to 5.

Perceptual-conceptual function. Perceptual-conceptual systems also function reciprocally with the environment. Deciding what to do and in what sequence is based on our perceptual knowledge of objects, places, and events. "To perceive is to monitor the environment and what happens in it in the service of guiding one's behavior. Perception depends on obtaining information about the environment from an array of potential stimulation" (Gibson and Spelke, 1983, p. 58).

Gibson and Spelke describe the concept of affordance as it is used to explain the reciprocal nature of the human being and the environment. Our perceptual systems extract information about the affordances of the environment. Affordances are what places, objects, and events mean to us functionally. "A floor affords support and can be walked upon. A wall is an obstacle that affords collision, but a doorway in the wall affords walking through. . . . Affordance is a functional term that emphasizes the utility of some aspect of the environment" (Gibson and Spelke, 1983). We select our goals and plan our movement sequences based on the affordances in our environment.

An important aspect of the concept of affordances is that perceptual systems have evolved in relation to the environment and directly provide invariant information about the properties of objects, places, and events. From birth, infants are able to actively explore and obtain knowledge about the affordances of their environments (Gibson and Spelke, 1983). Over time they learn about properties of objects, such as texture, shape, weight, and substance (rigidity, flexibility, deformability), and that what they do with objects depends not only on the object perceived as a whole but on the object's properties.

As a child develops, perceptions of the affordances of objects change. This can be illustrated by the common use of 1-inch cubes in infant tests. For the young infant a cube affords the action of grasping, then of banging or dropping for the effect produced. For the toddler, cubes are also perceived as affording building towers.

The quality and accuracy of motor skill depend on the matching of movement to the perceptual surroundings. Selecting goals and planning actions depend on perceptual knowledge and memory. Thus perception is an integral part of all facets of motor skill.

Memory

"Memory is the ability to store and use past experience" (Rosenblith, 1992, p. 372). Long-term memory is our store of knowledge and includes stored perceptions of objects, places, and events; motor actions; and the products of our thinking about and organizing what we know. All of our knowledge is stored in our memory, but the storage may last for varying amounts of time. Long-term memory is relatively permanent. Short-term memory is fragile and remains only for a brief period, which can be measured in minutes after information is processed. Memories as well as perceptions may be the subject of conscious attention. The part of long-term memory that is active (that of which we are aware at any given time) has been called *working memory*. Working memory comes into play in the recognition of a perceptual input and recall of perceptions or concepts, as well as in categorizing knowledge, reasoning, problem solving, and planning.

Of particular interest in a discussion of cognition and motor skill is the distinction between procedural knowledge or memory (knowing how) and declarative knowledge or memory (knowing that) (Mandler, 1983). When we show a child how to throw a ball, we are using our procedural knowledge or memory, and, as the child learns, he/she is storing procedural knowledge or memory. When a mother shows a child how to put on a shirt, she is using and teaching procedural knowledge. However, when a therapist teaches a mother an adaptive technique for teaching a child with a disability how to put on the shirt, a combination of procedural knowledge and declarative knowledge is used, the latter providing "facts" about the adaptations or principles of adaptation needed.

A primarily procedural memory system is central both to the storing of our actions and to perceptual processing (we recognize something without accessing facts of that recognition). It is probable that an infant uses both procedural and declarative organization of knowledge, though predominately the former. With development, declarative knowledge becomes increasingly predominant although adults continue to use procedural knowledge extensively (Mandler, 1983).

Thinking

We classify under thinking the higher-order mental processes acting on knowledge that has been encoded and stored in memory. These processes include the organization of the knowledge base into conceptual categories and the use of knowledge in reasoning, problem solving, goal selection, and planning.

Knowledge is organized through thinking. An infant not only perceives but forms concepts about objects, places, events, and actions. A concept is a unit of mental representation that designates a set of properties associated with each other (Clark, 1983). A word is a concept, but not all concepts can be expressed in words. Concepts are the reference point for categorization. An infant's first conceptual categories are perceptual (e.g., of visual forms) and can be demonstrated during the first year of life (Olsen and Sherman, 1983). Categorization involves abstraction of properties and selection of like properties among objects, places, events, and actions. The ability to classify

experiences is basic to intelligence and learning (Olsen and Sherman, 1983).

Knowledge has a reciprocal relationship with attention, perception, and memory. What is attended to, perceived, learned, and remembered forms the knowledge base. But that knowledge, organized into categories, in turn plays a role in what is attended to, learned, and remembered.

Knowledge is not only organized but used. The core of intelligence is in the allocation and adaptation of one's mental resources to a given task environment (Sternberg and Powell, 1983). Information needed to respond to environmental happenings is selected from the store of knowledge. Knowledge is used for the selection of a goal, a plan of action, prediction of the consequences of the action, and judgement about the monitored outcome. Planning involves identification of task requirements, adjustments to situational demands, and anticipation of events.

Knowledge is needed for understanding the task requirements for goal completion. In a discussion of goal-directed behavior in toddlers, Bullock and Lutkenhaus (1988) identified the following prerequisites. A general prerequisite is the understanding of means-end actions. Also the ability to maintain attention on the desired goal and to monitor progress toward the goal are needed. Remaining task-oriented requires "waiting or searching for appropriate opportunities to act, resisting distractions, overcoming obstacles, correcting actions and stopping action when a goal is reached" (p. 664). Even in the grasp of objects, the individual's goal related to the object is often the greatest determinant in selecting the particular type of grasp to be used (Napier, 1956).

Sequencing movements, particularly complex movements, places demands on problem solving. Rules must be developed by children for use of learned skills in a variety of situations (Elliott and Connolly, 1974). Such skills require activating, ordering, and refining the movement sequences that will allow for goal accomplishment. In this way skill development is viewed as reflecting problem solving (Bruner and Kozlowski, 1972).

In summary, of the basic cognitive processes in motor skill, it is clear that not all cognitive processes are implicated in the acquisition and execution of hand skills in children, but all hand skills require some level of one or more cognitive processes. The basic interrelated processes of attention, perception, and memory play a role in all skilled motor activity as they do in all of human behavior. Attention is essential to meaningful action. All actions take place within a perceptual environment. Motor skills are learned, that is, stored in memory. Knowledge and the use of knowledge determine the selection of actions. However, we need to learn much more about how these cognitive functions interact and influence the motor skill levels of the individual child.

Learning Motor Skills

Cognitive functioning is often reflected in an individual's ability to acquire new information and skills as well as to use previously learned information. Motor skills that require acquisition of sequences of movements for successful performance are particularly dependent on higher-level cognitive skills; in children the more basic motor skills may evolve with less dependence on understanding the goals of the movement. The acquisition of basic motor skills has been described in early studies (see Chapter 7). However, the classification of phases of mastering a new motor skill has been better described in adult learning, and we begin there.

Motor Skill Learning in Adults

The mastery of skilled movements or technical abilities in adults follows a process of fumbling and progressive adjustment until the actions become organized and self-regulated units (Paillard, 1960). The following three phases of this process have been described by Fitts and Posner (1967) based in large part on the findings from interviews with skill instructors. There is no distinct transition from one phase to another; rather, one phase merges gradually into another.

Cognitive phase. The first stage described is one in which cognitive requirements are high. At this time the individual learning the skill obtains information about the task and determines the order of movement for goal accomplishment. Conscious control of each movement is necessary, with close attention to cues and events that will later go unnoticed. The cognitive phase involves the selection of routines from prior experience, with these old routines put together into new patterns that are supplemented by new routines (Fitts and Posner, 1967).

Associative phase. In the second phase of skill learning more evidence of coordinated movement, reflecting the time and space demands of the task, is present, and visual cues are used less to guide the movements. Subroutines have now been learned, and errors of sequences and responses are gradually eliminated. This phase is a transition

from conscious control to a more automatic control, in which one movement cues another, and it is no longer necessary to recall each step in the sequence (Rosenbaum, 1991).

Autonomous phase. In the final phase the action sequences become automatic, and cognitive control becomes less direct. The actions can be carried out while attention is on other activities. The motor sequences are now a part of an entire motor program (Glass and Holyoak, 1986). Feedback has shifted from chiefly visual to chiefly proprioceptive, and vision is used primarily for vigilance and in refining movement (Paillard, 1960). In the autonomous phase movement is freer, graceful, quick, consistent, and efficient (Rosenbaum, 1991). The motor skill has reached the level that meets the characteristics of skilled movement as described above. Attention to movement details is reduced. At this time significantly less cognitive control over the movements is seen. This sequence suggests that cognition is important in early learning of a motor skill but has a decreasing role in skill refinement.

Motor Skill Learning in Children

The mastery of manipulative skills in the early years of life appears to follow the pattern of fumbling and progressive adjustments that occurs in adult motor skill learning (Paillard, 1960). The extent to which the development of motor skills in childhood follows that of the acquisition of motor skill by adults has not been established. The role of cognition in the development of complex motor skills that require learned sequences of movement is clear, but the role of cognition in the development of basic movement patterns such as reach may differ. However, there are certainly some similarities as well as some differences in the skill acquisition of adults and of even young children.

Similarities between adult and child motor learning. As in adult learning, the demands for cognition are particularly high in the early phase of skill learning in childhood. Even in the neonate, attention and perception, with vision predominating, are active in the conscious control of reaching.

The characteristics of complex motor skill development in children have many similarities to the learning of a new motor skill by adults. In learning a motor skill, movements are characterized by less and less variability and more automaticity, that is, with less attention to the movements (Sugden and Keogh, 1990). When skills are well learned, attention is given to the sequence of movements, rather than to individual movements (Elliott and Connolly, 1974). At that point a skill can be used in a variety of situations and even with long periods between occasions of use (Sugden and Keogh, 1990).

Glass and Holyoak (1986) suggest three ways in which basic skills such as grasp could be acquired. First, the varying objects seen by infants excite their curiosity, leading to many repetitions of attempts to grasp. Second, adults actively encourage repetition of goal-directed activity in infants. Finally, motor skills are learned under the guidance of the infant's mental representations. Self-activated visual representations form the basis for learning.

Differences in adult and child motor learning. In the first few years of life the basic patterns of manipulation are acquired. Later the learning of entirely new skills is rare; rather, new skills are modifications of old skills. Throughout childhood neural maturation plays an important role in skill development. However, Reid (1989) notes that cognitive factors must also be considered in understanding motor development, particularly in young children. Her study of 4- to 18-month-old children illustrates that movement patterns may be present but will not be used until the necessary cognitive skills have been developed. Explaining motor performance on the basis of neuromotor development alone is not sufficient (Reid, 1989).

The role of neural maturation accounts for a major difference between adult and child motor learning and is the reason for the great difference in the length of time needed to learn a motor skill. Fine motor skills continue to develop for many years after fundamental skills are acquired; adult level skill in manipulation of objects, and particularly tools, is not reached until adolescence (Gilfoyle et al., 1981; Connolly and Elliott, 1972; Exner, 1990a). Complex manipulation skills also have complex cognitive demands, and their development requires substantially more time than many other motor skills (Corbetta and Mounoud, 1990; Elliott and Connolly, 1974; Exner, 1990a). This long developmental period is probably at least partly due to the dependence of these skills on development in the areas of sensation, perception, and cognition (Lefford, 1970).

Facilitation of children's learning. It has been shown that a child's motor learning can be facilitated by adults. Vygotsky (1978, cited by Lochman, 1986) proposed that children are often able to accomplish skills in a social situation before being able to accomplish skills alone. The adults and other individuals who interact with a child often assist in this skill accomplishment by

affecting factors such as the child's attention, planning, and skills. In the same way, infants' sensorimotor skills may be facilitated by parent-child interactions (Kaye, 1982, cited by Lochman, 1986). Using this model, it may be suggested that when use of cognitive skills is supported and encouraged, motor skills may emerge more quickly.

Exner (1990b) conducted a study to determine how Vygotsky's concept of the zone of proximal development may apply to fine motor skills. In this study 3- and 4-year-old children were tested for their spontaneous use of in-hand manipulation skills. One week later they were given the same test of their manipulative skills but were provided with either verbal or visual (demonstration) cues. As a group, the children improved in their skill use when provided with cues, but the type of cue did not seem to affect their performances. Using Vygotsky's theory in interpreting the data, approximately 40% of the children showed a readiness for using more advanced in-hand manipulation skills when provided guidance by an adult. The other children did not demonstrate this readiness for using more advanced skills.

Cognitive characteristics of good infant learners. A study of the performance of gross and fine motor tasks of moderate difficulty by 13-month-old infants illustrated the relationship between cognitive development and motor skill development (Yarrow et al., 1982). The findings reflected a relationship between scores on the Bayley Developmental Scales and motor development in infancy. Competence in the task performance at 13 months was significantly associated with persistence in attempting the tasks. Competence and persistence were also each highly associated with performance on perceptual discrimination, spatial relations, problem-solving tasks, and the overall Motor Development Index. The authors also found that a measure indicating goal-directed behavior at 6 months of age was associated with the 13-month-old competence in performing the tasks. This suggests that competence in both motor and cognitive skills may be affected by the infant's emphasis on mastering environmental challenges at a very early age. The authors state that "infants who work assiduously at perfecting their skills may become more competent; in turn, competent infants derive greater satisfaction from working on skills, and thus are more likely to practice them. It does not seem to be simply a circular process, but a sequential and hierarchical one in which mastery motivation facilitates consolidation of skills and leads to emergence of new ones" (p. 140).

Cognition in the Development of Selected Motor Tasks

We have selected two developmental skills in childhood that illustrate the interaction of motor skill and cognition: object manipulation and movement timing.

Object Manipulation

Object manipulation, the use of skills in moving objects with the hands, is an early-developing fine motor behavior. The stages in the development of object manipulation illustrate its dependence on cognition as well as other aspects of development. Corbetta and Mounoud (1990) reviewed the progression of development. During the first 6 months of life the perception of visual and tactile stimuli is used to guide fine motor development as the infant develops an awareness of object placement in space. In the second half of the first year the infant adjusts actions of the hand in response to object characteristics such as size, shape, and surface qualities. By 9 to 10 months of age infants adapt their arm positions to horizontal versus vertical object presentation and shape their hands appropriately for convex and concave objects.

Several studies illustrated the developmental changes in the adaptation of young infants in their responses to differing perceptual attributes. Bruner and Koslowski (1972) studied infants to determine how fine motor skills change in response to the infants' recognition of the size of objects. They recorded the types of arm and hand movement made in response to presentation of two balls, one small and graspable and the other much larger. The infants, from 10 to 22 weeks of age, used a swiping motion with the larger ball and a movement of the hand(s) toward midline with presentation of the small ball. The differences were seen in babies even prior to their ability to effectively reach and grasp and therefore were not thought to depend on interaction with objects. This study indicates that young infants do perceive size differences and vary their motor responses accordingly.

Lochman, Ashmead, and Bushnell (1984) studied the emergence of the ability of 5- and 9-month-old infants to use appropriate hand orientations for grasping dowels presented in vertical and horizontal orientations. The older infants showed more appropriate hand orientation at the time of initial dowel contact than the 5-month-olds did. They seemed to be more effective in using visual information to adjust their hand orientations. The au-

thors interpreted the finding to indicate a developmental change in the ability of infants to integrate the perception of orientation of the dowel with their motor response.

Skill in performing two-handed activities lags substantially behind unilateral hand development. This may be because the relative complexity of using two hands requires greater attention and new problem-solving strategies (Corbetta and Manoud, 1990). For example, materials can be separated, combined, and made to work in relation to one another when both hands are used. Ramsay and Weber (1986) used Piaget's theory to explain the relationship between the development of two-handed skills and cognitive development. In stage five of the sensorimotor period, trial and error is used to solve problems. At this time the infants' management of both hands in completing a task that requires differentiation of roles for the two hands is characterized by a lack of an organized approach. The ability to sequence and time the movements of the two hands may depend on the ability to use foresight, which is seen in stage six of this phase.

Another illustration of the complexity of the developmental process is the finding of inconsistency in the performance of children. Hohlstein (1982) reported that infants between 4 and 12 months of age are inconsistent in the grasp patterns used even with no variance of object properties or use. A range of actions may be used at an early age, regardless of the task demands. The inconsistency may reflect the infants' difficulty integrating the sensory, perceptual, and cognitive requirements of activities, as well as their neuro-motor immaturity. A situational inconsistency in the use of well-developed motor patterns has also been observed when the motor demands of a task become too high. For example, children revert to an immature pattern of pronation when first attempting to cut with scissors (Gilfoyle and Grady, 1973). In a study of 40 3- and 4-year-old children, Connolly (1973) found that the children were able to use a well-developed power/precision grasp pattern on a writing tool but that they often reverted to a more immature pattern when the task became more difficult.

Exner (1990a) found that all basic in-hand manipulation skills and those that involve stabilization of materials in the hand during object manipulation were present in normal children before the age of 7 years, but that many of the children were inconsistent in their performances. She proposed that children's increase in the consistency of use of these skills during the preschool years is, in part, a result of their cognitive development. Cognitive development affects the child in two ways. First, it makes material handling and tool use desirable. Second, as the variety of grasp patterns or strategies for object manipulations are reduced for simple activities, the child can put effort into developing movement programs that comprise a number of individual movement skills.

Cognitive functioning is often reflected in an individual's ability to acquire new skill in the manipulation of objects as well as to use previously learned skills. Object manipulation that requires acquisition of a sequence of movements for successful performance is particularly dependent on higher-level cognitive skills. It appears as if integration of the sensory and perceptual components may be crucial in developing basic skills, with the cognitive aspects taking on more and more importance as developing skills become more complex. Such a view of skill development is not contradictory to the view presented earlier regarding the importance of cognition in early skill learning. With refinement of a skill sequence, after it is learned, cognition seems to play a decreasing role.

Studies of Movement Timing

Movement timing, together with spatial orientation, is critical to movement precision. Timing places high demands on the motor system for speed and efficiency, with concomitant high demands for attention and perception. Because reaction time and coincidence-anticipation are high-level skills, they have value for the study of attention and perception in motor performance.

Reaction time. Reaction time "provides an indication of an individual's speed in preparing a response, which for movement involves analyzing a situation followed by selecting and organizing a movement response" (Sugden and Keogh, 1990). It is not the time required for movement completion (that time is equated with movement speed), but it is the individual's processing time. To respond to a stimulus, the information must be encoded, comparisons must be made with prior situations or response options, a response must be selected, and finally it must be executed. Memory strategies have been identified as an area that influences children's ability to make a fast response (Chi, cited by David, 1985) but children can also be limited in how fast a reaction time is

possible due to their more limited ability to process several types of information simultaneously and to alter the focus of their attention.

A study by van der Meulen et al. (1991a) suggested that the production of fast arm movements to achieve a goal may be affected by poor attention. They found that children who were clumsy were not successful with their movement when they were not attending well and/or showed little effort in accomplishing the task. When the children did not have visual feedback, they performed more poorly; the researchers noted that decreased feedback may cause attention to be poorer and distractibility to be heightened. They also concluded that impaired motor control processes cause clumsiness and that children with these problems may be less able to efficiently use visual feedback (van der Meulen et al., 1991a).

Mentally retarded children have slow reaction times as compared to cognitively normal children and show more variability (are less consistent) in their reaction times than normal children. Reaction time is longer in children with more severe mental retardation than in those who show less cognitive limitation.

Coincidence-anticipation. Coincidence-anticipation is a second aspect of movement that depends on timing. Coincidence-anticipation is "the ability to produce a response which coincides with an external event. It reflects the performer's ability to interact with the environment, and it is critical in the development of motor competence . . . timing of the movement, rather than speed, is the critical factor. Cognitive processes in the form of strategies direct how the performer will use sensory information and guide the motor action" (Goodgold-Edwards and Gianutsos, 1991, p. 50). Bard, Fleury, and Gagnon (1990) note that coincidence-anticipation depends on spatial knowledge relative both to the object to be contacted and one's own body as well as the temporal component regarding when contact can or should be made. To be effective, individuals must also recognize and plan for the time they need for processing stimuli, the time they need to react, and their own speed of movement. The ability to deal with many issues in regard to the temporal aspects of movement is therefore a very important factor in infants' performance of skills. These temporal concepts may be more difficult to acquire than other concepts that reflect sensory or spatial relationships (Bard et al., 1990).

Coincidence-anticipation is affected by cognitive development, attentional development, use of memory, and strategies for handling information (Bard et al., 1990). These elements gradually become more and more effective, and coincidence-anticipation improves. Although infants can effectively determine moving objects through the visual system and basic skill in coincidence-anticipation is present at a young age, maturation of this aspect of movement skill requires a long period of time. Even 6-year-olds lack proficiency in integrating visual and motor skills (Bard et al., 1990). This may be due to their reliance on spatial rather than temporal cues. Increased skill in coincidence-anticipation is seen in children up to at least 10 to 12 years of age (Goodgold-Edwards and Gianutsos, 1991). Older adolescents and adults may show further development of coincidence-anticipation, particularly within very complex tasks (Bard et al., 1990). Certainly the high level of skill required in most sports continues to improve through adolescence and into adulthood.

Many children with identified clumsiness perform poorly or inconsistently on coincidence-anticipation tasks. However, researchers do not agree on the underlying dysfunction. Suggested problems have included slower processing resulting from inaccuracies in perceptual judgment (Sugden and Keogh, 1990); limitations in speed and precision of movement (Sovik and Maeland, 1986); and poor attentional control combined with poor motor planning, particularly with the need to modify motor plans during movement (van der Meulen et al., 1991b).

Coincidence-anticipation skill was assessed by Goodgold-Edwards and Gianutsos (1991) in 7- to 12-year-old children with and without cerebral palsy by using a computer task. Scoring involved documenting the amount of overshooting or undershooting of the target. The children with spastic cerebral palsy were much less accurate than were the normal children and generally "exhibited perceptual-motor match deficits beyond that expected on the basis of their primary motor or perceptual problem" (Goodgold-Edwards and Gianutsos, 1991, p. 78). These children varied their time of movement initiation in accord with the speed of the stimuli presented but were not successful in the adjustment of their movement time.

Coincidence-anticipation has also been studied with children who were mentally retarded as well as with young children who were considered normal (Sugden and Keogh, 1990). The findings with both groups were similar. The children showed little understanding of the amount of time that it would take an object to reach a particular point. These authors note that the difficulties in the mentally retarded children seem to be due to impairments in "central processing capabilities" (p. 108).

In summary, both reaction time and coincidence-anticipation involve measuring fairly simple motor actions but ones that must be timed in relation to an external stimulus. This area seems to have promise in delineating the degree of relationship between cognition and motion. For example, it may be found that accidents are more prevalent in some individuals with motor or cognitive problems.

Comment

Humans have very complex hands and can use their hands alone and with tools in highly skilled patterns (Connolly and Elliott, 1972). A variety of factors contribute to use of fine motor skills. Although refined tool use and fine manipulative activities depend on excellent finger control, Napier (1956) cautions that "it is in the elaboration of the central nervous system and not in the specialization [sic] of the hand that we find the basics of human skill" (p. 913). This elaboration of the central nervous system over the long period of the development of motor skills includes both the more motoric aspects of development found in the precision of spatially directed movement and timing and in the more cognitive aspects of attention, memory, object perception, planning, and problem solving. Movement timing and object manipulation both draw on the motor and cognitive systems, but the latter is especially interactive with higher levels of cognition.

Neuromotor maturation is essential to skilled hand use, but attention and goal direction must also be considered in age-related measurement of skill. The characteristics of precision and efficiency in motor skills develop slowly, as do the cognitive skills of attention span, problem solving, perceptual differentiation, and memory. We know that cognition and motor proficiency both improve in childhood, but we do not know the relative contributions of the processes at any given age. For example, the cognitive demands on simple grasp and release are minimal beyond infancy, but we do not know when children reach the speed and precision of adults.

THE PLACE OF MOTOR DEVELOPMENT IN COGNITIVE DEVELOPMENT

The importance of cognition in motor skill acquisition and development appears to be clear. However, the reverse has also been proposed: that perceptual motor activity is a mechanism for cognitive development. In the 1960s and 1970s, perceptual motor theory was influential in education and rehabilitation, and gross and fine motor activity programs were instituted with the expectation that improvement in cognitive ability would follow (for a review, see Cermak and Henderson, 1990). However, the perceptual motor theories have not been validated. This section addresses some of the theoretical issues of the role of the development of manipulation in the development of cognition, Some of the more recent studies that have addressed the impact of motor problems on cognitive development are also discussed. As will be seen, the results of studies are inconclusive.

Motor Activity and Cognitive Theory

Piagetian and Gibsonian Theory

In Piagetian theory infant motor activity plays a major role in cognitive development. Object manipulation is believed to be critical for the child's learning about object properties, particularly the characteristics that specify certain objects. The manipulation of objects is important as a way of facilitating mental activity, which is believed to be the key for learning object characteristics. Mental activity is believed to be more likely to occur when the child is actively involved in object manipulation than when the child is passive (Williams and Kamii, 1986; Gallagher and Reid, 1981).

Physical experience is also described as being important for logico-mathematical knowledge (that is, relationships between objects) (Williams and Kamii, 1986). Relationships among objects are believed to be understood better by young children when they are actively involved in placing them in these relationships. In older children such manipulation of materials for gaining physical knowledge and understanding relationships may not be necessary although it can be beneficial for them as well as for adults.

Gallagher and Reid (1981) discuss the implications of limited physical experience (seen in children with sensory, motor, and learning problems) on development of the children's cognitive skills. The Piagetian theorists suggest that children with

significant visual impairments and significant physical disabilities may have difficulty in initially acquiring knowledge of object properties but that their later development of abstraction about objects may be relatively normal. In contrast, other studies (Schmid-Kitsikis, cited by Gallagher and Reid, 1981) on learning disabled children who were dyspraxic (had difficulty organizing and sequencing movements) illustrated that, despite difficulty executing the tasks requested, they were able to explain the tasks' solutions.

Piaget considered that motor activity was necessary to the development of knowledge about the environment. The differing position taken by J. J. Gibson and E. J. Gibson is that "action is not 'prior' to perception . . . rather perceptual information is actively sought through coordinated systems of action, some of which are already functioning in this capacity at birth" (Lochman, 1986, p. 24). The Gibsons believed that our perception and action systems are designed for directly processing information about objects and the environment (Gibson and Spelke, 1983). Newborn infants are equipped with the capacity for learning about and differentiating within their perceived world.

Assumptions are that this perceptual knowledge is already present but that it is explored through activity. Neither of these positions considers how changes in motor functioning may be needed before more advanced perceptual knowledge can be readily demonstrated or acquired by the child. Motor control is apparently assumed to be static for the purpose of these studies yet is not a static function in infancy and childhood.

Extensive research in infant perception and memory has shown that Piaget underestimated the cognitive abilities of young infants, and it is now widely believed "that perceptual learning is a more important source of cognitive growth than Piaget gave it credit for"(Flavell, 1985, p. 39). However, it should also be noted that, although the Gibsonian and Piagetian theories differ in the relative importance given to motor activity, both positions emphasize the active role of infants in their own development, as exhibited in looking behavior and in reaching and mouthing behavior.

Reciprocity of Manipulation and Cognition

Although some of Piaget's interpretations of his observations have been called into question, his descriptions of early development were accurate, and his influence on and contribution to infant psychology endure (Flavell, 1985; Harris, 1983). He called attention to what now appears to be a reciprocity between manipulatory behavior and cognitive function.

Reciprocity has been proposed to describe the relationship between perception and fine motor skills and their connection to cognitive functioning. One suggestion is that orientation occurs first in the presence of a new object; exploration of the object for its perceptual characteristics occurs; and then manipulation of the object is used to gather further information. (Schneider et al., 1983). Williams (1990) stressed the importance of perception for initiating the movement activity but that the movement creates "new perceptual information, which helps to further guide ongoing eye-hand coordination activity" (p. 328). It appears that the control programs responsible for coordinating the sequence and timing of the motor actions may be related to perceptual-cognitive functioning.

The view that the two areas are mutually interdependent has been suggested by some authors. Fere (1887, cited by Connolly, 1973) implies this reciprocal relationship in his statement that "the hand is simultaneously an agent and interpreter of the growth of the mind" (p. 345). Sugden and Keogh (1990) propose that "movement skill . . . is a function of the neuromotor system and related information processing systems, which generally are identified as sensory, perceptual, and cognitive in nature. . . . Dynamic interactions among the systems determine the course and quality of movement skill development" (p. 2). Their descriptions do not indicate a unidirectional influence of one area on another. Apparently both motor and cognitive functioning must be at a high level for motor skills to be excellent.

Theoretic issues aside, the literature on fine motor and cognitive development appears to portray a strong association between hand use and cognitive development. As Williams (1990) said, "Eye-hand coordination is intricately involved in the young child's development; it provides the infant and toddler with a major tool for gathering information from the surrounding environment" (p. 327). It is probable that the critical relationship between cognitive and fine motor development is that information from the environment is vital to cognitive development and the hands are a major method of acquiring the information.

Impact of Motor Dysfunction on Cognitive Development

Piaget's theory generated extensive research on the relationship between motor activity and cognitive development. One approach to studying this relationship was to investigate the impact of a motor disability on general or specific cognitive skills. Other researchers have investigated the impact of cognitive limitations or development on motor abilities. It is generally agreed that gross motor development is not critical to the development of cognition. The relationship between fine motor development and cognition seems to be more important because reciprocity between hand skills and cognition appears to occur in normal development. However, as the following studies show, in most disability areas both cognitive and motor disabilities can occur, making it difficult to interpret the research.

Cerebral Palsy

To directly assess the influence of impaired mobility on acquisition of one aspect of cognitive development, Rothman (1986) studied children with and without cerebral palsy. The 60 children in this study were between 4 and 11 years of age, and all had normal intelligence. Piaget's "order of movement" task was given to all children. The children with cerebral palsy performed significantly more poorly than the normal children did. It was suggested that ordering movements may be limited in children with cerebral palsy as a result of their limited motor experiences, particularly at a young age.

Congenital Amputation

Kopp and Shaperman (1973) reported on the development of an infant born without arms who was not seen for treatment until he was 2 years old. At that time he received an extensive evaluation of his cognitive development. There was no evidence that he was in any way delayed. The child demonstrated learning and the development of knowledge without manipulation of objects. This does not negate the value of hand skills in focusing a child's attention and facilitating exploration. Rather, it supports the importance of visual exploration in learning and information processing (Kopp, 1974). It shows the adaptability of the human organism in the presence of severe disability.

Clumsiness

The effect of clumsiness on cognitive development has also been studied. Clumsy children have impaired control of individual gross and fine movements and movement sequences (Geuze and Kalverboer, 1987); skilled, purposeful movements are those affected (Gubbay, 1975). As a result daily living, home, school, and play skills are likely to be impaired (Dawdy, 1981; Hulme and Lord, 1986). Clumsy children have limited skills in the psychomotor area. They have impairment of visual-motor integration, speed, stability, and precision of movements and use of kinesthetic information to guide movement and difficulties with knowing the procedures for carrying out motor skills (Sovik and Maeland, 1986). For these reasons, clumsiness is "attributed to perceptual, central, or motor processing deficiencies" (Smythe and Glencross, 1986, p. 13).

To assess the effects of clumsy versus normal upper-extremity fine motor control on types of object interactions used, Kopp (1974) conducted a study with 8-month-old infants. All infants could use a radial finger grasp, but they were divided into clumsy and nonclumsy groups based upon their approach to reach and grasp. Clumsy infants were more likely to have difficulty with initiating an approach to the object presented, positioning the forearm, hand, and fingers for reach and grasp, and grasping effectively. They used more large arm movements and less object manipulation than the nonclumsy infants and spent more time visually regarding the objects than they did in all types of object manipulation combined. The coordinated group of infants showed significantly more exploration of objects, particularly more mouthing, and spent more time in object manipulation than in visual regard.

Kopp discussed the value of object manipulation in enhancing attention and providing information to infants. When fine motor movements are well controlled, the infant is believed to be able to attend to the object(s) without needing to focus attention on the motor control itself. An infant for whom object manipulation presents no problem may "demonstrate an extensive repertoire of object interactions because his attention can be focused solely on doing something with the object" (Kopp, 1974, p. 630). However, clumsy infants' use of visual skills to obtain information from the environment may be more advantageous for them because use of poor manipulation skills may actually contribute to distractions that could affect learning. It seems that greater attention to motor actions is needed by clumsy babies to increase the probability of success.

Clumsiness has often been associated with the presence of learning problems. However, learning problems are not always associated with clumsiness (Sovik and Maeland, 1986). In some clumsy children attention or visual perception is impaired,

but difficulty in doing tasks can cause poor attention; poor attention may affect motor skills but is not necessarily a characteristic associated with clumsiness (Dawdy, 1981; Levine et al., 1983).

In a longitudinal study of clumsy children from the ages of 6 to 16 years, Losse et al. (1991) found that motor and academic problems that were present in the early school years persisted into adolescence. Even the clumsy children who were performing well academically at 6 years of age were likely to have academic problems by adolescence. The most common problems were with handwriting, organization of information and materials, and performance in courses that required motor output to assess competence, such as in art, home economics, and science labs. Difficulty with handwriting is often cited as a common problem associated with clumsiness (Dawdy, 1981; Hulme and Lord 1986; Sovik and Maeland 1986; Levine et al., 1983). Sovik and Maeland (1986) described the increased prevalence of spelling, reading, and mathematical problems in clumsy children as compared with normal children. These areas of academic performance depend substantially on perceptual-cognitive skills.

Interpretation of studies of children who are clumsy is difficult because of the variability and complexity of their disabilities. The studies are inconclusive in respect to the need for motor skills in cognitive development. Clumsiness and poor ability in selected cognitive functions are associated in some but not all children.

Mental Retardation and Motor Skill Development

In an attempt to address the relationship between cognitive and fine motor skills, some authors have studied children with cognitive impairments and assessed their fine motor skills. Moss and Hogg (1981) studied fine motor skills in children with Down syndrome (n = 50) and normal children (n = 50), who ranged in age from 9 months to 44 months. The authors indicated that they believed it was important to study grasp, a skill that affects task performance, rather than the children's ability to complete the task. They suggested that variations in competence between those who have more skill and those who have less skill may be due to differences in grasp patterns and the ability of the children to anticipate requirements for task completion. Whereas the normal children showed greater use of mature grasps with increasing age and with smaller size pegs, the children with Down syndrome did not vary their grasps with peg size. Children with Down syndrome used more mature grasps with increasing age, but the oldest group of these children did not achieve the same level of competency as the normal children who were 6 months younger. The authors suggested that the difference in grasp patterns may be at least partly related to hand structure of the children with Down syndrome. Therefore they did not conclude that the fine motor delays were necessarily due to these children's cognitive delays.

The combination of a motor deficit and a cognitive deficit presents significant problems for a child. Findings of studies by O'Connor and Heremelin (1978) and Anwar (1986) have shown that children with Down syndrome have more difficulty with visual-motor skills than do other children with comparable mental retardation. It would be difficult to directly attribute these problems to the children's mental retardation. Many of these findings, if not all, could be attributed to the motor problem of poor stability that is associated with Down syndrome or the interaction of motor and cognitive problems. It is certainly likely that, regardless of the cause of the delay, the Down syndrome infants' lack of ability to accommodate their hands to objects and to explore them may interfere with their learning about key object properties. Perhaps a motor disability in conjunction with mental retardation interferes more significantly with acquisition of skills that require integration and planning than does a cognitive disability alone. Children who have more difficulty handling objects and do not have other good perceptual-cognitive skills that could be used to compensate for limited object manipulation in the process of learning about objects may have more severe problems than those who have problems in one of these areas.

Comment

Piaget's theory of the role of motor activity in cognitive development has had an impact on occupational and physical therapy as well as on education. We have reviewed these studies to show that, despite extensive research, there is little evidence supporting the *necessity* for either gross motor or manipulative ability in a child's cognitive development. However, this in no way diminishes the importance of manipulative hand skills in cognitive development. Children use their hands to learn; the control their hands give them in the

exploration of the environment is both motivating and facilitating. With limited hand use the child is more dependent on less efficient strategies and on the help of other persons in the learning process.

Perceptual and motor processing difficulties, then, not only affect motor performance but also can affect the child's ability to learn. However, it is difficult to establish a causal relationship between motor and learning problems (Losse et al., 1991). Studies in this area have primarily been conducted with descriptive and correlational methodology, not with experimental designs. When children have normal skills in most areas of development, relationships among the various aspect of development may be stronger than they are when children who fall outside the classification of normal are included. The previous studies of children with mental retardation and with motor problems clearly indicate that problems with motor and cognition occur together. However, they are not particularly helpful in clarifying the nature of this relationship or the relative dependence of one area on the other. Determining the interaction, however, is important because tests for many factors associated with learning and general cognition use motor output as a method of assessing performance (Sugden and Keogh, 1990).

This literature provides conflicting evidence related to the role of physical experience in the development of perceptual-cognitive skills. It may be that these cognitive skills can be acquired without a great deal of motor experience, but they are developed more slowly by children who have difficulty managing materials than by children who have normal motor skills.

CONCLUSIONS

Movement skill has been described as being goal oriented and made up of sequential movements that are organized in relation to spatial and temporal requirements. Attention is a prerequisite for all of the components of cognition. Perceptual skills are reflected in responses to the spatial and temporal features of movement as well as in the knowledge of objects, places, and events. Goal orientation implies that one is able to plan for and perceive the results of one's actions.

Cognitive development and motor development seem to have a reciprocal relationship, but with cognitive development having more significance for motor development than motor development for cognitive development. However, object manipulation skills, which, it has been suggested, reflect an infant's attention, seem to be the most efficient way for a baby to learn some object properties (such as texture and three-dimensional shapes).

It is hand function, not gross motor function, that seems critical in supporting cognitive development. The assumption that fine motor skills can reflect one's knowledge is implicit in most intelligence tests, which require demonstration of fine motor skills to complete many aspects of the performance component of the test battery. Fine motor skills are used to interact with objects and to indicate what one understands about objects. Tool use with the hands almost always requires cognitive development in regard to means-end relationships and in the expression of perceptual relationships of objects to one another and to one's own body. In contrast, fundamental gross motor skills seem to require little cognitive development for their emergence.

The significance of motor development for cognitive development has had much less study than has the study of the influence of cognition on motor development, and further study seems warranted. It should also be noted that the relationship between the two areas of development has generally not been studied in a causal manner because descriptive methodology has been used almost exclusively.

Much of the cognitive development research with normal infants and children assumes that the children have motor competence and that their motor skills are static; the significance of concurrent development of motor and cognitive skills is rarely addressed. Almost no literature addresses how infants and children with different degrees of motor skill may be affected in the acquisition of cognitive skills. Certainly, impaired hand use, as is seen in clumsy children and children with significant motor disabilities, seems to affect how children interact with objects and may even have an impact on the development of their attentional skills. Research with children who have cognitive limitations has indicated that gross motor skills are acquired without significant difficulty, but basic fine motor skills may be acquired more slowly than normal. Complex skills are clearly affected because the acquisition of skill sequences usually depends on cognitive processing. Once a sequence is learned, a cognitive limitation has less effect. Techniques for teaching motor skills that rely on teaching small elements of the skill and gradually linking these together appear to bypass the cognitive demands in early phases of skill learning.

This review has covered a number of topics related to the literature on the relationship between motor skills and cognition. Many aspects of this relationship are unclear, and we know little about how the relationship may differ for children with disabilities. We need knowledge of the differential impact of varying degrees and kinds of cognitive disability (attentional, perceptual, and conceptual) on the acquisition of motor skills and of the significance of motor problems for children's cognitive functioning. Such knowledge would be valuable in assessing children and planning interventions to maximize their skills.

REFERENCES

Anwar, F. (Ed.). (1986). *Cognitive deficit and motor skill.* London: Croom Helm.

Bard, C., Fluery, M., & Gagnon, M. (1990). Coincidence-anticipation timing: An age-related perspective. In M. Fleury, C. Bard, & L. Hay (Eds.). *Development of eye-hand coordination across the life span.* Columbia, SC: University of South Carolina Press.

Bruner, J.S., & Koslowski, B. (1972). Visually preadapted constituents of manipulatory action. *Perception, 1,* 3-14.

Bullock, M., & Lutkenhaus P. (1988). The development of volitional behavior. *Child Development, 59,* 664-674.

Cermak, S., & Henderson, A. (1990). Learning disabilities. In D.A. Umphred (Ed.). *Neurological rehabilitation.* St. Louis: Mosby.

Clark, E.V. (1983). Meanings and concepts. In P. Mussen (Ed.). *Handbook of child psychology* (Vol. II). New York: Wiley.

Connolly, K. (1973). Factors influencing the learning of manual skills by young children. In R.A. Hinde & J. Stevenson-Hinde (Eds.). *Constraints on learning.* London: Academic Press.

Connolly, K., & Elliott, J. (1972). The evolution and ontogeny of hand function. In B. Jones (Ed.). *Ethological studies of child behaviour.* London: Cambridge University Press.

Corbetta, D., & Mounoud, P. (1990). Early development of grasping and manipulation. In C. Bard, M. Fleury, & L. Hay (Eds.). *Development of eye-hand coordination across the life span.* Columbia, SC: University of South Carolina Press.

David, K.S. (1985). Motor sequencing strategies in school-aged children. *Physical Therapy, 65*(6), 883-889.

Dawdy, S.C. (1981). Pediatric neuropsychology: Caring for the developmentally dyspraxic child. *Clinical Neuropsychology, 111*(1), 30-37.

Elliott, J., & Connolly, K. (Eds.) (1974). *Hierarchical structure in skill development.* London: Academic Press.

Exner, C.E. (1990a). In-hand manipulation skills in normal young children: A pilot study. *Occupational Therapy Practice, 1*(4), 63-72.

Exner, C.E. (1990b). The zone of proximal development in in-hand manipulation skills of nondysfunctional 3- and 4-year-old children. *The American Journal of Occupational Therapy, 44*(10), 884-891.

Fitts, P.M., & Posner, M.T. (1967). *Human performance.* Belmont, CA: Brooks/Cole.

Flavell, J.H. (1985). *Cognitive development.* Englewood Cliffs, NJ: Prentice-Hall.

Gallagher, J.M., & Reid, D.K. (1981). *The learning theory of Piaget and Inhelder.* Austin, TX: Pro-Ed.

Geuze, R.J., & Kalverboer, A.F. (1987). Inconsistency and adaptation in timing of clumsy children. *Journal of Human Movement Studies, 13,* 421-432.

Gibson, E.J., & Spelke, E.S. (1983). The development of perception. In P.H. Mussen (Ed.). *Handbook of child psychology* (Vol. II). New York: Wiley.

Gilfoyle, E., & Grady, A.P. (1973). A developmental theory of somato-sensory perception. In A. Henderson & J. Coryell (Eds.). *The body senses and perceptual deficit.* Proceedings of Occupational Therapy Symposium on Somatosensory Aspects of Perceptual Deficits. Boston: Occupational Therapy Department, Boston University.

Gilfoyle, E.M., Grady, A.P., & Moore, J.C. (1981). *Children adapt.* Thorofare, NJ: Slack.

Glass, A.L., & Holyoak, K.J. (1986). *Cognition* (2nd ed.). Reading, MA: Addison-Wesley.

Goodgold-Edwards, S.A., & Gianutsos, J.G. (1991). Coincidence anticipation performance of children with spastic cerebral palsy and nonhandicapped children. *Physical and Occupational Therapy in Pediatrics, 10*(4), 49-83.

Gubbay, S.S. (1975). *The clumsy child.* New York: W.B. Saunders.

Harris, P.L. (1983). Infant cognition. In P.H. Mussen (Ed.). *Handbook of child psychology.* New York: Wiley.

Hohlstein, R.R. (1982). The development of prehension in normal infants. *The American Journal of Occupational Therapy, 36*(3), 170-176.

Hulme, C., & Lord, R. (1986). Clumsy children—A review of recent research. *Child: Care, Health and Development, 12,* 257-269.

Hutt, C. (1967). Effects of stimulus novelty on manipulatory exploration in an infant. *Journal of Child Psychology and Psychiatry, 8,* 241-247.

Katz, N. (1992). *Cognitive rehabilitation models for intervention in occupational therapy.* Boston: Andover Medical Publishing.

Klein, R.M. (1976). Attention and movement. In G.E. Stelmach (Ed.). *Motor control issues and trends.* New York: Academic Press.

Kopp, C.B. (1974). Fine motor abilities of infants. *Developmental Medicine and Child Neurology, 16,* 629-636.

Kopp, C.B., & Shaperman J. (1973). Cognitive development in the absence of object manipulation during infancy. *Developmental Psychology, 9,* 130.

Lecuyer, R. (1989). Habituation and attention, novelty and cognition: Where is the continuity? *Human Development, 32,* 148-157.

Lefford, A. (1970). Sensory, perceptual and cognitive factors in the development of voluntary actions. In K. Connolly (Ed.). *Mechanisms of motor skill development.* New York: Academic Press.

Levine, M.P. (1987). *Developmental variation and learning disorders.* Cambridge, MA: Educators Publishing Service.

Levine, M.S., Carey, W.B., Crocker, A.C., & Gross, R.T. (1983). *Developmental behavioral pediatrics.* Philadelphia: W.B. Saunders.

Lidz, C.S. (1987). *Dynamic assessment.* New York: Guilford Press.

Lochman, J.J. (1986). Perceptuomotor coordination in sighted infants: Implications for visually impaired children. *Topics in Early Childhood Special Education, 6*(3), 23-26.

Lochman, J.J., Ashmead, D.H., & Bushnell, E.W. (1984). The development of anticipatory hand orientation during infancy. *Journal of Experimental Child Pshychology, 37,* 176-186.

Losse, A., Henderson, S.E., Elliman, D., Hall, D., Knight, E., & Hongmans, M. (1991). Clumsiness in children—Do they grow out of it? A 10-year follow-up study. *Developmental Medicine and Child Neurology, 33,* 55-68.

Mandler, J.M. (1983). Representation. In P. Mussen (Ed.). *Handbook of child psychology* (Vol. II). New York: Wiley.

Moss, S.C., & Hogg, J. (1981). Development of hand function in mentally handicapped and nonhandicapped preschool children. In P.J. Mittler (Ed.). *Frontiers of knowledge in mental retardation.* Baltimore: University Park Press.

Napier, J.R. (1956). The prehensile movements of the human hand. *The Journal of Bone and Joint Surgery, 38B*(4), 902-913.

O'Connor, N., & Heremelin, B. (1978). *Seeing and hearing and space and time.* London: Academic Press.

Olsen G., & Sherman, T. (1983). Attention, learning, and memory in infants. In P.H. Mussen (Ed.). *Handbook of Child Psychology* (Vol. II). New York: Wiley.

Paillard, J. (1960). The patterning of skilled movement. In J. Field, H.V. Magoun, and V. E. Hall (Eds.). *Handbook of physiology.* Bethesda, MD: American Physiological Society.

Ransay, D.S., & Weber, S.L. (1986). Infants' hand preference in a task involving complementary roles for the two hands. *Child Development, 57,* 300-307.

Reid, D. (1989). A neo-Piagetian analysis of infants' visual-motor abilities. *The Occupational Therapy Journal of Research, 9*(5), 287-304.

Rosenbaum, D.A. (1991). *Human motor control.* New York: Academic Press.

Rosenblith, J.F. (1992). *In the beginning: Development from conception to age two.* London: Sage Publications.

Rothman, J. (1986). Conceptual development movement by youngsters with cerebral palsy. *Developmental Medicine and Child Neurology, 26,* 99-100.

Roy, E.A. (Ed.) (1985). *Neuropsychology studies of apraxia and related disorders.* New York: North-Holland.

Ruff, H.A. (1986). Components of attention during infants' manipulative exploration. *Child Development, 57,* 105-114.

Schneider, K., Moch, M., Sanfort, R., Auerswald, M., & Walther-Weckman, K. (1983). Exploring a novel object by preschool children: A sequential analysis of perceptual, manipulating and verbal exploration. *International Journal of Behavioral Development, 6,* 477-496.

Smythe, T.R., & Glencross, D.J. (1986). Information processing deficits in clumsy children. *Australian Journal of Psychology, 38*(1), 13-22.

Sovik, N., & Maeland, A.F. (1986). Children with motor problems (clumsy children). *Scandinavian Journal of Educational Research, 30*(1), 39-53.

Sternberg, R., & Powell, J. (1983). The development of intelligence. In P. Mussen (Ed.). *The handbook of child psychology* (Vol. II). New York: Wiley.

Sugden, D.A., & Keogh, J. F. (1990). *Problems in movement skill development.* Columbia, SC: University of South Carolina Press.

van der Meulen, J.H.P., Denier J.J., van der Gon, J.J., Gielen, C.C.A.M., Gooskens, R.H.J.M., & Willemse, J. (1991a). Visuomotor performance of normal and clumsy children. I. Fast goal-directed arm movements with and without visual feedback. *Developmental Medicine and Child Neurology, 33,* 40-54.

van der Meulen, J.H.P., Denier, J.J., van der Gon, J.J., Gielen, C.C.A.M., Gooskens, R.H.J.M., & Willemse, J. (1991b). Visuomotor performance of normal and clumsy children. II. Arm-tracking with and without visual feedback. *Developmental Medicine and Child Neurology, 33,* 118-129.

Williams, C.K., & Kamii, C. (1986). How do children learn by handling objects? *Young Children, 42*(1), 23-26.

Williams, H.G. (1990). Aging and eye-hand coordination. In M. Fleury, C. Bard, & L. Hay (Eds.). *Development of eye-hand coordination across the life span.* Columbia, SC: University of South Carolina Press.

Yarrow, L.J., Morgan, G.A., Jennings, K.D., Harmon, R.J., & Gaiter, J.L. (1982). Infants' persistence at tasks: Relationships to cognitive functioning and early experience. *Infant Behavior and Development, 5,* 131-141.

Development of Hand Skills

7

Grasp, Release, and Bimanual Skills in the First Two Years of Life

Jane Case-Smith

The development of hand skills is critical to the child's ability to play and explore, to perform daily living skills, and to function in life. Basic grasp and release patterns quickly mature into efficient manipulative skills in the first years of life. The purpose of this chapter is to describe the early development of grasp, release, and bimanual skills and the characteristics of each developmental phase and to define the factors that contribute to each phase of hand skills maturation. The first section briefly presents principles that underlie the development of hand skill. The second section describes the development of grasp, release, and bimanual skills. Finally, a third section provides an integrated description of hand skills and variables associated with hand skills development in the first 2 years of life.

DEVELOPMENTAL PRINCIPLES

The movements of the neonate are reflexive behaviors influenced by subcortical structures (McGraw, 1943, 1966; Andre-Thomas, 1964; Gilfoyle, Grady, and Moore, 1990). These reflexive behaviors are automatic reactions to sensory stimulation that result in neonates experiencing arm and hand movements over which they will later gain control. They are neurologic mechanisms that affect predictable patterns of posture and movement. Reflexes provide young infants with survival capabilities (such as sucking and rooting) and protective responses (such as avoiding response). Reflexes allow infants to experience a complete range of movement and tactile proprioceptive input. Reflexes and reactions are modified through interactions with the environment as infants assimilate the sensory feedback from reflexive movements (Gilfoyle, Grady, and Moore, 1990). In the first 6 months they become integrated into acquired or voluntary behaviors.

The sequence of hand skill development is driven by neurologic maturation and is influenced by the environment and the child's experience. McGraw (1943) describes a typical progress of maturation: (1) dominant reflexive responses, (2) inhibition of reflexes, (3) transitional behaviors, and (4) voluntary motor pattern and skill. This typical sequence varies in the timing of onset and completion of each phase but is remarkably invariant in the ordering of developmental motor patterns. The grasp reflex predominates for several months, prior to inhibition and the emergence of voluntary grasp. When cortical control begins to dominate over subcortical control of hand movement, the infant may demonstrate disorganized and confused movements (McGraw, 1941). Transitional behaviors mark the period when reflexes are inhibited and voluntary controlled movements begin to develop (Twitchell, 1970). The influence of the environment seems to be framed within individual capabilities of the child as determined by genetic makeup and neurologic integrity. Grasp and manipulation are learned and are differentially influenced by experience (Bushnell, 1985; Hay, 1979).

Coordinated movements are developed through sensory experience and feedback through the hand's surfaces (Halverson, 1937; McCall, 1974). The first grasping patterns of the neonates are driven by sensory input to the palmar surface. For most of the first year infant actions directly relate to sensory experiences, and movements are adapted based on sensory feedback. Grasp and hold patterns, which are first associated with proprioceptive-tactile input, become grasp and manipulate patterns guided by tactile, proprioceptive, and visual input (Bushnell, 1985; McCall, 1974).

By the end of the first year, infants initiate purposeful movements to experience space, to manipulate the environment, and to communicate with others (Bruner, 1970; Gilfolye, Grady, and Moore, 1990; McGraw, 1943). The 1-year-old child begins to handle and manipulate objects according to their functional purpose, in addition to their sensory qualities. The child's knowledge of the object's function guides the interaction with that object. Sensorimotor activity is important as an integrating mechanism for linking together the developmental progress of physical, intellectual, emotional, and social skills (Gilfoyle, Grady, and Moore, 1990; Holt, 1975; Flavell, 1963). Hand movement becomes an important way for the child to experience the environment and relates highly to functional abilities in all domains. During the second year and beyond, hand skills become highly associated with cognitive skills and the purposeful intentions of the child. While the hands continue to adapt to the sensory qualities of the objects held, movements are directed by the child's purposeful exploration and manipulation of the environment.

DEVELOPMENT OF GRASP, RELEASE, AND BIMANUAL SKILLS
Grasp

Reflexive Grasp

An infant's first grasp relates to the physiologic flexor muscle tone characteristic of the full-term neonate. Newborns tightly flex their fingers around a flexed thumb, only occasionally opening the hand in association with active extension of the trunk and/or arms. The neonate's fisted hand is consistent with the overall predominance of physiologic flexor tone that dominates upper and lower extremity movements. He/she frequently brings the fisted hand to the mouth when prone, pulling the hands toward midline while assuming an overall flexed position.

The first reflexive response of the arm and hand, termed the *traction response,* is demonstrated by the neonate when proprioceptive input or traction is applied to the arm. When the arm is pulled away from the body, synergistic flexion of the fingers, wrist, elbow, and shoulder results. As described by Twitchell (1970), stretch to the flexor and adductor muscles of shoulder is a sufficient stimulus for eliciting this response. In the first couple of weeks of life, the grasp reflex has not yet emerged. The neonate may posture with fisted hands, but responses to touch on the hands result in opening or partial opening.

It is not until the second to fourth week of life that the infant automatically closes the fingers around an object (or adult's finger) placed in his palm. This first *grasp reflex* requires that pressure (proprioception) as well as tactile input be applied to the palm and is accompanied with the traction response. A grasping reflex cannot be elicited in response to a visual stimulus.

By 4 weeks the grasp reflex can be elicited with a contact stimulus to the palm or fingers. A moving stimulus is most effective in producing this local grasp reaction, which is immediately followed by the traction response. By 8 weeks two distinct phases of the grasp reflex are observed. The first is the catching phase, which is an immediate flexion of the fingers and thumb. In the second or holding phase the finger flexion is sustained. This holding is intensified if the object is lightly pulled. The traction response declines at this time but can be elicited when the arm is pulled from the body (Twitchell, 1970).

By 3 to 4 months of age a *true grasp reflex* has developed and the traction response no longer automatically accompanies this response although dorsiflexion of the wrist continues to accompany the finger flexion. When an object is placed in the hand and is moved medially, the fingers flex in a sustaining grasp. A palmer grasp is observed with the fingers flexing tightly and pressing the object into the palm. At times greater pressure is observed from the ulnar fingers, which seem to develop active movement and strength before the radial fingers.

Transitional Reactions

The grasp reflex becomes altered at 4 to 5 months of age in that a contact stimulus to the medial side of the hand causes some supination. Twitchell (1965, 1970) terms this an *orienting* response. Soon after supination occurs with stimulation to the radial part of the hand, pronation can be observed with tactile input to the ulnar part of the hand. At this time fractionation of the grasp reflex begins. One or two fingers flex in isolation from the others, given specific stimulation of their volar surfaces.

At 5 to 6 months an *instinctive grasp* emerges, which combines the fractionated grasp and the orienting response (Twitchell). At this time the infant not only orients to the stimulus by adjusting his forearm but actually gropes for a tactile stimulus. Groping for the moving object that is touching the hand occurs without visual input and can be observed in the child who has visual impairment. The object is palpated before being grasped (Corbetta and Mounoud, 1990). Therefore instinctive grasp includes following a moving stimulus to secure it and then adjusting the hand's grasp to accomplish sustained holding of the object. Flexion of a single digit can be induced given isolated tactile contact. The instinctive grasp is a transitional behavior between primitive (reflexive) and mature patterns of movement, as the fractionated movements of the fingers and hand come under the infant's voluntary control (Gilfolye, Grady, and Moore, 1990).

Purposeful Grasp

The transitional behaviors described previously lead to the emergence of voluntary prehension (Gilfolye, Grady, and Moore, 1990). Between 4 and 6 months the infant develops control of grasp. Using both tactile and visual information, he/she becomes skillful in adjusting the hand to the object. The infant begins to use visual input to prepare the hand for grasp by opening and shaping the hand prior to grasp according to the object's size and shape (Corbetta and Mounoud, 1990).

These beginning abilities to grasp, orient, and adjust the hand to objects based on tactile and visual information signify the beginning of purposeful grasp. The infant becomes capable of using a variety of grasping patterns that are selected based on the affordances of the objects and his or her playful intentions. Initially the infant uses only a few grasping patterns and uses them indiscriminately. As the infant gains experience and matures, a wide variety of patterns can be observed. Halverson (1931) was one of the first to study grasping patterns in detail, using video recordings of infants 16 to 52 weeks of age. His observations and interpretations have contributed to developmental assessment and to our understanding of infant prehension patterns in the more than 60 years since his original research. While others have suggested revisions in the categories of grasp that he defined (Amman and Etzel, 1977; Gesell et al., 1940; Holstein, 1982; Illingworth, 1990), Halverson's findings remain valid for describing the development of grasp.

At 20 weeks most infants touch, but do not grasp, a cube placed before them. The infant who successfully secures the cube does so by pulling it to the other hand or the body and squeezing it against another surface. This *primitive squeeze* is therefore not a true grasp but is capturing the object against another surface (Halverson, 1931). According to Twitchell, successful grasp at this time would be instinctual and would require that the stimulus touch or be placed in the hand. Grasp automatically occurs when the object is moved through the hand.

Squeeze grasp (Figure 7-1) develops by 20 to 24 weeks. The infant presses the cube using total finger flexion against the palm. Because his/her proprioceptive system and motor control remain crudely developed, the cube is squeezed very tightly. Success in retaining the object is limited by his/her ability to adjust the object within the hand or differentiate finger movement. The thumb does not participate in this grasp and tends to lie in the palmar plane.

A *palmar grasp* is most frequently used by the 24-week-old infant. The palmar grasp is characterized by a pronated hand and flexion of all fingers around the object. The thumb may slide around the object passively rather than actively holding it (Figure 7-2). The pressure used to maintain a grasp of the object moves from the ulnar to the radial

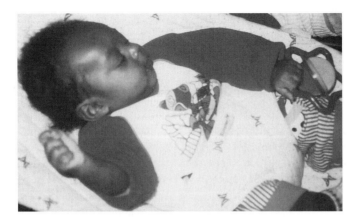

Figure 7-1. Squeeze grasp emerging (3 months).

finger pressing into the palmar surface of the hand. As the pressure of the grasp moves to the radial side of the hand, the thumb becomes active.

Finger and hand movements without object grasp contribute to the development of grasp (Halverson, 1931; Castner, 1932). The 4- to 5-month-old infant is often observed scratching the supporting surface when prone on elbows. The infant uses alternating finger flexion and extension of the digits together. Scratching may also occur on the caregiver's clothing when holding the infant upright against the shoulder. The scratching motion allows the infant to practice the full range of reciprocal finger flexion and extension. Scratching also provides the infant with rich tactile information about different texture surfaces.

Halverson (1931) observed rubbing of the hand on the surface as an additional method for obtaining tactile input in the infant at 16 to 28 weeks. As the infant continues to use scratching, finger movements become differentiated such that one or two fingers move in isolation of the others. Halverson observed pianoing or "raising and lowering of each finger alternately" on the table in infants 16 to 24 weeks of age. Pianoing appears to be an automatic movement rather than a purposeful isolated motion of each digit. As with other hand skills, isolated movements of the fingers occur first in these automatic behaviors, elicited by the sensory stimulation of the hand resting on a flat surface.

By 28 weeks the infant holds the object in a *radial palmar grasp* (Gesell and Amatruda, 1947) or what Halverson (1931) terms *a superior palmar grasp*. The radial fingers and thumb press the cube against the palm (Figure 7-3). Therefore, when held in a supinated hand, the object can be brought to and put into the mouth. The object can be banged against another surface, and the object becomes accessible for object transfer from hand to hand. The radial palmar grasp is a hallmark in

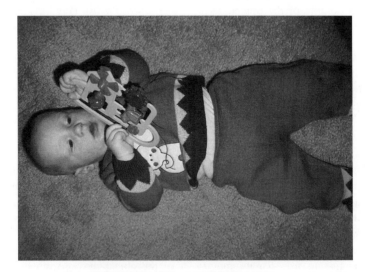

Figure 7-2. Palmar grasp (6 months).

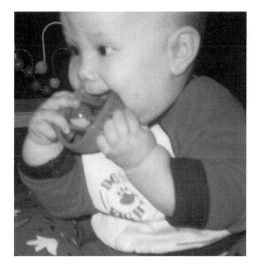

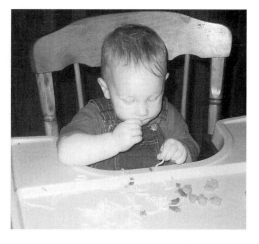

Figure 7-4. Radial digital grasp (8 months).

Figure 7-3. Radial palmar grasp (7 months).

grasp maturation because the infant now differentiates the sides of the hand, using the ulnar side to provide stability for the grasping movement and the radial side to prehend and hold the object. This early pattern signifies the initial development of radial fingers as the skill side of the hand.

Between 32 and 36 weeks the infant demonstrates grasp of the object in the fingers rather than the palm, and, by 36 weeks the infant exhibits a *radial digital grasp* (Gesell and Amatruda, 1947) or *inferior forefinger grasp* (Halverson, 1931). At this time the infant can prehend a small object between the radial fingers and thumb. With the object held distally in the fingers (proximal to the finger pads), the infant can adjust the object within the hand and as a result can use the object for various purposes while holding it (Figure 7-4). The adjustments allow for greater success in relating two objects or in bringing the object to the mouth for finger feeding. The movement of the object distally and to the radial fingers gives the infant greater control of the object and enables release control.

When the 36-week-old infant grasps a very small object (pellet size), a *scissors grasp* is used. Gesell and Amatruda, as edited by Knobloch and Pasamanick (1974), define a scissors grasp as prehension of a small object between the thumb and the lateral border of the index finger following a raking movement of the fingers. The hand is stabilized on a surface during this grasp, and the ulnar fingers are flexed to provide stability of the thumb and radial finger movement (Figure 7-5).

Forefinger grasp (Halverson, 1931) or *inferior pincer grasp* (Gesell and Amatruda, 1947) is observed at 40 weeks. This is a fingertip grasp in

which the infant stabilizes the forearm on the table as a base while grasping the cube. The fingers that prehend the small object are more extended than flexed. By 52 to 56 weeks the infant prehends and holds the object in between the thumb and forefinger tip. Successful prehension using a *superior pincer grasp* (Halverson, 1931; Illingworth, 1991) is achieved without the forearm stabilizing on the surface (Figure 7-6). At this time the fingers adjust to the size and weight of the object. The object is now in a position that it can readily be used in a play activity or as a tool. Because the infant no longer needs to stabilize to grasp, he/she can easily prehend objects from a variety of surfaces, in and on other objects. He/she can also use the index finger to turn or move the object before prehension to increase success in grasp. Along with increased accuracy in grasp at this time, by 1 year the infant requires less time to prehend an object, displaces the object less before grasp, and makes fewer adjustments to secure the object firmly in the hand.

By 60 weeks prehension is deft and precise. The child plans and uses grasping patterns that enable him/her to act on the object after prehension (Gesell and Amatruda, 1957). Fingertip grasp is used unless the object is large and heavy or the situation is one of stress for the child (such as being off balance or hurried). The hand is sufficiently differentiated to hold two cubes in one hand (Knobloch & Pasamanick, 1974). The child can independently move different parts of the hand (i.e., the radial and ulnar sides) and can control the action of isolated fingers.

Gesell described the grasp of an 18-month-old as enveloping rather than manipulative. At this age thumb opposition is good; however, the hand

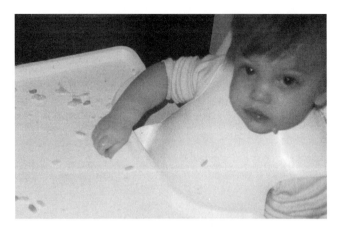

Figure 7-5. Scissors grasp (9 months).

remains primarily a prehender rather than a manipulator. Exploration of the object requires both hands and involves transferring and turning the object from one hand to the other (Figure 7-7). At this time the infant is able to adjust grasp to accommodate the weight and shape of the object. This enables holding a cracker without crushing it. The infant has increasing ability to differentiate the pressure used in finger flexion, indicating increased tactile and proprioceptive discrimination in addition to greater motor control.

In summary, by 24 months the child demonstrates increasing dissociation of the fingers, strength and control of the hand's arches, and sensitivity to the tactual properties of the object. These underlying hand skills enable the child to perform a great variety of functional skills (e.g., self-feeding, using a spoon, scribbling with a crayon, building a tower of three cubes, and turning pages of a book).

Release
Automatic Release

Object release matures after early grasping patterns are achieved. As with grasp, the first object release observed is a reflexive behavior. Finger extension is observed as the neonate withdraws and abducts the fingers in response to touch of the hand (Twitchell, 1970). This response, termed the *avoiding reaction,* is usually only a slight withdrawal of the neonate's hand. By 3 weeks and continuing to about 8 weeks, the avoiding response is easily elicited. When the dorsum of the hand is touched, the fingers abduct and extend. The hand may also pronate to withdraw from a contact stimulus. This response is elicited when the contact stimulus is lighter and more quickly applied than the firm palmar stimulation that elicits the grasp reflex.

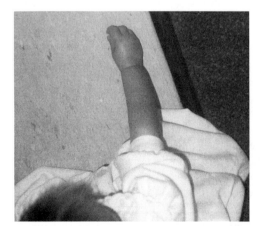

Figure 7-6. Superior pincer grasp (12 months).

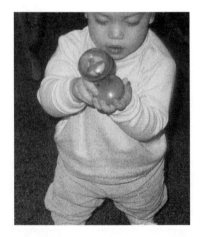

Figure 7-7. Turning and transferring an object (18 months).

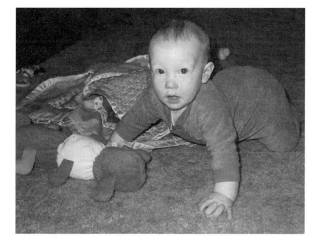

Figure 7-8. Weight bearing on hands (6 months).

Twitchell (1970) described an *instinctive avoiding response* that is similar in nature to the instinctive grasp response, in that it represents a transitional behavior between reflexive and voluntary responses. The instinctive avoiding response emerges between 12 and 20 weeks of age. It is characterized by pronation and adduction away from a stimulus on the hand's ulnar border and supination with abduction to stimulation of the hand's radial side. The instinctive avoiding reaction is fully developed by 24 to 40 weeks of age (Twitchell, 1965, 1970). At this time the infant withdraws from light contact stimulation, using a variety of hand movements, including flexion, extension, abduction, adduction, and rotation. Avoiding reactions are seen more frequently when the infant is irritable or when generalized tactile defensiveness is present. The avoiding response serves as an automatic mechanism to reinforce hand opening and facilitate finger extension to balance the effects of the grasp reflex. According to Gesell and Amatruda (1947), release requires inhibition of the flexor muscles with contraction of the extensors, which is a more mature, later developing neuromotor pattern. Cortical control over finger extension clearly develops after control of finger flexion and grasp.

From 5 to 6 months the infant begins a transition from reflexive to purposeful release. The infant demonstrates release accidently or involuntarily in association with movements, tactile stimulation to the hand, or contact with another surface. At 6 months release is observed during mouthing and bimanual play. The infant brings an object or finger food to the mouth with both hands and may release one or both once the object is stabilized in the mouth. When the infant holds an object with two hands, one hand may fall from the object.

Meanwhile, the infant practices finger extension in other activities. For example, the extended hand may be observed in patting the bottle. Additional facilitation of finger extension in the 6- (Figure 7-8) and 7-month-old (Figure 7-9) also occurs in the prone-on-hands position.

Purposeful Release

The first purposeful release is generally observed at 28 weeks. At this time the child transfers an object from one hand to the other. Initially object transfer is achieved by holding the object at midline with both hands and pulling it out of one hand into the other. Therefore the release is actu-

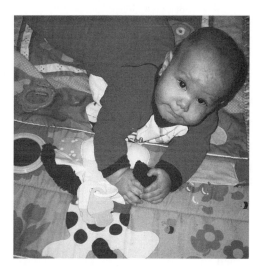

Figure 7-9. Weight bearing on hands (7 months).

ally a forced withdrawal accomplished by the opposite hand. During this same developmental period the infant releases an object on a table surface or another resisting (Gesell and Amatruda, 1947) or assisting (Ammon and Etzel, 1977) surface. Release with the assistance of another surface enables the child to roll the object from the fingers or remove it from the hand by inhibiting finger flexion (i.e., without active extension).

Between 40 and 44 weeks the infant demonstrates *active release* (Illingworth, 1990; Knobloch & Pasamanick, 1974). This first active release is often accomplished by flinging the object—combining elbow, wrist, and finger extension in a synergistic, ballistic movement. The infant now purposefully drops food and toys from his/her highchair and takes great pleasure in practicing this new-found skill. The object is released with the hand above the table surface, using full finger and thumb extension. Object-releasing activity is reinforced by the auditory and visual consequence of dropping the object. This new skill is also reinforced by the development of object permanence and the infant's interest in observing objects disappear and reappear.

By 52 weeks the infant demonstrates greater proficiency in releasing the object. With increasing control of finger extension, the infant begins to demonstrate graded hand opening when releasing. At this time he/she is practicing precision release for stacking one block on another or placing a form in its form space. Graded hand opening with controlled finger extension is first observed with the proximal hand base and forearm stabilized on a surface.

The need to stabilize a proximal hand or arm part on a surface to accomplish *controlled release* (for example, release cubes in a cup) continues through 18 months. In particular, more precise release, such as of a small object, requires the support of a stabilizing surface (Knobloch and Pasamanick, 1974). Release of a cube in building a three- cube tower is practiced, and, while generally successful, alignment of the cubes is imprecise. Typically, when stacking cubes or small blocks, the infant extends the fingers all at one time, using more extension than is required to actually release the object. The infant's release is graded rather than abrupt, and small wrist, forearm, and finger movements are used to adjust the positions of the cubes one on the other. Visual inspection during release is increasing, such that the hand can accurately place a cube or puzzle

piece. Perhaps the most important contribution to the infant's ability to place one object on another is internal stability of the arm while it is held in space, which allows the hand to act independently. By the end of the second year the child has well-developed internal proximal stability and smooth graded or incremental release patterns. He/she can open the hand partially while carefully monitoring whether the object is correctly placed. Therefore the infant is now able to adapt and adjust the hand opening according to the size, shape, and weight of the object. Controlled release in the 2-year-old enables the child to fit puzzle pieces into their form space, place small objects in a container, turn pages of a book, stack blocks, and manage a cup and feeding utensils. Object release continues to develop over the next 3 years with significant increases in steadiness, precision, dexterity, and speed.

Bimanual Skills

Early Development of Bilateral Arm Movements

Fagard (1990) indicated that bilateral arm movements are the predominant pattern of upper extremity movement throughout the first year of life. The infant grasps an object with specific motives for acting on that object. The behaviors observed after prehension, while varied, follow a developmental sequence. The sequence of bimanual skills observed during infancy relates to the infant's postural, sensory, perceptual, and cognitive development, as well as hand skill development.

The neonate exhibits both asymmetric and symmetric limb movements. Some of these are associated with the asymmetric tonic neck reflex; many appear to be random. Smooth, alternating arm and leg movements are most characteristic, with specific reflexive behaviors elicited by specific tactile input. The first bimanual reach toward an object may be observed at 2 months (White, Castle, and Held, 1964) although swiping at objects tends to be unilateral. By 3 months swiping increases and hand-to-hand interplay, without an object, is observed with hands clasped on the chest (Figure 7-10). The infant may involuntarily hold an object on the chest at midline, resulting from the clasping of the hands together. Most spontaneous arm and hand movements appear to be simultaneous and symmetric.

At 16 weeks this symmetry continues to predominate although one hand tends to lead the

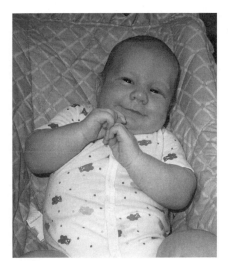

Figure 7-10. Hand play on chest (3 months).

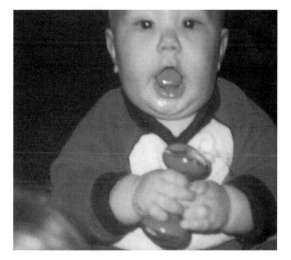

Figure 7-11. Bimanual holding with partial supination and wrist extension (7 months).

other. Usually the hands join together at midline, and the object is held between them. Almost universally, once the object is prehended, the infant brings it to the mouth or chest. The object may drop when transported to the mouth or may be captured against a body part. These behaviors are reinforced by the infant's drive toward symmetric midline movements at this age and the desire to experience oral sensation. Lack of internal trunk stability at 4 months also results in bringing both hands together around the object for distal stability.

The 20-week-old infant tends to use the simultaneous approach described earlier, in which both hands move toward the object at the same time. The infant attempts to prehend the object using both hands (Castner, 1932). Fenson et al. (1976) reported that, although the 5-month-old reaches for the object with two hands, he/she uses only one to grasp the object. The second hand may support the first after grasp is achieved, and often both hands bring the object to the mouth or hold it in space for visual inspection. Intermanual transfer has significantly increased (Rochat, 1989), although active purposeful release has not yet developed. Compared to 2- and 3-month-olds, 4- and 5-month-old infants demonstrate significantly better organized bimanual action with more holding and fingering of objects. The bilateral fingering behavior observed at this age has been described as grasping the object with one hand and touching it or scanning the object's surface with the other (Ruff, 1984).

Transitional Bilateral Skills

Between 24 and 28 weeks the infant approaches the cube most frequently with both hands, corralling it. During this developmental period first a simultaneous, then a successive bilateral approach is used. The infant initiates movement in the second hand as the first hand ends its approach (Castner, 1932).

Bilaterality versus unilaterality in approach seems to be determined by the object's size and the way it is presented. The 7-month-old uses a bilateral approach for large objects and a unilateral approach for small objects (Flament, 1975, as cited in Fagard, 1990). Other authors suggest that approach is determined by the external support provided for the infant's proximal stability during reach (Bushnell, 1985; Halverson, 1931). After grasping the object, the infant visually inspects it or brings it to the mouth. He/she may transfer it using the mouth as a stabilizer.

The 7-month-old uses primarily bilateral movements for object manipulation (Goldfield and Michel, 1986; Flament, 1975, as cited in Corbetta and Mounoud, 1990). At this time the infant demonstrates associated, rather than independent, bimanual movements. While the two hands act in concert, an increasing variety of exploratory and manipulative behaviors are observed (Figure 7-11). For example, the infant uses an extended index finger to poke or probe an object held in the other hand. This probing with one hand while holding with the other is a primary method of object exploration.

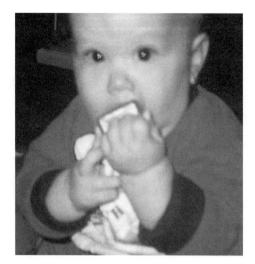

Figure 7-12. Mouthing a toy held in both hands (7 months).

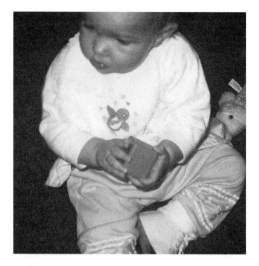

Figure 7-13. Two-hand cooperation in turning an object (10 months).

As previously mentioned, by 7 months the infant holds the object in the radial digits and actively transfers it from hand to hand, while visually and tactilely exploring it. Active supination and isolated wrist movements enable the infant to partially rotate or turn the object for visual inspection. These isolated movements are often mimicked by the other hand. Manipulation of the object at this time is limited to transfers from hand to hand or hand to mouth rather than within hand manipulation. Mouthing remains an important part of the infant's exploration (Figure 7-12).

After 7 months of age, infants begin to play with two toys at a time. The infant demonstrates banging of two objects together as the first indication of his or her capacity to associate objects (Corbetta and Mounoud, 1990). In the following weeks the infant adds to the repertoire of bilateral movements. In addition to visual inspection and hand-to-hand exchange, the infant waves toys in the air and bangs them on the table surface. Mouthing continues to be a significant behavior. However, by 9 months mouthing appears to be passive; that is, the mouth is an additional way to hold the object rather than a primary way to explore the object (Ruff, 1984). By 9 months the striking change in manipulation is not related to the development of any specific skill, but to the expanded range of behaviors observed. Halverson (1931) noted that 9-month-olds "exhibited all of the following behaviors: transfer, visual inspection, release and regain, bang it on the table, and hold it with both hands." Ruff (1984) found that

infants developed a different type of object rotation. The infant at 6 months rotated the object by rotating the wrist or supinating/pronating. By 9 months object rotation was primarily achieved by transferring it from hand to hand. This type of rotation was possible due to increasing control of the radial digits and ability to grade supination and pronation as the object moves from hand to hand (Figure 7-13). This two-hand cooperation in turning an object is evidence of beginning dissociation of symmetric arm movements.

Coordinated Bimanual Skills

Near the end of the first year a change is observed in the linkage between two-hand movement (Goldfield and Michel, 1986). Whereas 7-month-old infants move their hands in the same direction, 11-month-olds move them in complementary directions. This change marks the initiation of mature bimanual skills.

At 12 months the infant demonstrates significant increases in both dexterity with one hand and cooperative use of two hands together. Ruff (1984) observed an increase in fingering by 12 months, which she associated with an increase in the infant's abilities to simultaneously assimilate tactile and visual information. The two hands begin to demonstrate coordinated asymmetric roles. These complementary movements are observed as the infant simultaneously holds two objects or an object and a container. A typical bilateral pattern at this time is for one hand to be active (generally the preferred hand) and one hand to be passive or to support and stabilize the object (for example, one hand holds the container while the other removes a block inside). Bruner (1970) studied the success of infants in removing a toy from a toy box. He found that before 12 months infants are rarely successful in removing the object. Beginning at 12 months the hands work in cooperation; for example, one hand holds the bottle and the other unscrews the lid. With the advent of the second year, the infant begins to understand the function of certain objects, and with this new understanding a differentiated set of movements is established in object play. Hand skills increasingly become a reflection of the infant's cognitive and perceptual capabilities (see Chapter 6).

From 12 to 24 months the infant develops greater control of bimanual skills with increasing complexity and integration of motor patterns. Speed, accuracy, and dexterity increase. Proximal arm movements become dissociated from distal arm movements such that the infant can hold the hands in space to manipulate objects. He/she can also demonstrate controlled arm movement while maintaining grasp of an object (Exner, 1989). Many of the child's activities involve one hand manipulating and the other stabilizing the object. For example, the child begins to spoon feed while holding the bowl, scribble with a marker while holding the paper, bang with a toy hammer while stabilizing the target toy.

Between 18 months and 2 years the child learns a variety of bimanual skills that require control of simultaneous hand movements involving blended combinations of alternating stability and mobility (Gilfoyle, Grady, and Moore, 1990). Stringing beads, pulling off shoes, unwrapping a piece of candy are examples of skills in the repertoire of the 2-year-old that involve a sequence of bimanual movements in which the child simultaneously controls arm and hand stabilization and movement (Knobloch and Pasamanick, 1974). These bimanual movements can be asymmetric and dissociated, when the activity requires that two hands act together in different movements. Two-handed, simultaneous movement also represents a developmental step from the earlier pattern of one hand manipulating and the other stabilizing. Cooperative and complementary bimanual movements continue to be added to the child's repertoire of fine motor skills throughout the first decade of life. The complexity, speed, accuracy, and precision of the skills increase with experience, cognitive development, and neuromotor maturation.

Table 7-1 presents the developmental sequence of grasp, release, and bimanual skills. Although the developmental ages for the listed skills vary, the sequence of development tends to remain consistent across children. Therefore the months listed are approximate ages when the described skills are achieved.

AN INTEGRATED OVERVIEW OF HAND SKILL DEVELOPMENT

This section describes how posture, sensory system function, play, and cognitive development contribute to the early development of hand skills. It also provides a specific explanation of how the child's development of grasp, release, and bimanual skills relates to the development of play and cognitive skills.

First Quartile: Birth through 3 Months
Hand Skills

In the very young infant (neonate to 2 months old) reflexes dominate movements. Hand and arm movements are strongly influenced by tactile and proprioceptive input or by head position. It is not until the third month of life that reflexes diminish and purposeful visual motor coordination begins to develop. Practice of hand movements that the infant "instinctively" demonstrates allows the development of active range of motion and strength for object manipulation. Hand grasping at midline, visual regard of the hand, and instinctive grasp of an object are critical behaviors at this time that provide sensory experiences to the hand and promote the development of skill.

Contributing Factors

Posture. The 2-month-old infant primarily demonstrates asymmetric posturing, reinforced by the influence of the asymmetric tonic neck reflex (Gesell et al., 1940). In general, the asymmetric posture of the young infant limits his/her visual field and reinforces visual inspection of the hands (Bower, 1974). The 3-month-old has an emerging sense of midline, and in supine brings the head to midline and the hands toward midline (Figure 7-14). Symmetric weight bearing in prone and increasing head control contribute to establishing a sense of midline. Neck and shoulder stability is developing as a prerequisite for control of reach and hand movements in space.

Table 7-1. Development of grasp, release, and bimanual skills: birth through 24 months

AGE	GRASP	RELEASE	BIMANUAL SKILL
Neonate	Traction response	Avoiding reaction: hand opens with tactile stimulus to hand's dorsum	Smooth, alternating arm movements; reflexive arm responses to proprioceptive and tactile input
1 mo	Grasp reflex: local grasp reaction, followed by traction response	Avoiding reactions continue	Asymmetry of arm movements; reflexive arm responses to proprioceptive and tactile input
2 mo	Grasp reflex: catch and holding phases		
3 mo		Instinctive avoiding response; pronation and adduction from stimulus on ulnar side, supination, abduction from stimulus on radial side	Hands held together on chest, usually without object; symmetric, simultaneous arm movement
4 mo	True grasp reflex; primitive squeeze of fingers; diminished traction response; orienting response	Instinctive avoiding reactions continue; variety of hand movements used to avoid touch contact	Objects held with both hands at midline; symmetric, midline movements
5 mo	Instinctive grasp; squeeze grasp, gropes for tactile stimulus; adjusts hand to object	Release involuntary or accidental	Two-hand reach, with unilateral prehension; object transfer, hand to hand; Bilateral holding and fingering
6 mo	Palmar grasp; pronated hand and flexion of all fingers; adjusts hand using visual and tactile information	Object accidentally released in mouthing or bimanual play	Simultaneous, symmetric, bilateral approach with bimanual or unilateral prehension
7 mo	Radial palmar grasp; superior palmar grasp; differentiation of ulnar and radial sides stable; radial fingers hold object	Purposeful release; transfer of object from one hand to the other; release against a resisting surface	Successive bilateral approach with unilateral prehension; bilateral object manipulation; associated bimanual movements

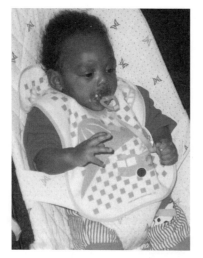

Figure 7-14. Hands toward midline (3 months).

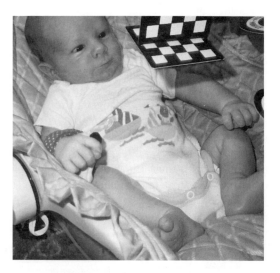

Figure 7-15. Visual regard (3 months).

Table 7-1. Development of grasp, release, and bimanual skills: birth through 24 months–cont'd

AGE	GRASP	RELEASE	BIMANUAL SKILL
8 mo	Radial digital grasp; inferior forefinger grasp; object held proximal to finger pads; ulnar side stable and radial fingers hold object	Purposeful release with assistance or resistance against a surface	
9 mo	Scissors grasp; able to hold small objects		Object rotation by transferring it hand to hand; plays with two toys, one in each hand, banging together; dissociation of symmetric arm movement
10 mo	Forefinger grasp; tip of thumb and forefinger used in grasp; grasping accuracy without stabilization	Active release; flinging of object by combining elbow, wrist, and finger extension; object release above surface	
11 mo			Complementary and cooperative bimanual movement
12 mo	Superior pincer grasp; tip of thumb and forefinger used in grasp; grasping accuracy without stabilization	Beginning of controlled release; remains imprecise	Coordinated, asymmetric movements; one hand stabilizes and one hand manipulates
15 mo	Deft and precise grasp; a variety of grasps used	Controlled release; increasing control when releasing	Beginning of two-hand tool use; continues pattern of one hand stabilizing and one manipulating
18 mo	Increasing dissociation, strength, and perception enable child to use tools and manipulate objects	Controlled release, increasing accuracy with limited precision of placement; tends to extend fingers all at one time	Asymmetric, dissociated bimanual skills; blended stability and mobility; alternating sequences of two-hand movements
24 mo		Greater precision and control of release; adjustment of hand opening according to object's size and shape	Increasing competence in two-hand tool use; increasing complexity in movement patterns; cooperation of two hands

Sensory. By the third month the head is held at midline, which frees the range of vision. During this same period the infant learns to control eye movements, and visual inspection becomes a key strategy for learning about the environment. Visual attention to specific events and objects indicates the infant's ability to focus and assimilate important information from the environment (Bower, 1974; White, Castle, and Held, 1964) (Figure 7-15). While visual attention becomes more discriminating, hand skills remain primitive in that the hand does not adapt to the specific sensory qualities of the object it grasps, and control of release has not been established (Figure 7-16).

The infant from birth through 3 months is often prone lying and has frequent opportunities for tactile/proprioceptive input to the hands and forearms. He/she presses into a prone propped position with head erect, resulting in deep proprioceptive input to the arms. Hand opening while weight bearing, prone-on-elbows, provides specific tactile input to the palms. Mouthing of the hand allows for tactile exploration of the hand and provides tactile/proprioceptive input to the hand. When the infant is supine, the hands find each other on the chest, clasping and engaging in mutual fingering. These tactile/proprioceptive experiences contribute to the development of grasp and release patterns, as do the visual experiences

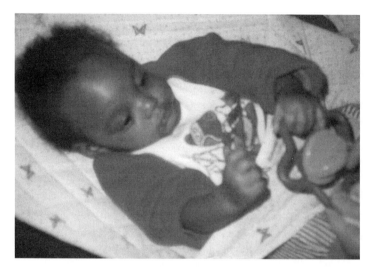

Figure 7-16. Unable to release object (3 months).

that contribute to the development of visually guided hand movements.

Play and cognition. Play at this time involves sensory experiences. The infant delights in the sensory experiences of touch, movement, and proprioception. The goal of generalized movements and reactions is to continue or to create sensory experiences. As the infant scratches the weight-bearing surface or the parent's shoulder, this behavior seems to be automatically reinforced by the tactile and proprioceptive input to the hand. When general swiping movements cause a mobile to move and make sounds, this sensory experience reinforces that action and the infant swipes at the mobile again. Visual exploration, mouthing, and tactile reflexes appear be the infant's primary methods for learning about the environment (Bower, 1974; Gesell et al., 1940). Generalized automatic and instinctive movements of the arms and hands soon come under the infant's cortical control in the following quartile.

Second Quartile: 4 through 6 Months
Hand Skills

In the period from 4 to 6 months, the infant makes remarkable strides in developing the visual motor system. The infant learns to reach toward an object, place hands on top of it, and rake the object toward the self. The infant exhibits a palmar grasp during this quartile with the object held at first by pressing the ulnar fingers into the palm and then by the radial fingers and palm. The palmar grasp that is the hallmark of this age is a crude grasp that does not allow the object to move within the hand. By 6 months the crude palmar grasp becomes a more functional palmar grasp, which is highly successful for obtaining objects and can accommodate different sizes and shapes. A palmar grasp is used regardless of the size of the object, such that even pellet-sized objects are raked into the palm of the hand. Control of release has not yet developed and occurs only against a resisting surface. The infant's reach becomes more accurate as he/she grasps everything within reach. Mother's hair and clothing become the targets of grasping efforts. Once the object is obtained within the hand, the infant frequently brings it to the mouth. At 4 and 5 months the forearms are pronated when reaching for and holding objects. By 6 months active supination increases, which allows the infant to hold the object in a position so that he/she can alternately mouth and visualize it.

Looking behaviors are primarily linked with fingering (Ruff, 1984; Rochat, 1989). This information is integrated with the tactile information obtained by mouthing the object (Gilfoyle, Grady, and Moore, 1990).

Contributing Factors

Posture. The predominant characteristic of the infant's posture between 4 and 6 months is symmetry. Head and hands come to midline, enabling a hands-together posture and visual inspection of both hands. As a result, the infant spends much of the time in hand-to-hand play, first on the chest and then in space at midline. Head and trunk control and postural stability change dramatically during this quartile. Thus the infant gains important axial support for reach and use of hands in space. Stability through the neck and shoulders helps the infant gain control of the arms; therefore in supported positions he/she can hold the arms in space while grasping an object.

The infant demonstrates increased postural control in the prone position, pushing onto extended arms and shifting weight side to side. When on elbows, the infant is able to lift one arm entirely from the weight-bearing surface for reach to an object. This complete lateral weight shift provides proprioceptive input through the hands across the palmar surface (Gilfoyle, Grady, and Moore, 1990). It also results in asymmetric sensory experiences. Prone positions help the infant strengthen arm and hand musculature and provide tactile proprioceptive information that appears important to the hand's perceptual development (Boehme, 1988) (Figure 7-17). Although the increased postural control of the 6-month-old supports symmetric movements of the arms in space, it does not appear adequate for skilled asymmetric or unilateral movements. In the following quartile, when trunk stability is sufficient for independent sitting, the infant develops an increased repertoire of arm and hand movements that includes both symmetric and asymmetric patterns.

Sensory. Sensory experiences continue to be a primary basis for movement. The infant delights in the sensory world and begins to integrate the information from more than one sensory system. Mouthing and fingering behaviors increase significantly in the second quartile of life (Rochat, 1984). Fingering behaviors are associated with visual inspection. At 4 and 5 months of age infants increasingly make successive oral and visual contacts with the object, thereby integrating information from two different sensory systems. Ruff and Kohler (1978) demonstrated that after 6-month-old infants tactually explore objects, they tend to visually prefer those objects. Their results provide evidence that the infant visually recognizes an object that was previously held and tactually experienced but not visualized. Sensory play at this time consists of mouthing, hand-to-hand fingering, and intense visual inspection. Proprioceptive input from weight bearing on hands in prone position may relate to the development of hand opening and the inhibition of finger flexion.

Play and cognition. Sensory experiences continue to dominate the child's play. Visual and auditory experiences have increased importance, and the infant demonstrates improved abilities to orient to and attend to visual and auditory information. Movements are motivated by the sensation that results, and attention is drawn to the immediate sensory experience. He/she begins to actively explore objects using specific movements to create sounds and visual effects. By 6 months the infant usually can purposely roll and initiate rolling to experience movement. Toys that react to simple movements are favorites in play. Rattles are good examples, in that almost any movement produces a sound, reinforcing the infant's play and exploration (Piaget, 1952). Toys that are activated by generalized responses continue to be preferred to those that require specific, more localized responses; for example, a mobile or rattle is preferred to a busy box requiring differentiated push, pull, and press of fingers (McCall, 1974).

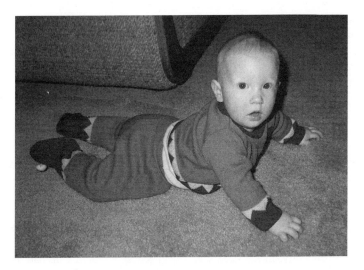

Figure 7-17. Prone position (6 months).

Third Quartile: 7 through 9 Months

Hand Skills

From 7 to 9 months the radial palmar grasp matures into a radial digital grasp. At 7 months the infant uses a radial palmar grasp with thumb abduction, pressing the object into the palm. By 9 months a radial digital grasp with the object held in the digits and the thumb opposing the digits has developed. Voluntary release is also initiated during this quartile and becomes an important part of the infant's repertoire of fine motor behaviors. Knobloch and Pasamanick (1974) emphasize the versatility observed in manipulation patterns at 7 months: "He grasps it, brings it to his mouth, withdraws it, looks at it on withdrawal, fingers it while he looks, looks while he rotates it, restores it to his mouth, withdraws it again for inspection, restores it again for mouthing, transfers it to the other hand, bangs it, contacts it with the free hand, retransfers it, mouths it again, drops it, rescues it, mouths it again" (p. 60). Hence the infant becomes capable of a long sequence of handling behaviors that incorporate a combination of visualizing and tactile exploration using the mouth and the hands.

Reach is accurately directed in the 7-month-old, and increased active supination is observed. The infant gains control of forearm supination while gaining control in the radial digits, positioning the object for visual inspection or entry into the mouth (Figure 7-18).

Toward the end of this quartile the infant develops an inferior pincer grasp. To achieve this prehension pattern, the infant's hand must be resting on the supporting surface for stability. A small object, such as a pellet, is grasped between the thumb and the radial side of the index finger using an adduction motion of the thumb. The first inferior pinch is usually accompanied with index finger probing (Gilfoyle, Grady, and Moore, 1990). The active use of the thumb in prehension initiates a lifelong pattern and enables the infant to successfully grasp objects of diminishing size.

Another important developmental milestone at this time is the grasp and manipulation of two objects simultaneously. At 7 months the infant can simultaneously grasp two objects, one in each hand. Beginning at 8 months, he/she delights in banging them together, signifying the first relating of two objects (McCall, 1974).

Contributing Factors

Posture. Gains in postural control allow the 7-month-old to sit independently. In the next sev-

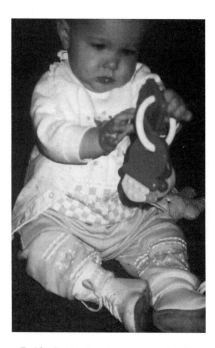

Figure 7-18. Supinating forearm to visualize object (9 months).

eral months sitting becomes a favorite play position because the hands are free to hold objects, and the infant can control weight shift forward or to the sides to obtain objects. Increased axial control seems to support the use of one-hand reach and to support bimanual fingering (exploration) of an object held at midline. Trunk rotation has developed in fully supported positions (that is, rolling from supine to prone and prone to supine) and begins to develop in sitting positions (Gilfoyle, Grady, and Moore, 1990). Related to these skills, the infant demonstrates crossing the midline and begins to use the hand in crossed lateral space.

The infant also assumes the quadruped position and may begin to creep. The on-hands-and-knees position results in frequent weight bearing on the hands. This position tends to be dynamic and mobile, thereby providing tactile and proprioceptive input across the hand (Figure 7-19). The frequency of play in prone position (in and out of quadruped) strengthens the arms and hands. The infant shifts weight across the hands in a diagonal direction while moving from quadruped to side sitting (Boehme, 1988). Strengthening of the arms also occurs through pulling to stand and supporting himself while erect.

Sensory. The role of vision in guiding manipulation has an increasingly important role in this quartile and then throughout development. Whereas tactile input had primary influence on

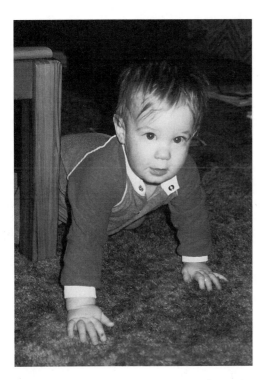

Figure 7-19. Hands-and-knees position (8 months).

grasp and manipulation, vision becomes a primary sense for guiding the infant's manipulation. Mc-Call (1974) reported an increase in manipulation with visual regard at 8½ months. Ruff (1979) found that, while fingering increased in the 9-month-old, it seemed to relate to the tactile properties of the object, and looking behaviors did not increase significantly. Castner (1932) observed that the duration of regard increased at 8 and 9 months, as did the infant's accuracy in reach and grasp of a pellet.

Although manipulation with visual regard increases during this time frame, active mouthing decreases (McCall, 1974). This active mouthing appears to be replaced with fingering. The increasing importance of vision in manipulation complements rather than diminishes the importance of the tactile system. The infant is now able to integrate visual and tactile information, using both senses simultaneously to learn about the object's properties (Corbetta and Mounoud, 1991; Ruff, 1984). Intermodal transfer of tactile and visual information (visual recognition of an object after handling it without vision) becomes possible at this age (Ruff and Kohler, 1978; Steele and Pederson, 1977).

Proprioceptive perception becomes more discriminating during this quartile. Changes in dis-crimination of the object's weight and shape enable the child to hold a cracker without crushing it and lift an object with the appropriate amount of force (see Chapter 3).

Play and cognition. During this quartile the infant spends much time in object exploration. Interest in and awareness of the environment increases, as described in the previous section. Visual and tactile exploration of objects predominates. These exploratory behaviors are characterized by a rich variety of manipulative skills. Cause and effect are well established, and rather than repeating the same actions on a toy, the infant tries new strategies to create different reactions (Piaget, 1952). Play includes imitation of actions observed, including toy manipulation. The physical properties of the object guide responses, since the infant does not yet understand the specific functional uses of objects. The infant begins to bang objects together and place one object in proximity to another. These behaviors signal the advent of tool usage and specific actions of one object in relation to another (Bruner, 1970).

Fourth Quartile: 10 through 12 Months
Hand Skills

In this quartile the infant demonstrates important changes in prehensile and manipulation skills (Knobloch and Pasamanick, 1974). These skills include controlled object release, grasp of very small objects, increased relating of two objects together, and functional use of objects. Neuromotor, cognitive, and perceptual abilities develop concurrently to complement and reinforce each other through the play behaviors of the infant. The infant now uses fingertips and distal portions of the fingers when precision grasp is required. The thumb actively opposes the index finger in a precise and deft pincer grasp. The radial portion of the hand is consistently used in skillful manipulation with the ulnar fingers flexed for increased hand stability. Maturation of the pincer grasp enables the infant to prehend pellet-sized objects and to successfully grasp small objects from a variety of surfaces. The infant now has control of hand opening and can release the object with controlled finger extension. This release no longer requires the support of a resisting surface. The infant first uses this skill to achieve interesting auditory and visual effects of the object dropping and later uses this skill to place objects in, on, or near each other. Release

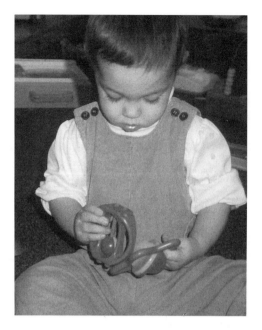

Figure 7-20. Object turning with visual exploration (12 months).

of medium-sized objects is more accurate than release of large or small objects (e.g., release of the pellet remains difficult) (Gesell et al., 1940). The infant uses two hands together in new ways. In addition to symmetric hand movements, the infant begins to stabilize with one hand and manipulate with the other. This pattern is used to combine two objects or to explore a held object using index probing (Figure 7-20). Object rotation and transfer occur frequently and are complemented with a range of exploratory behaviors including shaking, turning, banging, dropping, pressing, and pushing (Halverson, 1931; McCall, 1974).

Exploratory behaviors are refined in that they better match the sensory qualities of the object (Ruff, 1984). Increased perception and understanding of object shape and size with increased control of isolated finger movements enable the infant to approach an object with the hand shaped according to those characteristics. Active supination and dominant use of the radial fingers during manipulation allow the child to visualize the object while manipulating it. Increased precision of grasp and control of release enable the child to more accurately relate to objects. For example, he/she now can release a cube in a cup (Illingworth, 1991; Gesell et al., 1940). When high levels of precise release are required—placement of one cube on another—the infant generally remains unsuccessful.

Contributing Factors

Posture. Postural stability increases such that the infant has greater control of arms in space while sitting independently. The internal stability of the arm allows the 12-month-old to prehend a small object using a superior pincer grasp (that is, use a pincer grasp without stabilizing the arm on the surface). Postural stability is an important factor in the development of accurate and well-directed reach (Knobloch and Pasamanick, 1974). With increasing trunk stability and rotation the infant is able to reach out of reach to the body's contralateral side. Postural stability also enables the child to reach overhead and behind when sitting.

Weight-bearing experiences continue to provide heavy work for the upper extremities. Creeping is usually the primary form of mobility. The infant may rise into the hands-and-feet position (bear crawling), resulting in heavy work for the arms. Fast creeping over a variety of surfaces provides important tactual and proprioceptive input to the hands.

Sensory. At 12 months the infant continues to use vision as a primary guide to object manipulation. The infant can visually recognize the physical properties of the object and act on it appropriately. For example, by 12 months the infant immediately bangs and hits a rigid object and squeezes or presses a spongy object (Gibson and Walker, 1984, in Corbetta and Mounoud, 1991). Fingering and hand-to-hand manipulation become the primary modes for exploring the sensory qualities of an object (Ruff, 1984). Integration of senses continues and the infant becomes increasingly able to recognize objects visually that had been explored only through the tactile sense.

Play and cognition. The cognitive milestone in hand skill development in this quartile is that the infant develops understanding of the object's functional purpose, thereby attempting to use objects for the function that they are intended. As a result, the spoon, which previously was used to make noise in banging, now is viewed as a utensil for bringing food to the mouth. While early attempts to spoon feed generally fail, the intent is clear. For the first time the infant's repertoire of manipulative skills increases, in accordance with functional capabilities of the object more than its sensory qualities. The infant pushes a truck, pulls a toy dog on a string, lifts a telephone receiver to the ear, rolls a ball, lifts a brush to the head. All of these movements are based on emerging cognitive understandings, as functional play begins to pre-

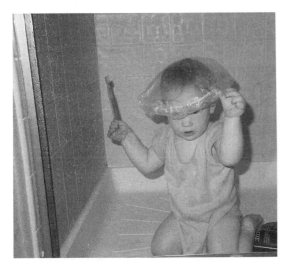

Figure 7-21. Infant (12 months) imitating movements observed in adults.

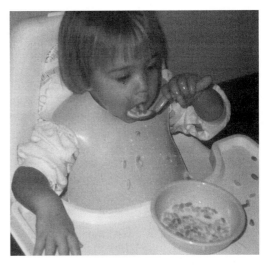

Figure 7-22. Spoon feeding (18 months).

dominate over sensory play. The child's interest in relating two objects also results in more advanced unilateral and bilateral skills. Endless repetitions of putting objects in a container and placing one object next to another create interesting results for the infant and at the same time refine releasing skills. New skills in imitation are a basis for developing additional manipulation skills as the infant attempts new movements that he/she observes others perform (Figure 7-21).

Second Year: 13 through 18 Months
Hand Skills

Based on the groundwork of the first year of development, the infant refines the learned manipulative patterns and combines them into more complex and longer play sequences. Although the object is consistently held in the radial fingertips, the hand's grip is relatively stationary, and the infant manipulates the object by transferring it from one hand to the other rather than manipulating it within one hand. The hand can now hold two blocks, indicating dissociation of the two sides of the hand and isolation of finger movement. The same independent finger movements are demonstrated in object release, which becomes more accurate, allowing the infant to stack three cubes by 18 months. To place the third cube, the child demonstrates internal arm stability with controlled hand mobility.

Controlled independent movements of the wrist and forearm while grasping are observed as the infant correctly places puzzle pieces and uses a spoon. Tool use increases markedly, for example,

first use of a crayon to scribble and a spoon to feed (Figure 7-22). This first functional tool use is characterized by a static grip on the utensil with the active motion occurring at proximal joints (shoulder, elbow, and wrist). As described in the first part of this chapter, bimanual skills increase in variety and frequency.

Contributing Factors

Posture. By 13 months the child's balance and postural stability are sufficient for upright ambulation. Trunk rotation and pelvic stability are noted in smooth transitions from floor sitting to standing and from standing back to sitting. Postural control can now support hand manipulation with arms in space, as observed in stacking blocks, placing objects in a container, and toy exploration. Now that upright ambulation is the child's consistent form of mobility, upper extremity weight-bearing experiences become limited and the hands no longer are critical for support, resulting in increased emphasis on their role in manipulation (Figure 7-23).

Sensory. Hand skills are no longer driven by sensory exploration as the functional use of objects becomes the prime motive for manipulation. The child continues to integrate visual, tactile, and proprioceptive sensations by practicing perceptual motor skills, demonstrating increased abilities to use information from these sensory systems to correct and refine movements. Thus increased precision of movement is due to increased perceptual ability as well as improved motor skill.

The child can now recognize the tactile and auditory properties of the object through visual

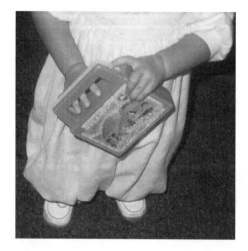

Figure 7-23. Holding and manipulating an object while standing (15 months).

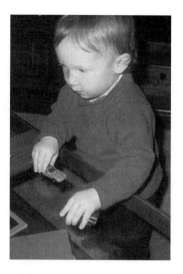

Figure 7-24. Functional play with a toy car (15 months).

inspection and therefore approaches an object with an appropriate response, for example, shaking a rattle, squeezing a sponge, crumpling paper, or using more force to lift a large object.

Play and cognition. Cognitive abilities have a tremendous influence on the development of hand skills at this time. The maturity of manipulative skills supports the development of play schemata. Both increase in complexity and sophistication. The functional purpose of toys determines the toddler's response: dialing the phone, turning the music box, unzipping a zipper, scribbling with a crayon, or pushing a car (Figure 7-24).

With an increased interest in relating multiple objects, the child fills a container with small objects, places one object on or next to another, and scoops food with a spoon. These relational play

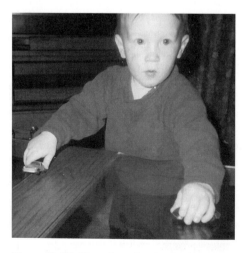

Figure 7-25. Use of two hands simultaneously (15 months).

activities often require stabilizing the toy or object with one hand while manipulating with the other. The child's understanding of cause and effect and object permanence results in increased interest in switches, hinges, push buttons, and pop-up toys. Switches require elaboration of the prehensile patterns developed and new combinations of arm and hand movements. Most play activities now require bimanual skills, and the child is able to use hands together simultaneously or reciprocally (Corbetta and Mounoud, 1990) (Figure 7-25).

The child engages in longer and more complex play sequences that require new combinations of hand skills. Pushing, pulling, probing, rotating, and turning are combined into a new repertoire of play behaviors (Nicholich, 1977). With new understanding of tool use, the child engages in play activities that require mobility of the proximal arm and stability of the hand for grasping of the object (Exner, 1989). The functional use of some objects, such as a cup, requires a series of combined mobility and stability of the arm and hand (Figure 7-26). The functional play that characterizes the child at this age correlates with an increasing purposefulness in manipulation. While the child continues to explore objects to learn their sensory properties, he/she often "uses" objects for their specific function as part of a purposeful play activity.

Second Year: 19 through 24 Months

Hand Skills

The significant changes that occur by the end of the second year are associated with the child's

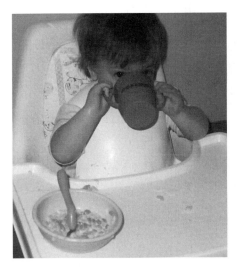

Figure 7-26. Functional use of an object: cup drinking (18 months).

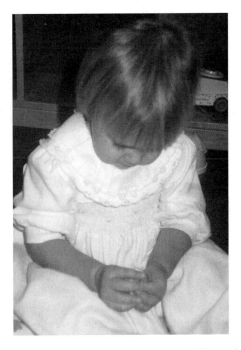

Figure 7-27. Blended mobility and stability and use of isolated finger movement (21 months).

ability to blend mobility and stability into more complex motor patterns and integrate sensory information with motor skill. The 24-month-old is capable of building a six-cube tower by precisely centering each cube and slowly releasing it, using gradual extension of individual fingers. This same careful placement of objects is observed with simple puzzle pieces that match a form space. The precision increases due to a blending of stability and mobility in the arm and hand that allows movement of a single digit or at one joint while the rest of the arm holds a stable position. The coordination of mobility and stability allows for endless combinations of movement patterns, many of which are observed throughout the life span (Figure 7-27).

The child now frequently uses utensils in play and self-care activities. Pencil grasp has moved from a palmar grasp to a supinate palmar and in some children to grasp within the fingers (Schneck and Henderson, 1990). By 3 years most children demonstrate a static tripod grasp of the pencil. Many children at 24 months grasp the spoon using the fingers in a supinated hand position. Tasks that require precision are performed with fingertip grasp, and those that require power, the palmar grasp.

In addition to these changes in dexterity, the child at 24 months demonstrates improved perceptual-motor integration that allows him/her to assimilate and imitate a circular stroke, match a form to a form space, hold an object with appropriate pressure, place and release an object with accuracy, and demonstrate beginning eye-hand coordination in ball play. All of these skills indicate

an increased ability to integrate sensory experience and make accurate motor responses or adaptations to those sensory inputs (Connolly, 1987).

Contributing Factors

Posture. Postural control is excellent by 2 years as the child begins to concentrate on speed, strength, balance, and endurance. Postural stability of the child at 24 months enables use of the hand with control in all positions and planes around the body. Although dexterity diminishes when the child is in a less stable position (such as half kneel), postural stability in typical sitting and standing positions is sufficient for control of a great range of manipulative skills (Figure 7-28).

Sensory. Improved sensory discrimination and integration enable the child to demonstrate increased variety and control of perceptual-motor skills. By 24 months the child is able to assimilate multimodal sensory information and make appropriate adaptive responses. Success in perceptual-motor skills such as stringing beads and simple dressing tasks indicates the child's ability to integrate and use sensory information.

Play and cognition. The child's play continues to focus on concrete, functional activities with toys. Play sequences increase in length and complexity (Fenson and Ramsey, 1980). Symbolic play begins about the same time that language develops, between 16 and 20 months. At first the

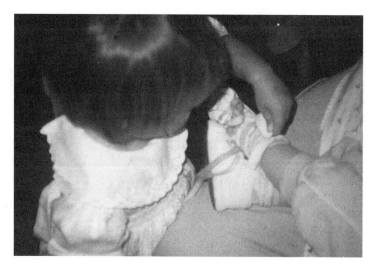

Figure 7-28. Superior pincer grasp while standing (21 months).

infant demonstrates self-play that is centered around or directed toward the self (Fenson et al., 1976). The child's play might consist of simulating eating, drinking, or sleeping. Between 19 and 24 months the child's symbolic play becomes directed to objects. This decentered play involves acting on dolls or teddy bears, feeding them, putting them to bed, combing their hair. The hand skills to perform such actions are complex and require that a series of related movements be linked together. These play activities are thus an integrated combination of bimanual skills, most of which require that one hand holds and the other acts on the object.

The child uses utensils with competency. He/she now has sufficient control of crayon or pencil grasp to make a vertical stroke. Self-feeding is more successful because the child does not turn the spoon as it enters the mouth. Spoon feeding and early drawing skills are made possible by integration of sensory and perceptual information into blended patterns of mobility and stability.

CONCLUSION

Hand skills undergo tremendous developmental changes in the first 2 years of life. From simple grasping patterns the child develops elaborate manipulative skills. Hand skills evolve from reflexive, stereotypical patterns that are automatic to an almost infinite variety of hand and finger combinations for manipulating objects and acting on the environment.

A number of variables support the child's development of hand skills. Increased postural stability and control support increased arm and hand control. Increased sensory discrimination and integration promote the development of perceptual hand skills. Increased cognitive understanding promotes play schemata based on functional use of objects. The child holds objects first in the palm, then in the fingers, and finally in the fingertips. As he/she holds objects more distally, coordination of two hands together evolves, enabling the child to achieve greater competence and skill in play and interaction within the environment.

REFERENCES

Ammon, J.E., & Etzel, M.E. (1977). Sensorimotor organization in reach and prehension. *Physical Therapy, 57,* 7-14.

Andre-Thomas, A.J. (1964). The neurological examination of the infant. In *Clinics in developmental medicine, No. 1.* Philadelphia: JB Lippincott.

Boehme, R. (1988). *Improving upper body control.* Tuscon: Therapy Skills Builders.

Bower, T.G.R. (1974). *Development in infancy.* San Francisco: Freeman.

Bruner, J.S. (1970). The growth and structure of skill. In K. Connolly (Ed.). *Mechanisms of motor skill development.* New York: Academic Press.

Bushnell, E.W. (1982). Visual-tactual knowledge in 8, 9½, and 11 month old infants. *Infant Behavior and Development, 5,* 63-75.

Bushnell, E.W. (1985). The decline of visually guided reaching during infancy. *Infant Behavior and Development, 8,* 139-155.

Castner, B.M. (1932). The development of fine prehension in infancy. *Genetic Psychology Monographs, 12,* 105-193.

Connolly, K., & Dalgleish, M. (1989). The emergence of a tool-using skill in infancy. *Developmental Psychology, 25*(6), 894-912.

Corbetta, D., & Mounoud, P. (1990). Early development of grasping and manipulation. In C. Bard, M. Fleury, & L. Hay (Eds.). *Development of eye-hand coordination across the life span.* Columbia, SC: University of South Carolina Press.

Exner, C. (1989). The development of hand skills. In P. Pratt & A. Allen (Eds.). *Occupational therapy for children.* St. Louis: Mosby.

Fagard, J. (1990). The development of bimanual coordination. In C. Bard, M. Fleury, & L. Hay (Eds.). *Development of eye-hand coordination across the life span.* Columbia, SC: University of South Carolina Press.

Fenson, L., Kagan, J., Kearsley, R.B., & Zelazo, P.R. (1976). The developmental progression of manipulative play in the first two years. *Child Development, 47,* 232-236.

Fenson, L., & Ramsay, D.S. (1980). Decentration and integration of the child's play in the second year. *Child Development, 51,* 171-178.

Flavell, J. (1963). *The developmental psychology of Jean Piaget.* Princeton: Van Nostrand.

Gesell, A., & Amatruda, C.S. (1947). *Developmental diagnosis.* New York: Harper & Row.

Gesell, A., Halverson, H.M., Thompson, H., Ilg, F.L., Castner, B.M., Ames, L.B., & Amatruda, C.S. (1940). *The first five years of life.* New York: Harper & Brothers.

Gesell, A., Thompson, H., Amatruda, C.S. (1934). *An atlas of infant behavior: A systematic delineation of the forms and early growth of human behavior patterns. Volume One: Normative Series.* New Haven: Yale University Press.

Gibson, E.J., & Walker, A.S. (1984). Development of knowledge of visual-tactual affordance of substance. *Child Development, 55,* 453-460.

Goldfield, E.C., & Michel, G.F. (1986). The ontogeny of infant bimanual reaching during the first year. *Infant Behavior and Development, 9,* 81-89.

Halverson, H.M. (1931). An experimental study of prehension in infants by means of systematic cinema records. *Genetic Psychology Monographs, 10,* 107-286.

Halverson, H.M. (1937). Studies of the grasping responses of early infancy. I, II, III. *Journal of Genetic Psychology, 51,* 371-449.

Hay, L. (1979). Spatial temporal analysis of movements in children: Motor programs versus feedback in the development of reaching. *Journal of Motor Behavior, 11,* 189-200.

Hay, L. (1990). Developmental changes in eye-hand coordination behaviors: Preprogramming versus feedback control. In C. Bard, M. Fleury, & L. Hay (Eds.). *Development of eye-hand coordination across the life span.* Columbia, SC: University of South Carolina Press.

Hohlstein, R.R. (1982). The development of prehension in normal infants. *American Journal of Occupational Therapy, 36*(3), 170-176.

Holt, K. (1975). Movement and child development. In *Clinics in developmental medicine.* Philadelphia: JB Lippincott.

Illingworth, R.S. (1991). *The normal child: Some problems of the early years and their treatment* (10th ed.). Edinburgh: Churchill-Livingstone.

Knobloch, H., & Pasamanick, B. (1974). *Gesell and Amatruda's developmental diagnosis: The evaluation and management of normal and abnormal neuropsychologic development in infancy and early childhood.* Hagerstown, MD: Harper & Row.

McCall, R.B. (1974). Exploratory manipulation and play in the human infant. *Monographs of the Society for Research in Child Development, 39,* 155.

McGraw, M.B. (1941). Neural maturation as exemplified in the reaching-prehensile behavior of the human infant. *The Journal of Psychology, 11,* 127-141.

McGraw, M.B. (1943). *The neuromuscular maturation of the human infant.* New York: Columbia University Press.

Nicolich, L. (1977). Beyond sensorimotor intelligence: Assessment of symbolic maturity through analysis of pretend play. *Merrill-Palmer Quarterly, 23,* 89-102.

Piaget, J. (1952). *The origins of intelligence in children.* New York: Norton.

Rochat, P. (1989). Object manipulation and exploration in 2- to 5-month-old infants. *Developmental Psychology, 25*(6), 871-884.

Ruff, H.A. (1984). Infants' manipulative exploration of objects: Effects of age and object characteristics. *Developmental Psychology, 20*(1), 9-20.

Ruff, H.A., & Kohler, C.J. (1978). Tactual-visual transfer in six-month-old infants. *Infant Behavior and Development, 1,* 259-264.

Schneck, C., & Henderson, A. (1990). Descriptive analysis of the developmental progression of grip position for pencil and crayon control in nondysfunctional children. *American Journal of Occupational Therapy, 44*(10), 893-900.

Steele, D., & Pederson, D.R. (1977). Stimulus variables which affect the concordance of visual and manipulative exploration in six-month-old infants. *Child Development, 48,* 104-111.

Twitchell, T.E. (1965). Normal motor development. *Journal of the American Physical Therapy Association, 45,* 419-423.

Twitchell, T.E. (1970). Reflex mechanisms and the development of prehension. In K. Connolly (Ed.). *Mechanisms of motor skill development.* London: Academic Press.

White, B.L., Castle, P., & Held, R. (1964). Observations on the development of visually directed reaching. *Child Development, 35,* 349-364.

Zelazo, P., & Kearsley, R. (1980). The emergence of functional play in infants: Evidence for a major cognitive transition. *Journal of Applied Developmental Psychology, 1,* 95-117.

8

Object Manipulation in Infants and Children

Charlane Pehoski

The hand is a wonderful tool that has as its primary purpose the exploration and manipulation of objects. The development of the hand in the service of object manipulation follows a long course. It is one of the ways children experience success and the perception of competence. Bruner (1973) points out that competence includes not only social interaction but also mastery over objects.

How the child gradually gains control over the hand to manipulate objects is the theme of this chapter. Infancy appears to be a time when reach is perfected and the basic grasp patterns are developed. At first the infant can manipulate objects only by waving the arm and moving the wrist since the object is held in a power grip that fixes it in the hand (Napier, 1956). Gaining the ability to transfer an object hand to hand greatly expands the actions the infant can produce with the object. But it is the appearance of a precision grip (pad of radial fingers to pad of thumb) that marks a major change in the eventual skills of the hand. Landsmeer (1962) indicates that the purpose of a precision grip is to "operate the object with precision by means of the fingers." As we will see, the perfection of this skill covers a long developmental period. Voluntary release (such as releasing an object in a predetermined place) also develops in late infancy and is an important component to skilled object interaction. Like object release, many of the basic components for skilled hand use are seen during infancy, but their perfection takes many years. As an example, the child must learn to control the release of an object so he/she can place it with skill and accuracy. In-hand manipulation skills, or the movement of an object in the hand after grasp, need to be acquired, and although the infant has the rudiments of two-hand use, the ability to plan the movements of both hands at the same time is not yet present.

This chapter discusses what is known about the development of these components. There are many gaps in our understanding of the changes that are happening and how these might have an impact on the child's gradual mastery of the physical world. Given the importance of object manipulation to human behavior, it is interesting that so little has been done to study this motor skill. In looking at what has been written, we divided the children into four age groups: infancy (neonate to 12 months), toddler years (12 months to 2 years of age), preschool/early childhood years (3 to 6 years of age), and the older child. In addition, themes that might help us understand the direction skilled hand use is taking at each of these stages are also explored.

One last note, the hand is the tool of the mind. It is the mind that directs and guides the hand. Object exploration or manipulation is the result of our desire to master the physical world. In infancy the basic drive to explore the world is present and, although the infant's physical skills are limited, these skills are used to gain information about object properties. It is very probable that this drive sets the stage for all future object exploration and the continued drive toward mastery.

OBJECT MANIPULATION DURING INFANCY

Manipulation implies that the movement of the object is done to achieve some purpose or goal, that is, that the individual is consciously engaged in the activity and directing the action. By this definition, there was a time when researchers would not have considered studying object "manipulation" in the very young infant. Neonates and young infants were considered to be primitive beings dominated by reflexes that would gradually be integrated so the infant could engage the world. More recent research has been guided by the belief that infants are born curious and with a drive to explore their universe, admittedly within the limitations of their physical capabilities. As an example, if properly supported and alert, neonates will reach toward a

visually captured object (Bower, Broughton, and Moore, 1970; von Hofsten, 1982). Although this behavior has been termed prereaching (Trevarthen, 1974) or prefunctional (von Hofsten, 1982), it is voluntary and has a purposfulness not seen in more reflexive behaviors.

Movements Used in Object Exploration By Infants

We are therefore born with the drive to reach out and explore the physical world. Even as a neonate, the infant uses primitive motor skills to begin this process. Although the neonate may be able to accomplish a primitive form of reach, he/she does not yet have voluntary control over the grasp of an object but will hold an object placed in the hand. For the young infant the mouth also appears to be an instrument of grasp or exploration. Rochat (1987) looked at the neonate's use of the hand and the mouth to explore or differentiate object properties. He addressed this question by looking at the reaction of neonates to a soft or rigid object placed in either the mouth or the hand. Newborn infants (49 to 96 hours of age) were presented with either a soft foam or rigid plastic tube, which was placed in their hand for grasp or in their mouth for sucking. The tubes were attached to a transducer, which was able to monitor the amount of pressure the infants applied to the two different objects. When grasped with the hand, the hard object was associated with significantly more squeezes than the soft object. When it was placed in the mouth, the reverse was seen. Obviously the infants were responding to differences in the flexibility of the object. The author suggests that the hand appears to be more concerned with the graspability of an object and the mouth with suckability. He also states that this "supports the idea of an early detection of what objects afford for functional action"; that is, the hand and the mouth are tuned from the very beginning to actively explore an object's functional properties.

The object manipulation of the infant under 4 months of age is of necessity limited since reach and grasp are still quite primitive. Yet if an object is placed in the infant's hand or the infant happens to grasp an object once in contact with it, some attempts to explore the object's characteristics appear to be present. At this age all objects are held static in a palmer grasp or a power grip (Napier, 1956). Therefore all manipulation of the object must come from the shoulder, elbow, or wrist since the object is fixed in the hand. This is particularly true when two-hand use is not yet present (the object can not yet be transferred hand to hand).

Based on the observation of infants from 1 month to about 10 to 12 months of age, Karniol (1989) proposed 10 stages in the early object exploration of the infant (see box opposite). Three of these stages were related to the infant under 4 months. If an object was placed in the hand of a 2- to 3-month-old infant, the earliest engagement Karniol noted was that the infant would rotate or twist the wrist but only if the object happened to be visible to the infant. If the hand was not visible, the object was dropped.

The next actions to develop in Karniol's schema were translation movements, or a deliberate effort to change the location of an object by moving the arm toward or away from the body. Often this involved bringing an object to the mouth or was combined with rotation. Karniol feels that these movements assist the infant in combining changes in the retinal image of the object with proprioceptive feedback from the arm.

The third method of engagement that Karniol observed in the very young infant was a movement she called vibration. She defines this as rapid, periodic movements of an object by repeated bending of the arm. If the object produced noise, the motion might be maintained or be more vigorous. If the object did not make noise, it might be translated, rotated, and visually examined before being dropped. Therefore it would appear that the very young infant will manipulate objects if they are placed in the hand, but this manipulation is limited to movements of the arm and wrist.

At about 4 months of age the infant still uses a mass grasp on objects, but reach is becoming more functional. It is also important that the infant can now bring both hands together to engage the object at midline. This ability expands the action that can be taken on objects and is a necessary first stage of "complementary two-hand use" (Bruner, 1970). Midline behavior is facilitated by changes in the general control of the arm and the body itself. There is better balance in the trunk and neck flexor and extensors, so the head is held in midline and the child can tuck the chin to better observe the hands. By 4 months the child can also lie on his/her back and bring the hands together up into the space above the body (Bly, 1980). This ability to bring the two hands together is used by the infant in exploring objects.

Ten Stages in the Development of Object Manipulation in Infancy

ONE TO THREE MONTHS
Stage 1: Rotation: An object is moved by twists of the wrist.

Stage 2: Translation: Movements of the arm that change the location of an object by increasing or decreasing the distance from self.

Stage 3: Vibration: Repeated, rapid bending motions of the arm as the object is held.

THREE TO FOUR MONTHS
Stage 4: Bilateral hold: The object is held passively in one hand as the other hand holds or does something else to another object.

Stage 5: Two-handed hold: Single object held with both hands.

Stage 6: Hand-to-hand transfer: An object held in one hand is transferred to the other.

FIVE MONTHS
Stage 7: Coordinated action with single object: One hand holds the object stationary and the other hand does something to it (e.g., strokes a doll or pulls at the hair).

SIX TO NINE MONTHS
Stage 8: Coordinated action with two objects: Manipulation of two objects, each held in a separate hand, such as hitting two blocks together.

Stage 9: Deformations: The object is made to change shape such as tearing paper or pressing a toy to make a sound.

Stage 10: Instrumental sequential actions: The sequential use of two hands in obtaining a goal, as demonstrated when the infant lifts a cup to obtain a cube.

Data from Karniol, R. (1989). The role of manual manipulative stages in the infant's acquisition of perceived control over objects. *Developmental Review, 9,* 222-225.

At 3 to 4 months, Karniol (1989) adds bilateral hold and two-handed hold to the list of options available to the infant; that is, the infant can hold an object while the other hand does something else or hold the object using two hands. In a study of the object manipulation and exploration of 2-, 3-, 4-, and 5-month-old infants, Rochat (1989) saw an increase in mouthing in the 4- to 5-month-old infants over the 2- to 3-month-olds, a behavior he found significantly associated with two-handed grasp. Two-hand support for an object may there-fore assist the infant's attempts to mouth objects, increasing the likelihood of this form of exploration occurring. Once midline engagement of the hands is developed, manipulation is also assisted by allowing one hand to hold and the other to explore the surface of the object with the fingers. Rochat (1989) also saw an increase in this fingering behavior in his 4-month-old subjects.

Further object exploration is possible around 5 to 6 months of age, when the infant is able to transfer an object hand to hand. This is an important complementary two-hand use stage. Karniol (1989) indicates that, when this action is first seen, the infant often rotates the wrist and bends the arm with the object in one hand and then transfers it to the other hand and repeats the action. In recording the infant's exploratory actions during a 90-second segment with a toy, Rochat (1989) found that the 5-month-old infants in his study transferred the toy a mean of three times, whereas the 2-, 3-, and 4-month-old infants transferred the toy a mean of less than once per trial. Therefore, like Karniol's infants, Rochat's infants began to incorporate hand-to-hand transfer into their exploratory play at about 5 months of age.

By 6 months of age infants now have a variety of actions at their disposal by which they explore and manipulate objects. They can mouth, look, rotate, wave, bang, finger (run the fingers over the surface of an object), and transfer the object hand to hand. But grasp at this stage is still dominated by a power grip. The thumb may be opposed to the finger when picking up an object such as a block (Halverson, 1931), but, when a smaller object is grasped, the fingers and thumb work together so the object is raked into the hand. By 9 to 10 months a major change occurs, and infants can now isolate the movements of the index finger and thumb from other movements of the hand and fingers. They can poke with the index finger and pick up a small object in a precision grip between the radial fingers and the thumb (Bayley, 1969; Folio and Fewell, 1983). When studying 6-, 9-, and 12-month-old infants, Ruff (1984) found an increase in fingering behavior in the older infants (running the fingers over the surface of an object), a function she felt was facilitated by the increased independence of the fingers and increased coordination of the two hands. Grasp of an object, such as a cube, has also changed; the cube can now be held with the fingers acting independent of the palm, so the object no longer needs to be pressed against the palm but can be held out on the finger

surface (Halverson, 1931). The ability to move the object out onto the finger surface, the development of a precision grip, and the beginning of the differentiation of individual fingers are critical to the further development of skilled manipulation by the hand.

Another important development during this period is the beginning of controlled release. As an example, it is also at about 9 to 10 months that infants can release a cube into a cup (Bayley, 1969; Folio and Fewell, 1983).

Therefore, since infants' exploratory actions become more refined as they gain better control over the motor abilities, the variety of actions that can be taken on an object increases. Infants use these motor skills to explore the properties of the objects they grasp. That is, infants' actions with objects are not purely random but have the characteristics of true exploration.

Exploratory Nature of Infant Object Manipulation

Steele and Pederson (1977) looked at the difference in manipulation with changes in object properties in 6-month-old infants. They measured the amount of visual fixation on the object as well as the amount of manipulation. Manipulation in this study was defined as any contact between the infant's hand and the object. No attempt was made to further define the type of manipulation. Familiar objects the infant had previously manipulated and novel objects were used. The authors found an increase in looking and manipulating with novel over familiar objects and also an increase in manipulation to changes in shape and texture but not to color. Of these two variables, texture elicited more manipulative behavior from the infants than changes in shape. The authors concluded that "the results indicate that an object that presents different tactile sensations is necessary to produce different manipulative behaviors" (p. 109).

Ruff (1984) also looked at how infants responded to different object characteristics. In this study, infants of 6, 9, and 12 months of age were presented with two sets of blocks that varied in color and pattern; more importantly, they also varied in surface texture and shape. Of interest was the observation that the infants tended to adjust their manipulative behavior to the different physical characteristics of the objects; that is, they mouthed and transferred the object more in the shape series and did more fingering in the texture series (such as blocks with bumps and depressions).

In addition, with increasing familiarity with an object, these exploratory actions on the object decreased. This included looking, handling, rotating, transferring, and fingering. One behavior—banging the object—did not decrease over time. The author suggests that this activity may represent a play behavior unrelated to object exploration. This was also found by Ruff et al. (1992), who further suggest that certain types of mouthing may not be related to true object exploration.

Object Exploration by The Mouth and Hand

In early infancy object exploration by both the mouth and hand is a major component in the infant's interaction with objects, particularly the infant 7 months of age and younger. Ruff et al. (1992) indicate that in their study mouthing behavior peaked at about 7 months of age and comprised 27% of the time the infant was engaged with an object. This fell to 17% for 11-month-old infants. Ruff (1984) suggested that the decrease in mouthing may be due to a better haptic system becoming available in the hand.

Ruff et al. (1992) looked at the exploratory behavior of both the hands and the mouth in 5- to 11-month-old infants. They describe what they called active mouthing and distinguish this from more general actions of objects in the mouth. Active mouthing was defined as movements of the object in the mouth by the hand (such as being turned in the mouth) or when the mouth moved over the object. The authors found a significant association between active mouthing and then immediately looking at the object, but not other forms of object-mouth interaction (such as just holding the object in the mouth). After a bout of active mouthing the infant would immediately pause to look at the object. They hypothesized that mouthing with looking might serve an exploratory or information-gathering function. To study this further, they presented infants with familiar and novel objects and noted the forms of exploration used in the two situations. They found that mouthing with looking and manual actions such as turning the object, transferring hand to hand, and fingering all declined as the infant became familiar with the object but returned when the infant was presented with a novel toy. They, therefore, suggest that these actions are truly exploratory and a means of gathering information about objects. Other actions, such as mouthing without looking, banging, and waving, did not significantly decline

in frequency as the infants became familiar with the object, and they indicate that these actions may therefore serve some other function.

Role of Vision in Infant Object Manipulation

Up to this point we have discussed changes in the motor system that provide the infant with mechanisms by which object manipulation and exploration can happen. We have also indicated that even at the youngest ages infants appear to use the motor skills available to them to explore object characteristics. Also important to the object exploration of infants is consideration of the role vision plays in driving and supporting this behavior.

Blind infants are significantly delayed in their object exploration when compared with sighted peers. Fraiberg (1968) indicated that blind infants do not spontaneously bring their hands to midline for mutual fingering, as seen in the 4-month-old sighted child. She argued "that there is good reason to believe that the mutual fingering games and the organization of the hands at midline are largely facilitated by vision and that the tactile engagement of the fingers requires simultaneous visual experience to insure its pleasurable repetition" (p. 281). She also indicated that the hands of the blind infant do not explore objects, but serve primarily to bring the object to the mouth.

It would therefore appear that, for the normally sighted infant, vision is an important motivator that leads the hand into space and serves to facilitate grasp and manipulation. As indicated above, Karniol (1989) found that when a 2-month-old infant grasped an object, he/she would also rotate it but only if the hand could be seen. If the hand was out of visual regard, the object would be dropped. In his study of 2- to 5-month-old infants, Rochat (1989) looked at what infants did first with an object. Did they immediately bring it to the mouth or did they first bring it to the eyes to look at it? (The infants were all seated in slightly reclining infant seats). He found that at 2 to 3 months over two thirds of the infants first brought the object to the mouth. At 4 to 5 months the majority of the infants first brought the object into the field of vision for inspection. This was particularly true of the 5-month-old infants, where visual exploration was used first in 90% of the sample.

Hatwell (1987) stated that after 5 months manual activity is closely controlled by vision. She indicated that at this age manual inspection is so tightly linked to vision that, if the infants cannot see their hands, their performance is greatly curtailed. As an example, some of the infants she tested refused to close the hand on an object when the hand was hidden under a screen. The 5- and 6-month-old infants did not attempt to remove the screen or fuss but simply did not close their hand on the object. Some older infants 7 to 15 months of age did attempt to remove the screen, and, when this was not possible, they began to fuss. In all, she indicated that 60% of the infants could not be tested on an intermodal haptic task using a screen to shield the hands from vision. It was not until 20 months that 80% of the infants accepted the screen.

Rochat (1989) also indicated that fingering of an object by infants may be linked to vision. In one study using 2-, 3-, 4-, and 5-month-old infants, the author found a significant interaction between fingering and looking. To test this interaction further, he studied a different set of 3-, 4-, and 5-month-old infants as they manipulated objects in dark and light situations. The dark situation was accomplished using an infrared light and a video camera sensitive to this light. He found that fingering was dramatically decreased in the dark situation, whereas the incidence of mouthing and hand-to-hand transfer remained the same in the two experimental conditions. The author indicated that early fingering therefore appears to be linked to vision and depends on this modality. Alternately, mouthing appears to be independent of vision, and in this study early hand-to-hand transfer also did not appear to depend on vision.

It would therefore appear that, at least in younger infants, vision is an integral part of the process of grasp and manipulation and in fact may be the early motivator for object exploration and drive some of the more refined manipulative actions such as fingering of an object.

Handling Multiple Objects

Effective object manipulation also requires that the infant solve the problems of how to deal with more than one object at a time. Bruner (1970) attempted to look at what he called "taking possession of objects" by presenting infants with a small toy and then presenting a second toy to the same hand. If the infant did not make an attempt to secure the second toy, it was then held at midline. After two toys were grasped, the infant was handed a third and fourth toy and the child's

solution to this multiple object problem observed. Bruner found that the 4- to 5-month-old infants had difficulty managing two objects. Often, as the infant's attention was attracted to the second toy, the toy in hand would be dropped. The 6- to 8-month-olds were able to solve the two-toy problem by transferring the initial toy to the other hand and then grasping the second toy.

Solving the problem of three objects required a different strategy that was not seen until 9 to 11 months; that is, when offered the third object, the older infants "stored" one of the objects he/she had been holding on the table or lap. But half the infants of this age then retrieved the stored object immediately. They did not appear to be able to inhibit the drive to pick up what they saw or could not delay this process. By 12 months the infants had the solution of this problem well "in hand." They not only transferred the first object to the other hand in anticipation of receiving the second object but also anticipated the third and fourth by storing the toys in hand in the lap or the arm of the chair. By 15 to 17 months the infants also stored by handing objects to the parent or to the examiner. By 12 months and older, therefore, infants have learned to deal with several items at one time.

Summary and Therapeutic Implications

As infants gain increasing control over the movements of the arm and the hands, they also increase the options available to them for object exploration. In the very young infant objects are fixed in the hand, and exploration is limited to movements of the arm and wrist. An important expansion of the actions available to infants comes when they can bring both hands together and eventually transfer an object from one hand to the other. The infant can now wave, bang, mouth, transfer, rotate, and run fingers over an object's surface. The ability to manage more than one object at a time is also an important aspect of object interaction, and infants appear to gradually accomplish this skill over the first 12 months of life. During this period infants also develop two other extremely important skills: (1) control over voluntary release or placement of an object and (2) the ability to use a precision or refined pincer grip. This latter skill is critical to the further development of object manipulation by the hand.

From a therapeutic point of view, it is important to note that changes in object properties seem to elicit different manipulative behaviors from infants. As an example, changes in shape appear to generate more transferring and rotation activities, and changes in texture more fingering and possibly an increase in the duration of manipulation. Often parents and others who interact with infants see the infant's mouthing, turning, and handling of objects as random motions. But as indicated, at least some of these movements appear to be meaningful attempts to explore object properties. This is important information to consider when evaluating and planning programs for a child. Pointing out to a parent or caregiver how the infant changes manipulative strategies with changes in object properties can help them appreciate the infant's competencies and the importance of these actions to the infant's learning. Providing the infant with a variety of objects that differ in shape and texture may well facilitate this process.

In observing infants, it is also important to note when they do not show the variety of exploratory behaviors appropriate for their age. As indicated, waving, banging, and some forms of mouthing may not serve the same exploratory functions as activities such as transferring hand to hand, fingering, rotating, and active mouthing. Ruff et al. (1984) state that

the infant who does not finger, rotate, and transfer objects very much has less opportunity to learn about object properties. We can speculate that the less infants learn about object properties the less they will engage in categorization of objects. Any deficit in categorization should affect early language development. In this way it is possible for manipulative exploration of objects to contribute directly to an infant's cognitive development (p. 1173).

Several studies (Nelson, 1979; Ross, 1985; Ross, Lipper, and Audel, 1986; Ruddy and Bernstein, 1982; Thun-Hohenstein et al., 1991) have found preterm infants to score lower than term infants on eye-hand and fine motor items of developmental tests. Kopp (1976) found preterm infants to differ significantly from full-term infants on the duration of exploratory activity. In another study (1974) this same author found a greater percentage of preterm infants (age corrected for prematurity) to be clumsy in object manipulation when compared to term infants (70% of the preterm infants and 19% of the term infants). The clumsy infants were also noted to spend less time manually exploring objects and more time in visual exploration.

Ruff et al. (1984) also studied the manipulative abilities of preterm and term infants. They divided the preterm infants into high- and low-risk groups depending on the infants' early medical history. They then compared these two groups to a group of full-term infants (preterm infants' age, corrected for prematurity). They found a significant decrease in the incidence and amount of fingering, transfer, and rotation of objects in the high-risk group compared to the two other infant groups.

The quality of an infant's object interaction can therefore provide important observational information and assist in providing caregivers with suggestions for an infant's continued development. Infants learn about their physical world through their manipulative actions. These activities offer the infant an opportunity to experience a sense of success and mastery and may provide experiences on which later cognitive strategies can be based. These experiences may not be readily available to the physically handicapped infant, and this child needs to be assisted through proper positioning and the selection of appropriate toys.

The role of vision in guiding infant exploration has also been noted. In young infants it may be a driving force, motivating them to interact with the objects in their world. Infants with poor vision or those who seem to lack a good link between the eyes and the hand (such as an infant or child who does not appear to watch what the hands are doing) should be provided assistance in object manipulation.

OBJECT MANIPULATION DURING THE TODDLER YEARS

Compared to those of the infant, the manipulative skills of the toddler show great strides in development. Unfortunately, we know this more from intuition than actual research. Toddlers can do more than "grasp" an object—they are beginning to be able to manipulate the object in the fingers and the hand. Release of an object has also improved, and these two skills allow the child to interact effectively with smaller objects. It is also at this age that children start to demonstrate complementary two-hand use, greatly expanding their manipulative abilities. Each of these areas will be explored.

Beginning of In-Hand Manipulation

In discussing the fine motor abilities of the 12-month-old child, Gesell et al. (1940) stated that the child's "prehensory patterns are approaching adult facility. . . . fine prehension is deft and direct." That is, the child has a neat pincer grasp and can use it with skill. As indicated, this is an important achievement for the child, but these prehensory patterns must be changed to manipulatory patterns for true hand skill to develop. As an example, 12-month-old infants can pick up a small object such as a Cheerio very well, but if provided with several Cheerios in the hand, their manipulatory skills are challenged. Young children generally solve this problem by bringing the entire hand to the mouth rather than moving the object within the hand. Therefore one of the tasks in the next few years is to take the "deft and direct" prehension patterns they have learned and develop the capacity to manipulate objects in the fingers and in the hand.

Exner (1989, 1990, 1992) has called this ability in-hand manipulation, or the adjustment of an object in the hand after grasp. The purpose of these adjustments is to allow more efficient placement of the object in the hand for use or for voluntary release. Three components of this skill have been defined. One is the ability to move an object from the fingers to the palm, or the palm to the fingers (such as picking up a coin and placing it in the hand and then moving the coin from the hand to the fingers for placement in a bank or purse). Exner refers to these as translation movements. Another component is the ability to rotate the object in the pads of the fingers, either through simple rotation, where the object is rolled or turned in the fingers, or more complex rotation movements. In more complex rotation movements the object is generally rotated at least 180 degrees, and the movement requires independent action of the fingers and thumb. The third component is shift, or the movement of an object in a linear direction on the finger surface. The thumb often performs most of this movement with reciprocal movements of the radial fingers such as moving a pencil after it has been grasped so the fingers are closer to the point (Exner, 1990a). In addition, these activities can also be accomplished while another object is stabilized in the hand. An example of a palm-to-finger movement with stabilization is when several small objects are held in the hand and one of them is moved to the fingers for placement, such as when one of several Cheerios is moved from the palm to the fingers for placement in the mouth. Children in the toddler years are not yet adept at all components of in-hand manipulation.

In her original pilot study, Exner (1990) looked at the in-hand manipulation skills of 90 children between the ages of 18 months to 6 years 11 months. The developmental trend in these skills indicated that moving an object like a small peg from the fingers to the palm for storage, then moving it back out to the fingers, and simple rotation were three of the easiest tasks and were accomplished by at least half of the 18-month-old to 2-year-old children in her study. Other tasks, such as the complex rotation of a pen in the fingers so the point is in a position for use, were more difficult and not accomplished until the preschool years (Table 8-1). Exner (1990) indicates that skills which do not involve simultaneous stabilization of materials during in-hand manipulation activities are easier than those where the child must control both sides of the hand (ulnar side to hold and radial side to manipulate).

Exner (1992) also indicates that the amount of individual finger movements required for a task may make one component of in-hand manipulation more difficult than another; that is, the ability to move an object such as a peg from the fingers to the palm is a relatively easy task since the fingers tend to work as a unit. Rotating a pen in the fingers for use, however, requires the sequencing of individual movements among the radial fingers and the thumb. Although the 12-month-old child has the ability to isolate the index finger and can use the index finger or radial fingers and thumb to pick up a small object, there is reason to believe that further isolation of finger movements is still difficult for the child under 3.

As an example, Stutsman (1948) looked at the ability of young children to make a fist and wiggle the thumb without moving the fingers. She states that this task "appears rather suddenly at 33 months." Gesell et al. (1940) also talked about the ability to wiggle the thumb (or voluntarily isolate the movements of the thumb) as being a skill observed in 2-year-old children. The ability to move the fingers individually seems to come later. When Stutsman (1948) asked young children to oppose each finger to the thumb, she found that this was possible for only three children between 30 and 36 months of age. By 36 to 41 months 35% of the children accomplished the task, but it was not until 42 to 47 months that 50% of the children were successful. It would appear that isolated movements of individual fingers are difficult for children 3 years of age and under, and this may be a major deterrent to the ability to accomplish deft and direct manipulatory patterns of objects in the fingers.

Another factor that may limit the toddler's in-hand manipulation skills is the force of the grip used to hold an object. When the grip strength was measured as children and adults picked up a small

Table 8-1. Pilot study on the development of in-hand manipulation skills in children 18 months to 6 years of age

AGES (YEARS)	SKILLS OBSERVED IN 50% OR MORE OF SUBJECTS
1.5-2.0	Finger-to-palm translation using small pegs
	Complex rotation with jar lid placed upside down on table
2.0-2.4	Palm-to-finger translation when a key was placed in the palm of the hand
	Palm-to-finger translation with a small peg
	Simple rotation with jar lid on jar
	Simple rotation with small peg
	Complex rotation with peg-like toy dolls
	Finger-to-palm translation with stabilization with small pegs
	Shift with palmar stabilization with eraser placed in a small box
2.5-2.9	Complex rotation with small pegs
3.0-3.4	Shift when page turning
	Finger-to-palm translation with stabilization using a 1½ inch cube and other medium-sized objects
3.5-3.9	Simple rotation of pen (tip oriented ulnarly)
4.0-4.4	Shift of pen after tip oriented ulnarly
4.5-4.9	Shift of pen after tip oriented radially
5.0-5.4	Palm-to-finger translation with stabilization with small peg
	Complex rotation of pen after tip oriented radially
5.5-5.9	No new skills demonstrated
6.0-6.4	Complex rotation with palmar stabilization with small peg
6.5-6.9	No new skills demonstrated

Modified from Exner, C. E. (1990). In-hand manipulation skills in normal young children: A pilot study. *Occupational Therapy Practice, 4,* 68. Additional data from Exner, C. E.. Personal communication.

object between the thumb and index finger, children were observed to use greater grip force than adults (Forssberg et al., 1991; see also Chapter 3). This was particularly true for children 5 years or younger. When the steps necessary to prepare to lift this small object were also carefully measured with instruments sensitive to changes not observable to the eye, it was found that it took longer for young children to prepare to lift the object. Children 8 months of age (the youngest group of infants studied) to 18 months demonstrated a significantly longer time from when the lead finger/thumb touched the block to when the second finger/thumb arrived. Small children were also noted to contact the object several times before a stable grip was established, and they also had a tendency to push down as they were gripping. Forssberg et al. (1991) indicated that this preparatory stage was three times longer in infants under 10 months and about twice as long in children under 3 years.

Therefore, if young children have difficulty isolating finger movements, are slow in preparing for a grip (at a micro level), and also tend to grip objects harder in their fingers than adults, in-hand manipulation skills that require the grasp and release of an object and the coordination of these

movements among different fingers are going to be quite difficult or impossible. As an example, fasteners on clothes, particularly buttons, require manipulation skills by the fingers. For many children under 3 years of age, this is a difficult task. Another task that requires isolated movements of the fingers is the ability to move a pencil or writing implement in a dynamic tripod grip (Rosenbloom and Horton, 1971). This is also difficult for many children under 3 years of age (Rosenbloom and Horton, 1971; Saida and Miyashita, 1979). Despite these limitations, the toddler is beginning to experiment with simple in-hand manipulation tasks such as picking up and storing several objects in the hand. As the child gains more control over the movement of individual fingers and refines the force of grip, these functions improve.

Control Over Object Release

The child between 12 months and 2 years of age is also gaining control over the release of objects. This is an area that has not been widely studied, even though Gesell et al. (1940) state that release is "one of the most difficult prehensile activities to master in early life." These authors point out that it is the inability to release a cube properly that often causes the infant to fail when attempting to build a two-block tower. At 2 years of age, when the child can build a tower of several blocks, the child may press rather than place the block, often with enough force that the structure falls. The authors also note that, even at 3 years of age, the child may still have difficulty with release on more delicate tasks. For instance, the child may pull the lace out when the hand is pulled away while lacing shoes. Controlled release is an important component of object manipulation. In many in-hand manipulation tasks the object is grasped and then repositioned by delicate grasp-release movements of the fingers. The development of this ability, particularly the ability to release without the need to press down or use a supporting surface and to remove the fingers from the object surface with correct timing, is an area for valuable future research.

Complementary Two-Hand Use

An important skill that develops between 12 months and 2 years of age is complementary two-hand use (Bruner, 1970). As indicated in the previous section, the infant's ability to use two hands in the manipulation of an object greatly expands the exploratory options available. But being able to hold an object in each hand, or even the ability to hold an object in one hand while acting on this object or manipulating another, does not take advantage of the potential skill achieved when *both* hands are active at the same time. This requires that the child be able to program or motor plan different but complementary actions with the two hands. This ability is more than just programming a holding function for one hand and a doing function for the other. It involves the monitoring of active movements of both hands at the same time. There is reason to suspect that this skill is not present until 2 years of age. To look at the development of complementary two-hand use, we need to step back and briefly look at the younger infant to observe the transition to higher-level activities.

Bruner (1970) studied the early acquisition of this skill in infants 6 to 17 months of age. He presented the infants with a box that required them to hold open a sliding, transparent lid to obtain a toy. Bruner found that the 6- to 8-month-old infants in his study would tend to just bang or claw at the lid itself. In fact, this activity often appeared to distract the infant from the toy, and banging

became the main activity of interest. He indicated that this behavior was also common in 9- to 11-month-old infants. In addition, another very common behavior of infants of this age was to open and close the lid, becoming distracted by this activity and not attempting to retrieve the toy. Another behavior that was seen in these younger infants was the opening of the lid with one hand and then slipping the same hand into the box with the other hand not participating at all. At 12 to 14 months the infants added another approach to the solution of the problem—to raise the lid with one or two hands and go after the toy with the free hand but to let go of the lid during the retrieval attempt. Even at 17 months, which was the oldest group of infants studied, the activity was not yet well mastered.

Ramsay and Weber (1986) used a similar task in looking at this skill in 12- and 13-month-old infants compared with 17- and 18-month-olds. They found their infants to be a bit more competent than Bruner's (1970), which in part may have been related to differences in the testing apparatus. Ramsay and Weber also had a box with a transparent lid, but this lid was hinged and lifted rather than pushed open. Another difference was that the transparent lid in Ramsay and Weber's study was furnished with a white knob. This may have provided the children with a clue as to how to solve the problem. Ramsay and Weber state that in their study use of only one hand was rare and seen only in the younger age group. The most common method of approach was to lift and hold the lid with one hand and to retrieve the toy with the other hand. They found this approach to be used an average of 50% of the time in the 12- to 13-month-old children and 78% of the time in the 17- to 19-month-old group. The younger children also used a strategy in which both hands would open the lid, and then one hand would hold as the other hand retrieved the toy. This was seen an average of 37% of the time in the younger group and only 12% of the time in the older infants. Another strategy that was used almost equally by both groups of infants was to lift the lid with one hand, then transfer the hold of the lid to the free hand, and to retrieve the toy with the hand that originally opened the lid (used 13% of the time by the younger infants and 10% of the time for the older group).

Ramsay and Weber (1986) also looked at whether the right or left hand was used to reach for the toy. In the younger age group 74% of the time it was the right hand that reached for the toy. The left hand appeared to have the more passive role of holding open the lid. In the older children the left hand appears to have assumed more importance. The left hand was used to reach for the toy 57% of the time, and the right hand was used 43% of the time. The authors indicate that this change in the active use of the left hand in the older children might reflect the progressive ability of the dominant hemisphere to control the sequencing of movements for both the right and left hand. That is, by 17 months to 19 months it would appear that the child can accomplish a holding task with one hand while reaching or doing something else with the other hand. Of interest was the gradual emergence of both hands having an equal opportunity to participate in the "doing" component of the activity rather than a tendency for this action to be completed by the right hand, a function that Ramsay and Weber suspected might be related to the development of bilateral control of sequenced movements by the right hemisphere (hemisphere implicated in praxic or sequencing of motor movements). One wonders if this is a transition step to the next level of skill, the ability to sequence or plan movements of *both* hands at the same time.

Stutsman (1948) has commented on this function in children. She states that the "inability to perform different movements with the two hands at the same time seems to be characteristic of the child under 36 months of age." One of the tasks she presented to young children was to give them a long string attached to a toy that was lying on the floor. The child was instructed to pull in the string to attempt to get the toy. Unsuccessful attempts included walking over to pick up the toy or only yanking the arm back to partially move the toy forward. The problem was correctly solved only when the child managed to pull in the string hand over hand to obtain the toy. She found that 90% of the 30- to 35-month-old children in the normative sample were able to solve the problem, 60% at 24 to 29 months, but only 22% at 18 to 23 months. In discussing this task she states, "This test should rank among those tests for young children which tend to show the growing ability to successfully use the two hands" (p. 168).

Another task that requires complementary use of two hands is bead stringing. Often young children who are unsuccessful on this task seem to have the idea of how to proceed but have difficulty with the complementary two-handed use aspect of the task. They place the string correctly into the bead but then do not seem to know how to transfer the activity between the two hands to complete the

task. Almost all studies place the successful accomplishment of bead stringing at 2 years of age (DuBose and Langley, 1977; Gesell et al., 1940; Folio and Fewell, 1983). As an example, in the *Peabody Developmental Motor Scales* (Folio and Fewell, 1983) the ability of young children to string three beads is examined. The authors found that this task could be accomplished by only 16% of the 18- to 23-month-old children in the normative sample, but by 70% of the children between 24 and 29 months of age, a significant change in behavior over a relatively short time. It would appear that something has happened that allows this task to be successfully completed. It is probable that a major factor in this success is the emergence of complementary two-hand use.

Summary and Therapeutic Implications

The child at 12 months to 2 years of age has made marked strides in the development of the control necessary for refined object manipulation by the hand when compared to the infant. The child is beginning to develop in-hand manipulation skills, which will be facilitated as the child gains increasing ability to isolate the movements of individual fingers and when the force of grasp is better controlled. The child has also gained marked control over the release of objects when compared to the infant, and the child can now use both hands together in a complementary fashion.

Children at this age enjoy picking up and manipulating small items; once they are past the mouthing stage they will appreciate the opportunity to explore their ability to pick up and hold several small objects in their hand. Besides having large dolls or trucks available to play with, the child can also be furnished with small trucks and dolls that require more delicate movements of the hand. Release can also be practiced by standing up small peg dolls in a row.

This is also a time when complementary two-hand use is developing and the child may enjoy the opportunity to practice these skills. Placing items in a purse or bag necessitates interaction between the two hands, since the activity is often not successful unless the holding hand is also active during the process. Bilateral hand skills also make dressing oneself possible. Children can now coordinate the use of two hands to pull up their pants or put on a sock.

Object size needs to be considered. Exner (1990a) found that the manipulative abilities of small children were affected by the size of the objects presented. She found that, in general, tiny (1/2-inch peg) or medium (1-inch cube) objects were more difficult to handle than an object such as a key. Connolly (1973) also found differences in children's grip patterns based on differences in object size. Newell et al. (1989) looked specifically at the effect of object size in relation to hand size in children 3 years 3 months to 5 years 4 months when compared with adults. The subjects were asked to pick up boxes of varying size (0.08 to 24.2 cm) and place them in another slightly larger box. The authors found that young children and adults predominantly use the same grip pattern when the object is scaled to the size of the hand. Object size should therefore be a part of the thinking when planning activities for small children.

OBJECT MANIPULATION IN THE PRESCHOOL AND EARLY CHILDHOOD YEARS

Three through 6 years of age appears to be a time when the child is gaining control over the intrinsic movements of the hand. One of the major changes seen during this period is the continued emergence of in-hand manipulation skills. This ability will greatly expand the activities the child can accomplish. For example, between 3 and 7 years the child learns to deal with the fasteners on clothes, cut, paste, and manipulate a writing instrument. These tasks require both the cooperation between the two hands and the ability to manipulate objects in the fingers and hand.

Studies of In-Hand Manipulation

One of the representative manipulative skills that has been studied during this age period is buttoning. Stutsman (1948) indicated that no child in her normative sample who was under 23 months of age was able to manage the button on a one-button strip, and only 9% at 24 and 29 months successfully completed this task. This is not surprising given what we have previously discussed about the difficulty children of this age have in differentiating the movements of individual fingers. She found a major change in the ability of the 30- to 35-month-old children. In this age group 72% of the sample was successful.

Despite the 30- to 35-month-old children's ability to perform the task, their efficiency or speed was markedly different from that of older children. For example, Stutsman found that it took an average of 170 seconds for the children in her

30- to 35-month-old sample to button two buttons, whereas 12 months later, at 42 to 47 months, the children completed the task in 34 seconds. Folio and Fewell (1983) found similar results when they asked children to button and unbutton one button in 20 seconds. Only 2% of the normative sample at 30 to 35 months could accomplish the task, whereas at 48 to 59 months 65% of the children were successful. Therefore, despite the ability of many 2½-year-old children to accomplish buttoning, the speed with which the activity is performed is so slow as to preclude it from being functional. The question is: Are the younger children slower because the movements themselves are not as efficient or is it that they are using a different method than older children? Is speeding up only a matter of getting faster or is it also a process of learning more efficient strategies?

Pehoski (1994) looked at this question using an in-hand manipulation task and found that, at least on this task, both aspects of performance changed. She asked 153 children between the ages of 3 years and 6 years 11 months to turn over 10 small pegs in a pegboard using only one hand (a complex rotation task). A group of adult subjects were also presented this task to establish a standard against which the children's performance could be judged. All the children sampled were able to accomplish the task, but the time they took for completion and the methods they used in performing this activity differed among the age groups. The time for completion decreased with age, but even at 6 years 11 months the children were significantly slower than an adult population. Of the age groups of children tested, the 3-year-olds were by far the slowest group and differed significantly from the other age groups.

Perhaps of more interest was the finding that the methods the children used to accomplish this task differed not only between the age groups of children but also from adults. In the sample of normal adults, Pehoski found that all the subjects used the same method to perform this task. Each of the adults picked up the 10 pegs and rotated them using a series of individual movements of the two radial fingers and the thumb. The methods used by the sample of children were more varied, and often the children mixed the use of more than one method in the 10 repetitions of this task. Many of the children were able to demonstrate use of the adult method, but they also used two other approaches when solving this problem. One was to use an external surface against which the peg was turned, such as holding the peg against the chest as it was rotated. Inadvertent use of the other hand was also considered as using an external surface. The other method was to rotate the arm before picking up the peg so that the peg was turned through the derotation action of the arm, thereby excluding or simplifying the use of individual finger movements. Use of the adult method increased with age, although even at 6 years this method was used only 80% of the time.

Of interest was the marked change to an adult method seen in the 48- to 53-month-old children. The 3-year-olds in the sample relied heavily on the use of an external surface when turning the peg. This method was used an average of 40% to 50% of the time by the two youngest age groups. By 48 to 53 months this method had fallen to 25%, and the predominant method used was that of the adults (used 70% of the time). That is, by 4 years of age the children were rotating the peg in the fingers and used this method as the predominant solution to the problem.

As part of this same study Pehoski (1994) also asked her subjects to complete another complex rotation task. In this task the subjects were asked to turn a peg over and over in the fingers and to complete as many rotations as possible up to 10 rotations. All the adults easily accomplished this task. The 3-year-old children had a great deal of difficulty and were able to complete only a mean of one or two rotations, whereas the 4½-year-old children were able to accomplish a mean of almost seven rotations (6.45 rotations). By 6 years of age the mean number was eight or nine rotations. Therefore 4 years of age again appears to be a period of marked improvement in the ability to manipulate or rotate an object in the fingers.

Factors Contributing to the Improvement of In-Hand Manipulation Skills

What are the aspects that are changing to allow an increase in speed and a more consistent, adult method of performance? The adult method of turning over a peg using only one hand requires the differentiation and change in performance between the two radial fingers and the thumb. As an example, the thumb and index finger hold the peg while the middle finger pulls on the bottom of the peg to begin the 180-degree turn. To complete the turn, the middle finger and thumb must now hold the peg as it is pushed around by the index finger. As discussed, the ability to differentiate the movements of the individual fingers (such as the ability

to sequentially oppose the fingers to the thumb; Stutsman, 1948) seems to appear at about 42 to 47 months of age. Once present, there is a gradual increase in the speed of these movements. As an example, the *Peabody Developmental Fine Motor Scales* (Folio and Fewell, 1983) looks at the ability of children to oppose each finger to the thumb within 5 seconds. It was found that this task could be accomplished by only 22% of the 42- to 47-month-old children, but by 48 and 59 months 72% of the children were successful. The ability to isolate individual fingers of the hand and the ability to perform this activity with speed would appear to be a requisite skill for efficient in-hand manipulation activities and may be one of the reasons children 4 years of age and older are better at in-hand manipulation skills than 3-year-olds or younger children.

Physiologic changes are also occurring that may assist this process. The ability to perform individual finger movements is the result of corticospinal input (Lawrence and Kuypers, 1968; Lawrence and Hopkins, 1976; see also Chapter 1). Yakoviev and Lecours (1967) found that the myelination of this tract was completed by 3 years of age, but Koh and Eyre (1988) found that an increase in conduction velocity continued until 11 years of age; that is, the rate at which input travels in this tract increases through 11 years of age and would therefore appear to assist in the efficiency or speed of movements.

Manipulating an object such as a peg in the fingers, rotating a pencil so the tip is in the correct position to write, and turning a small bead in the fingers to orient the hole for stringing all require a grip that is sufficient to keep the object from being dropped but also light enough to allow the object to be moved. In the study by Forssberg et al. (1991) mentioned previously, children were noted to use significantly greater grip force than adults when picking up a small object. In adults the force of the grip is matched to the properties of an object (such as its weight and frictional qualities), and determining this force is related to tactile feedback from the hand (Westling and Johannson, 1984). Adults use just enough force to provide a small margin of safety so the object does not slip out of the fingers. If the adult's fingers are anesthetized, eliminating the tactile feedback that monitors the frictional conditions between the object and the fingers, the ability to adjust the grip force is compromised. Therefore tactile feedback or sensory-motor loops are necessary for the successful accomplishment of this skill. It is also interesting to note that Westling and Johannson (1984) found that the adults in their study with the greatest manual dexterity were also those who employed the smallest safety margins.

Evans, Harrison, and Stephens (1990) have looked at the maturation of cutaneous reflexes in children. To do this they stimulated the cutaneous nerve of the index finger and monitored the EMG response while the first dorsal interosseous muscle was actively contracting. The authors did not observe a full adult-like EMG response until the early teen years. As an example, the adult EMG response to digital nerve stimulation has three components: an initial increase in muscle electrical activity, followed by a decrease, and finally a second, prominent increase. The last of these components, referred to as the E2 component, is felt to require the integrity of the dorsal columns (tract carrying discriminative somatosensory information to the cortex). In the Evans et al. (1990) study the E2 component was not seen until 4 years of age, and then there was a gradual increase in the number of children who demonstrated this aspect of the response until 12 years of age, when all children exhibited an E2 response. Of further interest was the finding that children who did not demonstrate an E2 component were more likely to perform poorly on a test of rapid finger movements. Therefore the appearance of this component of the cutaneous reflex response may be implicated in the speed of finger movements.

Summary and Therapeutic Implications

Children between the ages of 3 and 6 years are making rapid improvement in their ability to manipulate objects in the fingers and in the hand. This is still a difficult task for many 3-year-old children, and an activity such as buttoning buttons is just beginning to be done with enough speed to make the task functional. Other activities, such as rotating a small object in the fingers, is still difficult for the 3-year-old, and the child is likely to substitute another method for the movements of the fingers (such as rotating the object against an external surface). Four years may be a time of marked change in these abilities, particularly the complex rotation of an object in the fingers. It is at this age, Pehoski (1994) found, that children tend to switch from using an external surface when rotating a small peg, to accomplishing the task in the fingers. It is also at this age that children are able to

demonstrate the ability to maintain this performance and rotate the peg several times. Five- and 6-year-old children continued to show improvement in these skills although this improvement was not as marked (the difference in improvement between the 4-, 5-, and 6-year-old subjects was not statistically significant).

Of interest is that several other functions also appear to be changing around 4 to 5 years of age. As an example, Forssberg et al. (1991) found that after 5 years there was no significant difference in the grip force between a population of adults and a population of children when the subjects were asked to pick up a small object between the index finger and thumb. As indicated, the regulation of the grip force rate on this task has been linked to tactile mechanisms. Evans et al. (1990) found that an important component of the cutaneous reflex is not present until 4 years of age and that the appearance of this component maybe linked to the speed of sequential finger movements.

The strength of the grip force and the ability to rapidly sequence the movements of the fingers are important components in the manipulation of an object in the fingers or the hand. Vision can guide the hand to the target, but tactile mechanisms will guide the object in the hand. Nature may well have a rule that says, "Use whatever mechanisms you can to manipulate an object, but whatever you do, don't drop it!" This rule is ensured by tactile mechanisms that detect even minor slippage of a held object and tell the motor system to increase or adjust the grip (Johannson and Westling, 1987). If these mechanisms are immature, generally increasing the grip force or holding an object more tightly than would be necessary may be one way of compensating for this skill. In Pehoski's study (1994), when children were asked to rotate a peg and replace it in the board, dropping the peg was not a common finding. No child dropped more than one of the 10 pegs, and approximately half the children dropped no pegs at all. When working with children, a tendency for objects to be dropped from the fingers should be noted. When this is felt to be excessive, one possible area to consider is the integrity of tactile-motor mechanisms.

Another point to note when evaluating children is that most tests for children in the preschool/early childhood years do not include items that assess in-hand manipulation skills. The evaluator may therefore wish to add tasks of this nature, particularly for the child who is 4 years of age and older, so these skills can be observed.

OBJECT MANIPULATION IN OLDER CHILDREN

Information on the object manipulation of older children is difficult to find. Both Exner (1990) and Pehoski (1994) found that 6-year-old children had not yet achieved either the consistency or speed of an adult population. We know intuitively that object manipulation improves beyond 6 years of age. (However, how many of us would want a 10-year-old to paint our kitchen cabinets or are happy with the resulting mess after a group of 12-year-olds make pizza in the kitchen?) Some of the changes we see in older children are the result of improved judgment and the ability to delay gratification (a 10-year-old might race through the painting of the kitchen cabinets in a desire to see the finished project, not only to get the job done). But we would also expect there to be changes in the actual use of the hand.

Denkla (1973, 1974) looked at the ability of 5-, 6-, and 7-year-old children and of 8-, 9-, and 10-year-olds to rapidly oppose each of the fingers to the thumb and also to rapidly tap the index finger and thumb together. She found a significant increase in speed among the 5-, 6-, and 7-year-old children on these tasks but not between the 8-, 9-, and 10-year-olds. There was therefore a relative plateau in the speed of performance in the children over 8 years of age. On other tasks, such as the Upper Limb Speed and Dexterity subtests of the Bruininks-Oseretsky Test of Motor Proficiency (Bruininks, 1978), children would appear to continue to improve their speed after 8 years of age.

Speed alone is not enough; accuracy is also improving as well as the timing of motor acts. One form of timing has been called coincidence-anticipation, or the ability to time a movement with another moving object. Bard, Fleury, and Gagnon (1990) suggest that this skill may improve linearly with age until it levels off at around 15 years. But the authors also state that "further progress is sometimes noticed beyond this age in tasks with high degrees of stimulus uncertainty and motor-response difficulty, thus placing a greater burden on decision and motor processes" (p. 292). Coincidence-anticipation may be one of the reasons a 10-year-old might make more of a mess out of painting the kitchen cabinets than an adult. The child might have more difficulty timing the movement of a brush loaded with paint from the can to the cabinet door before paint drips from the brush.

There may also be changes in higher-order grasp patterns in older children. As an example, in a study of normal 3- to 6-year-old children, Schneck and Henderson (1990) found that 27.5% of the 6-year-old children used a grip on a pencil other than a dynamic tripod grip. In a sample of normal adults Bergman (1990) found this figure to be 12%, possibly indicating that some children may still change their pencil grip pattern after 6 years. Ziviani (1983) also saw changes in pencil grip in older children. In looking at the pencil grip of children 6 years 8 months to 14 years of age, she found a significant difference in the amount of flexion at the proximal interphalangeal (PIP) joint of the index finger. Younger children used more flexion than older children, a factor Ziviani feels may be related to the amount of pressure being exerted while writing.

A final area in the literature that indicates continued changes in older children is in complementary two-hand use. As the child grows, the complexity of bimanual task that can be completed expands as well as the efficiency between the two hands. Brumi (1972) looked at the abilities of 5-, 8-, and 10-year-old children to string beads, wind a string on a spool, and clap the hands. The author found that the older children tended to keep one hand stable while the other moved (for example, in winding the thread both hands did not rotate in mirror image of each other). Fagard (1990) suggests that one of the changes that is happening in older children is an increasing ability to do *asymmetric* tasks with the hands. One factor that she suggests may be assisting this process is improved interhemispheric communication.

There are probably many other areas where older children surpass their younger counterparts in object manipulation. As indicated, this is not an area that has been well studied, and the information is hard to summarize. We do know that children get faster with age, and in particular the timing of movements improves. Bilateral hand skills also become more complex and efficient. The force of grasp during an activity such as writing may also change, and it is interesting to speculate that this may be related to the continued maturation of cutaneous reflexes.

CONCLUSION

Efficient object manipulation depends on several factors. There is the necessity to be able to differentiate the movement of individual fingers and to perform this action with speed. Manipulation skills also depend on a grip force that is sufficient to keep the object from dropping, but loose enough so that the object can be moved with ease. This ability is apparently dependent on tactile mechanisms. In addition, an object must also be released with skill and with the appropriate timing. The ability to use the hands together is also important. Without the ability to plan and use both hands together in a complementary fashion, the function of the hands would be severely limited. Maturation in each of these abilities assists the child's mastery over objects and striving toward competence.

There is still much that is not known about the developmental course and changes in development that emerge as the child becomes more competent. We need more information on how normal children develop manipulative skills. As an example, we know very little about the beginning of in-hand manipulation. There are no studies on the development of controlled release, a process that probably follows closely on how children grasp objects. The gradation of pressure as a child picks up, puts down, and manipulates objects deserves further study, as does how the force of grasp affects higher-level skills, such as holding a pen and writing. These are only a few of the areas needing future research. Object interaction is an integral part of human behavior yet it is an area that has been poorly studied. A more complete understanding of this area of development would help both the evaluation and the treatment planning of children felt to have difficulty in achieving competency in object interaction.

REFERENCES

Bard, C., Fleury, M., & Gagnon, M. (1990). Coincidence anticipation timing: An age-related perspective. In C. Bard, M. Fleury, & L. Hay (Eds.). *Development of eye-hand coordination across the life span.* Columbia, S.C.: University of South Carolina Press.

Bayley, N. (1969). *Bayley scales of infant development.* New York: Psychological Corporation.

Bly, L. (1981). The components of normal movements during the first year of life. In D.S. Slaton (Ed.). *Development of movement in infancy.* Chapel Hill, N.C.: University of North Carolina Press.

Bower, T.G.R., Broughton, J.M., & Moore, M.K. (1970). Demonstration of intention in the reaching behavior of neonate humans. *Nature, 228,* 679-681.

Bruininks, R.H. (1978). *Bruininks-Oseretsky test of motor proficiency.* Circle Pine, Minn.: American Guidance Service.

Brumi, H. (1972). Age changes in preference and skill measures of handedness. *Perceptual and Motor Skills, 34,* 3-14.

Bruner, J.S. (1970). The growth and structure of skill. In K.J. Connolly (Ed.). *Mechanisms of motor skill development.* New York: Academic Press.

Bruner, J. (1973). Organization of early skilled action. *Child Development, 44,* 1-11.

Connolly, K. (1973). Factors influencing the learning of manual skills by young children. In R.A. Hinde & J.S. Hinde (Eds.). *Constraints on learning.* London: Academic Press.

Denckla, M.D. (1973). Development of speed in repetitive and successive finger movements in normal children. *Developmental Medicine and Child Neurology, 15,* 635-645.

Denckla, M.D. (1974). Development of motor coordination in normal children. *Developmental Medicine and Child Neurology, 16,* 729-741.

DuBose, R.F., & Langley, M.B. (1977). *Developmental activities screening inventory.* New York: Teaching Resources.

Evans, A.L., Harrison, L.M., & Stephens, J.A. (1990). Maturation of the cutaneomuscular reflex recorded from the first dorsal interosseous muscle in man. *Journal of Physiology, 428,* 425-440.

Exner, C.E. (1989). Development of hand function. In P.N. Pratt & A.S. Allen (Eds.). *Occupational therapy for children.* St. Louis: Mosby.

Exner, C.E. (1990). In-hand manipulation skills in normal young children: A pilot study. *Occupational Therapy Practice, 1,* 63-72.

Exner, C.E. (1992). In-hand manipulation skills. In J. Case-Smith & C. Pehoski (Eds.). *Development of hand skills in the child.* Rockville: American Occupational Therapy Association.

Fagard, J. (1990). The development of bimanual coordination. In C. Bard, M. Fleury, & L. Hay (Eds.). *Development of eye-hand coordination across the life span.* Charleston, S.C.: University of South Carolina Press.

Fenson, L., & Kagan, J. (1976). The developmental progression of manipulative play in the first two years. *Child Development, 47,* 232-236.

Folio, M.R., & Fewell, R.R. (1983). *Peabody developmental motor scales.* Allen, Texas: DLM Teaching Resources.

Forssberg, H., Eliasson, A.C., Kinoshita, H., Johansson, R.S., & Westling, G. (1991). Development of human precision grip. I. Basic coordination of force. *Brain Research, 85,* 451-457.

Fraiberg, S. (1968). Parallel and divergent patterns in blind and sighted infants. *Psychoanalytic Study of the Child, 23,* 264-301.

Gesell, A., Halverson, H.M., Thompson, H., Ilg, F.L., Castner, B.M., Ames, L.B., & Amatruda, C.S. (1940). *The first five years of life.* New York: Harper & Row.

Gibson, E.J., & Walker, A.S. (1984). Development of knowledge of visual-tactual affordance of substance. *Child Development, 55,* 453-460.

Halverson, H.M. (1931). An experimental study of prehension in infancy by means of systematic cinema records. *Genetic Psychological Monographs, 10,* 107-285.

Hatwell, Y. (1987). Motor and cognitive functions of the hand in infancy and childhood. *International Journal of Behavioral Development, 10,* 509-526.

Johansson, R.S., & Westling, G. (1984). Role of glabrous skin receptors and sensorimotor memory in automatic control of precision grip when lifting rough or more slippery objects. *Experimental Brain Research, 66,* 141-154.

Karniol, R. (1989). The role of manual manipulative stages in the infant's acquisition of perceived control over objects. *Developmental Review, 9,* 205-233.

Koh, T.H., & Eyre, J.A. (1988). Maturation of corticospinal tracts assessed by electromagnetic stimulation of the motor cortex. *Archives of Diseases of Children, 63,* 1347-1352.

Kopp, C.B. (1974). Fine motor abilities of infants. *Developmental Medicine and Child Neurology, 16,* 629-636.

Kopp, C.B. (1976). Action-schemes of eight-month-old infants. *Developmental Psychology, 12,* 361-362.

Landsmeer, J.M. (1962). Power grip and precision handling. *Annals of Rheumatic Disease, 21,* 164-170.

Lawrence, D.C., & Hopkins, D. A. (1976). The development of motor control in the rhesus monkey: Evidence concerning the role of corticomotoneuronal connections. *Brain, 99,* 235-245.

Lawrence, D.G., & Kuypers, H.G. (1968). The functional organization of the motor system in monkey. I. The effects of bilateral pyramidal lesions. *Brain, 91,* 1-14.

Napier, J.R. (1956). The prehensile movements of the human hand. *The Journal of Bone and Joint Surgery, 38,* 902-913.

Nelson, M.N. (1979). Bayley developmental assessment of low birthweight infants. In T.M. Field, A.M. Sostek, S. Goldberg, & H.H. Shumen (Eds.). *Infants born at risk: Behavior and development.* New York: SP Medical and Scientific Books.

Newell, K.M., Scully, D.M., Tenenbaum, F., & Hardiman, S. (1989). Body scale and the development of prehension. *Developmental Psychology, 22,* 1-13.

Palmer, C. (1989). The discriminating nature of infants' exploratory actions. *Developmental Psychology, 25,* 885-893.

Pehoski, C. (1994). *In-hand manipulation skills in normal children 3.0 to 6.11 years of age.* Unpublished doctoral dissertation, Boston University, Boston.

Ramsay, D.S., & Weber S.L. (1986). Infants' hand preference in a task involving complementary roles for the two hands. *Child Development, 57,* 300-307.

Rochat, P. (1987). Mouthing and grasping in neonates: Evidence for the early detection of what hard and soft substances afford for action. *Infant Behavior and Development, 10,* 435-449.

Rochat, P. (1989). Object manipulation and exploration in 2- to 5-month-old infants. *Developmental Psychology, 25,* 871-884.

Rosenbloom, L., & Horton, M.E. (1971). The maturation of fine prehension in young children. *Developmental Medicine and Child Neurology, 13,* 3-8.

Ross, G. (1985). Use of the Bayley Scales to characterize abilities of premature infants. *Child Development, 56,* 835-842.

Ross, G., Lipper, E., & Auld, P.A. (1986). Early predictors of neurodevelopmental outcome of very low-birthweight infants at three years. *Developmental Medicine and Child Neurology, 28,* 171-179.

Ruddy, M.G., & Bornstein, M.H. (1982). Cognitive correlates of infant attention and maternal stimulation over the first year of life, *Child Development, 53,* 183-188.

Ruff, H. (1984). Infants' manipulative exploration of objects: Effect of age and object characteristics. *Developmental Psychology, 20,* 9-20.

Ruff, H., McCarton, C., Kurtzberg, D, & Vaughan, H.G. (1984). Preterm infants' manipulative exploration of objects. *Child Development, 55,* 1166-1173.

Ruff, H., Saltarelli, L. M., Capozzoli, M., & Dubiner, K. (1992). The differentiation of activity in infants' exploration of objects. *Developmental Psychology, 28,* 851-861.

Saida, Y., & Miyashita, M. (1979). Development of fine motor skill in children: Manipulation of a pencil in young children aged 2 to 6 years old. *Journal of Human Movement Studies, 5,* 104-113.

Schneck, C.M., & Henderson, A. (1990). Descriptive analysis of the developmental progression of grip positions for pencil and crayon control in nondysfunctional children. *American Journal of Occupational Therapy, 44,* 893-900.

Siegel, L.S. (1981). Infant tests as predictors of cognitive and language development at two years. *Child Development, 52,* 545-557.

Steele, D., & Pederson, D.R. (1977). Stimulus variables which affect the concordance of visual and manipulative exploration in six-month-old infants. *Child Development, 48,* 104-111.

Stutsman, R. (1948). *Guide for administering the Merrill-Palmer scales of mental tests.* New York: Harcourt, Brace & World.

Thun-Hohenstein, L., Largo, R.H., Molinari, L., Kundu, S. & Duc, G. (1991). Early fine motor and adaptive development in high-risk appropriate-for-gestational-age preterm and healthy term children. *European Journal of Pediatrics, 150,* 562-569.

Trevarthen, C. (1974). Psychobiology of speech development. In E.H. Lenneberg (Ed.). *Language and brain: Developmental aspects. Neurosciences Research Program Bulletin, Volume 12,* Boston: Neuroscience Research Program.

von Hofsten, C. (1982). Eye-hand coordination in the newborn. *Developmental Psychology, 18,* 450-461.

Westling, G., & Johansson, R.S. (1984). Factors influencing the force control during precision grip. *Experimental Brain Research, 53,* 277-284.

Yakovlev, P.I, & Lecours, A. (1967). The myelogenetic cycles of regional maturation of the brain. In A. Minkowski (Ed.). *Regional development of the brain in early life.* Oxford: Blackwell.

Ziviani, J. (1983). Qualitative changes in dynamic tripod grip between 7 and 14 years of age. *Developmental Medicine and Child Neurology, 25,* 778-782.

CHAPTER

9

Hand Preference and Its Development

Elizabeth A. Murray

Handedness has been defined to mean that "the arms and hands are asymmetrical in use and function so as to reliably favor one hand or the other across a range of skillful acts" (Harris & Carlson, 1988, p. 301). Hand preference is seen when an action requires complex, coordinated sequences of movements involving the distal muscles.

Handedness refers not only to which hand is preferred (left versus right) but also to the degree of preference or the extent to which each hand is used for a range of tasks (McManus, 1985). Methods of evaluating hand preference range from self-report of preferred hand (Silva and Satz,

1979) to complex questionnaires with many items to manual preference tests, in which a person is observed performing a variety of tasks that either are unimanual or require a lead hand. One of the most commonly used assessments of hand preference is the Edinburgh Inventory (Oldfield, 1971). In this assessment subjects are asked which hand they prefer for a variety of activities, such as writing, throwing, using a spoon, and opening a box. Based on the proportion of items they perform with each hand, a person can be classified as right-, left- or mixed-handed, meaning that some activities are performed with the right hand and some with the left hand. (In young children this condition is described as not showing a hand preference [Tan, 1985]). Alternatively, individuals may be labeled as demonstrating a strong hand preference (meaning all or nearly all items are performed with one hand) or weak hand preference. In this case, even though the majority of items are performed with one hand, a significant proportion are performed with the other. "Significant" is defined differently by different researchers; there are no universally accepted rules for determining whether a person demonstrates strong or weak handedness. Additionally, a person who does not use the same hand consistently for individual items (such as hammers) may be described as displaying ambiguous handedness (Satz, Soper, and Orsini, 1988). Thus classification of hand preference varies tremendously because studies use different measures, categories, and rules of classification.

Annett (1970) found that the items in which children were least likely to switch preference over time were hammering, writing, using a tennis racquet, throwing, striking a match, and using a toothbrush. Based on activities such as these, the incidence of left-handedness is generally estimated to be 10% to 15% of the general population (Porac and Coren, 1981). Sex differences in hand preference have been noted; from 1% to 4% more females than males are right-handed (Harris and Carlson, 1988).

Healey, Liederman, and Geshwind (1986) performed a factor analysis on a handedness inventory that contained 55 items. Four factors emerged. Factor 1, which accounted for over 71% of the variance, included actions such as writing and drawing, which require fine motor movements that are continually modified. Factor 2 accounted for nearly 4% of the variance. It included actions that are localized to the hand and/or arm and require minimal modification once begun. Examples of such movements are pointing to an object in the distance and snapping the fingers. Factor 3 included performing a cartwheel and holding a baseball bat. These items require coordination of the arms and trunk and also do not require continuous modification. Factor 3 accounted for nearly 2.5% of the variance. Throwing a ball or a dart at a target were two items included in Factor 4, which accounted for almost 2% of the variance. These items involve movement of proximal muscles but require more precision of movement as well as eye-hand coordination. Healey et al. (1986) suggest, then, that handedness is composed of these different factors and that hand preference may vary, depending on the activities used to measure it. A person may show a preference for the left hand when performing continuous fine motor movements but prefer the right hand for activities that require coordination of the trunk and arm.

THEORIES OF HAND PREFERENCE

Psychologic Theories

Early theories suggested that hand preference was purely learned and that children were merely imitating their parents when demonstrating a preferred hand. However, since young children tend to imitate in mirror-image fashion (Gesell and Ames, 1947), one might then expect that hand preference would alternate from generation to generation. Blau (1946) suggested that preference for the left hand was a result of "emotional negativism" and that a child indicated a rejection of his/her parents by

using the hand opposite to their preferred hand. The preponderance of evidence to date, however, indicates that hand preference is biologically based.

Genetic Theories

Left-handedness does tend to run in families. Left-handed mothers, in particular, are more likely to have left-handed children (Annett, 1981). Also, natural children in a family with left-handers show a higher incidence of left-handedness, whereas this pattern is not seen in adopted children (Rice, Plomin, and DeFries, 1984).

One of the most popular theories on the inheritance of hand preference has been developed by Annett (1981). She hypothesizes what she calls a right shift factor. In her model, inheritance of this factor results in both localization of speech in the left hemisphere and a shift in the distribution of skilled movements to the right, resulting in a bias toward a strong right hand preference. Those who do not inherit this factor are more evenly balanced between the right and the left hand for skilled tasks, such as writing. Environmental factors and social pressure play a stronger role on the development of a preferred hand for those without the right shift factor. Annett further suggests that the right shift factor is expressed in utero shortly before birth. Factors that adversely influence brain growth at this time may both inhibit this shift and result in developmental disabilities, thus helping to explain the increased incidence of left-handers in persons with these disabilities (Annett, 1981; Annett and Kilshaw, 1984). Although Annett has presented a substantial amount of research to support her hypothesis by demonstrating that the proportions of hand preference in large samples fit her model, others suggest that distributions of asymmetry in hand skill fit into two normal curves, one with a right shift and one with a left shift (McManus, 1985; Tapley and Bryden, 1985). Still others hypothesize a left shift factor, with left-handedness being inherited and right-handedness being due to environmental influences (Corballis and Morgan, 1978).

Pathology

Many of those studying hand preference believe that at least some left-handedness is the result of pathology. Bakan has suggested that all left-handedness is a result of brain injury due to birth stress that results in neurologic insult. He conducted surveys of college students, asking them to indicate their hand preference, whether they knew of any difficulties in their birth, and what their order of birth was in their family. Bakan used birth order as an indicator of perinatal stress, assuming that first deliveries, as well as fourth and later births, would pose the greatest risk (Bakan, 1971, 1977; Bakan, Dibb, and Reid, 1973). The surveys indicated that a significantly higher proportion of left-handers were the products of potentially stressful births. Most subsequent studies, however, have not supported Bakan's findings (Levander, Stalling, and Levander, 1989; Nachson and Denno, 1986; Ounsted, Cockburn, and Moar, 1985; Tan and Nettleton, 1980) although Harris and Carlson (1988) point out that other factors related to birth order, such as maternal age and mode of delivery, may be related to pathology. However, these authors also report that extensive studies of prenatal, perinatal, and neonatal risk factors have not found an association between risk factors and left-handedness in normal children. They suggest that, when left-handedness is a sign of pathology, it is most likely not the only sign. In support of this argument, Ross, Lipper, and Auld (1987) found that, in 4-year-old children with a history of very low birth weight, when compared to a group of normal children, a higher incidence of mixed or left hand preference occurred only in those with cognitive and/or language deficits.

Satz and colleagues (Satz, 1972; Satz et al., 1988) have suggested that left-handedness may result from early left-sided brain lesions, which may result in a shift in hand preference as well as other cognitive and motor problems. The shift in handedness depends on the area of and degree to which the left hemisphere is damaged. Satz emphasizes that only some cases of left-handedness are a result of pathology.

Perhaps the most interesting theory of left-handedness has come from Geshwind and Galaburda (Geshwind, 1983; Geshwind and Galaburda, 1985a, 1985b). In studies of right- and left-handed subjects living in Glasgow, Geshwind observed an increased incidence of learning disorders, as well as autoimmune disease, in the left-handers. Geshwind has hypothesized that testosterone in utero may explain these findings. During fetal development the right hemisphere matures earlier than the left hemisphere (Best, 1988). Geshwind has theorized that in some cases the presence of testosterone may further slow the growth of the left hemisphere, either because an excess is produced or because the fetal tissue is overly sensitive to it. As a result of this decreased growth, correspond-

ing regions of the right hemisphere develop more rapidly. Thus, depending on when the slowing of development of the left hemisphere occurs, the result may be that handedness is shifted to the right hemisphere. One also might expect this slowing of growth to affect later neuronal development of language centers of the left hemisphere, possibly resulting in learning problems. Geshwind has implicated testosterone because of the higher frequency of both left-handedness and learning disorders in men than in women. However, since both male and female fetuses are exposed to testosterone in utero, females may be affected by testosterone in a similar manner.

Geshwind recognized that there may be a genetic predisposition to factors, such as increased sensitivity to or production of hormones, that may thus result in left-handedness. Additionally, due to her own genetic endowment, a mother may create an anomalous hormonal uterine environment.

Some studies (Bemporad and Kinsbourne, 1983) have provided support for Geshwind's theory. However, others have not been able to replicate his findings. Satz and Soper (1986) have criticized Geshwind's Glasgow studies. They point out that learning disabilities were determined only by subject report. They also question his definition of left-handedness (performing all items on a hand preference questionnaire with the left hand) as too restrictive.

Asymmetry

Some authors (Brown and Wolpert, 1990; Morgan, 1977) suggest that hand preference is related to mechanisms that result in various anatomic asymmetries, including direction of hair whorling and location of the heart. These asymmetries, including hand preference, are seen as evolutionary. Evidence cited includes mirror twins, or identical twins in which one is left-handed and the other is right-handed. However, as Geshwind and Galaburda (1985b) have pointed out, there are few cases of identical twins in which the heart is on the right side of the body (situs inversus). They suggest that left-handedness in these cases is either a result of pathology or a lack of inheritance of the right shift factor, as postulated by Annett.

HAND PREFERENCE AND DEFICITS

As mentioned earlier, the proportion of left-handers in the general population is estimated to be between 10% and 15%, depending on the measure used (Porac and Coren, 1981). However, it has been suggested that an even higher proportion of left-handedness is associated with several different deficit conditions, including epilepsy (Harris and Carlson, 1988; Hecaen and Ajuriaguerra, 1964), learning disorders (Geshwind and Galaburda, 1985a), mental retardation (Bradshaw-McAnulty, Hicks, and Kinsbourne, 1984), and infantile autism (Colby and Parkinson, 1977; Soper et al., 1986).

Cognitive Deficits

The incidence of left-handedness is reported to be approximately 10% to 15% of the general population. However, this figure may be higher among clinical populations with mental retardation. Ross, Lipper, and Auld (1987) compared 4-year-old children with IQs below 85 to a group of normal controls. Of the children with below average IQ, 19% were left-handed, compared with 11% of the control children. They reported that the increase appeared to be primarily among the children with more severe mental retardation. In another study, Hicks and Barton (1975) found only 13% of persons with mild-to-moderate mental retardation were left-handed, whereas 28% of those with severe-to-profound mental retardation showed a left hand preference. In contrast, Lucas et al. (1989), in a study of institutionalized adults with mental retardation, reported no significant difference in the proportion of left-handers based on severity of retardation.

Studies of normal subjects have, in general, found no difference between left- and right-handers in overall intelligence (Hardyck and Petrinovich, 1977; Hardyck, Petrinovich, and Goldman, 1976). Additionally, studies assessing language abilities have generally noted no differences in handedness between subjects with language impairments and normal controls (Bishop, 1990; Neils and Aram, 1986). Lucas et al. (1989), however, found an increased incidence of left-handedness in adults who had both mental retardation and additional language impairments. They hypothesized that this finding reflected left hemisphere impairment.

There is some suggestion of an association between left-handedness and giftedness. Hardyck (1977)) analyzed IQ scores of 7688 children in grades 1 through 6. He noted a slight increase in left-handers at both the lower and upper extremes of intelligence. Hardyck suggested that the presence of more left-handers at the upper range of intelligence balanced out those at the lower end, thus making the differences between left- and right-handers "not noticeable" when group averages are used. Benbow (1986) has found the proportion of left-handers among 13-year-olds who are verbally or mathematically gifted to be nearly 20%. Others have suggested that left-handers may have special talents in areas such as art and music (Geshwind and Behan, 1982).

Some have suggested that the consistency of hand preference is more strongly associated with cognitive abilities. In a study by Soper et al. (1987) of institutionalized adults with mental retardation, approximately 45% were found to show ambiguous handedness, compared with 10% who were left-handed. In a longitudinal study, hand preference of children was measured at 6-month intervals from 18 to 42 months. The children were then tested on a variety of measures, including intelligence, at yearly intervals from 5 to 9 years of age. Girls who had demonstrated consistent hand preference performed significantly better than girls whose hand preference had varied from one assessment to the next. (No similar difference was seen in the boys.) Furthermore, Whittington and Richards (1987) assessed the hand preference of 11,000 children at ages 7 and 11. Those children who changed hand preference between these two times scored lower than children with consistent preference on a variety of cognitive measures. Kinsbourne (1988) also found an excess of mixed hand preference in children with learning disabilities, and other researchers have pointed out that ambiguous handedness is prevalent in individuals with infantile autism (Satz et al., 1984, 1988; Soper and Satz, 1984)

Motor Deficits

It has been suggested that left-handers may be clumsier than right-handers although this idea is controversial. In fact, left-handers are known to have an advantage at certain sports (McLean and Ciurczak, 1982). Tan (1985) assessed the gross motor abilities of 4-year-old children whom she classified as right-handed, left-handed, or showing no hand preference based on a manual preference test. Results indicated no differences between right- and left-handers in gross motor skills. However, the children with no hand preference were significantly poorer than the other two groups in this area.

Bishop (1984, 1990) hypothesized that children who were pathologically left-handed would show particularly poor performance with their right hand. She assumed that mild neurologic abnormalities of the left hemisphere could result in clumsiness in the right hand, thus forcing preference in the left hand. Bishop found left hand preference to be more common in children with the poorest performance with the nonpreferred hand, thus supporting her hypothesis. Furthermore, these children also demonstrated more speech problems than the other children in her studies. Gillberg and his associates (1984) also found clumsiness in the nonpreferred hand to be more common in left-handers than right-handers. In contrast, Rudel, Healey, and Denckla (1984) observed no differences between left- and right-handed children for either hand when imitating repetitive finger and hand movements, such as finger tapping and forearm rotation.

An interesting study of fine motor skills in children with hemiplegia was conducted by Hiscock and her associates (1989). They reasoned that, if most children were meant to be right-handed, then children with right hemiplegia, presumably a result of left hemisphere lesions, would be forced to use what should have been their nonpreferred hand. In contrast, children with left hemiplegia should still have adequate use of their preferred right hand. Thus they predicted that children with right hemiplegia should do more poorly than children with left hemiplegia on unilateral fine motor tasks. Their findings, based on 30 right-hemiplegic and 27 left-hemiplegic children, confirmed their prediction, although they noted that the children with right hemiplegia were more variable in their performance. They suggest that this variability may be related to the location and severity of the lesion.

Why Is Hand Preference Associated with Deficits?

Most researchers now agree that the increased incidence of left-handedness in certain clinical populations is due to brain pathology that affects the left hemisphere. Satz has stated that the increase in the proportion of left-handers in some deficit populations is due to early left-sided brain injury that results in pathologic left-handedness in a child who was genetically predispositioned to become right-handed. Although right-sided lesions would be expected to occur as frequently as left-sided ones, these would result in a change in handedness only in those predisposed to being left-handed, which is a small percentage of the population. Satz states that, in populations with deficits such as epilepsy and mental retardation,

approximately 10% are natural left-handers (as would be predicted by the proportion in the general population) and another 7% to 10% are pathologic left-handers (Satz, 1972; Satz et al., 1984, 1988; Satz and Soper, 1986).

Geshwind and his associates theorize that the increased incidence of left-handers in many deficit populations can be explained by the slowing of growth of the left hemisphere in utero by testosterone. The anomalous development of the left hemisphere can lead, in turn, to deficits in cognition, and, in particular, language abilities (Geshwind, 1983; Geshwind and Behan, 1982; Geshwind and Galaburda, 1985a, 1985b). Geshwind and his associates also hypothesize that depressing the development of the left hemisphere facilitates right hemisphere development and possibly results in the development of special talents in left-handers. They note that left-handers are said to excel in areas that rely heavily on spatial abilities, such as architecture and mathematics.

The major difference between the two theories described previously is whether all left-handedness is the result of pathology, as Geshwind would imply, or whether there are two different types of left-handedness, only one of which is due to pathology. This question is as yet unanswered. (See Harris and Carlson, 1988, for a detailed discussion of this issue.)

Hemispheric Specialization in Left-Handers

There is evidence that many left-handers do show different patterns of hemispheric specialization than right-handers. Although studies indicate that the vast majority of right-handers have a consistent pattern of language functions lateralized to the left hemisphere and visual-spatial abilities controlled mainly by the right hemisphere, left-handers appear to be much more variable. Research on both normal left-handers and left-handers who are known to have sustained a unilateral head injury suggests that, although many show a pattern of hemispheric specialization that is similar to that of right-handers, possibly 30% to 40% have either a more bilateral representation of language skills or language primarily lateralized to the right hemisphere (Harris and Carlson, 1988). Furthermore, autopsies have found less anatomic asymmetry in the brains of left-handed subjects (Galaburda et al., 1978).

It is important to note that not all atypical patterns of hemispheric specialization result in functional deficits (Liederman, 1988). Furthermore, most of the findings of increased incidence of disability in left-handers are based on clinical populations. When left-handers and right-handers in the general population are compared, there appears to be no difference in school performance or in intellectual ability.

DEVELOPMENT OF HAND PREFERENCE

The development of hand preference in infants and young children has become a focus of research in the past 15 years (Harris and Carlson, 1988). Before that time the predominant view of hand preference was that it was not consistent until 8 to 10 years of age (Belmont and Birch, 1963; Gesell and Ames, 1947).

Preference in Infants from Birth to 30 Months

Until recently it was assumed that infants under 1 year did not display a preference for either hand. Rather, they reached for objects to the left with their left hand and objects to the right with the right hand. Bruner (1969) referred to this phenomenon as the "midline barrier" that infants seldom crossed. However, recent research indicates that hand preference may be apparent in even young infants.

Two different methods have been used as measures of hand preference in infants from birth to 30 months. The first is analyzing the orientation of the head when the infant is in the supine position. In the second method the hand used by the infant in various activities is recorded.

Head Orientation When Supine

The earliest measure thought to indicate later hand preference is the direction toward which a newborn or young infant prefers to turn the head when lying supine. This preference is present at birth and continues through the first 2 to 3 months of life (Hopkins et al., 1990; Liederman and Coryell, 1981; Michel, 1981). Most studies suggest that approximately 70% to 90% of young infants demonstrate a bias toward the right side (Harris and Carlson, 1988).

Although this bias is clearly toward the right for the majority of infants, there is a question of whether it actually reflects hand preference. Determining if supine orientation predicts future hand preference requires longitudinal studies. In one

study Michel and Harkins (1986) measured the direction of head orientation preference of 20 infants and compared this measurement to hand preferences in reaching at intervals up to 2 years of age. Eighteen of the infants demonstrated stable hand preference, and the preferred hand was predicted by the direction of early head orientation. Michel suggests two explanations for their findings. One is that the infants have more opportunity to view one hand and thus develop better eye-hand coordination with that hand. The alternative explanation is that the same underlying factor determines both handedness and head orientation.

Related to supine head orientation is the asymmetric tonic neck reflex (ATNR). In the classic form of the ATNR the head is turned to one side, the arm and leg on that side are extended, and the opposite arm and leg are flexed. Gesell and Ames (1947) suggested that "the earliest manifestations of human handedness are in some way bound up with the phenomenon of the tonic neck reflex." In their longitudinal study of hand preference they included observation of the number of times each infant assumed the ATNR to the left and to the right when lying supine. They reported that, out of 19 infants, all seven who showed a preponderance of the ATNR to the right were right-handed at age 10. Only four out of the nine who assumed the ATNR to the left more frequently than to the right were left-handed at 10 years. Gesell and Ames concluded that the asymmetric tonic neck reflex is predictive of later hand preference but that there were significant exceptions. It does appear, based on their data, that the ATNR may be a better predictor of right than left hand preference.

Hand Use

Most studies that analyze preference in hand use in infants employ structured tasks in which objects are presented to the infant's midline and/or to both the left and right of midline with equal frequency. The type of hand use varies. Some studies analyze visually directed reaching, whereas others define hand use as the hand that manipulates the object. Still others use objects or activities that require bimanual activity, in which one hand stabilizes an object while the other hand investigates it. Hand preference in these cases is defined as the hand that explores the object. Studies either use a cross section of infants at different ages or study the same infants over time. Results of these studies have been inconsistent. Several studies (Gesell and Ames, 1947; Ramsay, 1985) indicate fluctuations in hand preference during the first year, with infants at times preferring one hand over the other and at other times showing no preference or tending to reach for and manipulate objects with both hands together. Gesell and Ames (1947) studied hand preference in children from 8 weeks to 10 years of age by recording the amount of time that the children spent contacting an object, either unilaterally or with both hands, in a structured situation. (For children ages 2½ and older they also included analysis of play at school.) They noted no hand preference for infants at ages 8 and 12 weeks. At 16 to 20 weeks there appeared to be a preference toward the left hand for touching objects. Thereafter, in the first year hand preference varied between left, right, and bilateral. Additionally, seven infants were selected for longitudinal study. Of these seven, six eventually became right-handed. Analysis of their hand preference over time indicated a high degree of variability during the first 2 years.

Ramsay and his associates (Ramsay, 1985; Ramsay and Willis, 1984) noted that a preference for manipulation with the right hand coincided with the onset of babbling. This preference disappeared within 3 to 4 weeks and then appeared again. They also noted a high degree of variability within individual infants, and they felt their data supported the findings of Gesell and Ames (1947).

Carlson and Harris (1985) tested 32 infants every 3 weeks from 24 to 39 weeks of age and again at 52 weeks. Although they noted an increasing proportion of reaches with the right hand over this period, they also noted much variability in the infants.

Others (Michel, Ovrut, and Harkins, 1986; Young et al., 1983) suggest that handedness can be observed early on. Young and his associates (1983) reviewed 17 studies of hand preference for reaching and manipulation in young infants (up to 4 months). Right hand preference was found in 13 of the 17 studies. They concluded that the right upper limb is preferred for directed activities from early infancy. In contrast, Ramsay (1980) observed no hand preference in infants at age 5 or 7 months. A right bias appeared only in 9-month-olds. His findings were supported by Peters (1983), who reported no preference in 6-month-olds but a right preference in infants at age 12 months.

Michel, Ovrut, and Harkins (1991) used a variety of activities to measure reaching, manipulation, and bimanual activities in 6- through 13-month-old infants. They noted a relatively stable preference for the right hand that increased with

age. Cornwell and her associates (1991) found similar stability of hand preference in girls at ages 9, 13, and 18 months. In a longitudinal study of 49 children by Archer and her associates (1988) nearly 75% of the children demonstrated a clear hand preference for manipulation and bimanual activities at 18 months. Approximately 70% of these children had the same hand preference at ages 24 and 30 months. Archer and her associates suggest that handedness is determined by at least 18 months in most children.

Some of the variations in hand preference may be because infants change rapidly, both motorically and cognitively, yet the same tasks are used at a variety of ages. "The appearance of stability or instability in infant handedness may depend more on the types of sensorimotor skills assessed than on any inherent variability in the infant's handedness" (Michel et al., 1985).

Although a task such as reaching may be used to assess hand preference at a variety of ages, the purpose of reaching may be different. For example, young infants may reach for a crayon to place it in the mouth, whereas the older infant may reach with the aim of manipulating it (Cornwell et al., 1991). Additionally, the attributes of the object used may have an effect. Gesell and Ames (1947) noted that reaching for a pellet brought out more consistently unilateral responses than did reaching for a bell.

Based on their research, Michel and his associates (1986) indicated that hand preference for visually guided reaching appears at about 4 to 5 months. Hand preference for object manipulation does not become apparent until at least 6 months, and it is not until 12 to 13 months that hand preference emerges when performing complementary bimanual actions, in which one hand supports an object so that it can be explored or used by the other.

It is important to note that most of these studies measure hand preference in structured settings, with specific materials that are placed either at midline or at precise positions to the left and right of midline. Little has been done to look at spontaneous hand use in unstructured or semistructured settings. One study (Rice, Plomin, and DeFries, 1984) assessed hand use of 272 infants at 12 months and again at 24 months in a naturalistic play setting. Only 10% of the children demonstrated a preference for one hand at 12 months. This figure rose to 30% at 24 months. (The direction of hand preference was not reported.) In another study 22 infants ranging in age from 6 months to 2½ years were videotaped for 8 hours per day over 11 days. Both frequency and duration of hand use were recorded for each hand. For the group as a whole, the right hand was used more frequently and for longer durations. Unfortunately, no information is given about hand use in individual subjects or about differences between younger and older infants (Provins, Dalzeil, and Higginbottom, 1987).

It appears, then, that a preference for one hand can be seen in many infants although this preference may fluctuate over time and is not seen in all infants. Right hand preference predominates, but not to the degree seen in the adult population. Furthermore, hand preference at this age does not mean the consistent use of one hand but rather that one hand is used more frequently than the other. These variations may be due in part to changes in both fine motor and cognitive abilities. Additionally, Carlson and Harris (1985) describe what they refer to as the principle of minimal effort, which may compete with hand preference. All things being equal, it takes less effort for an infant to reach for an object on the left side with the left hand than to cross over with the right hand (possibly due to the relative shortness of the infant's arms and limited trunk rotation).

Children from 30 Months to 7 Years

In children from 2½ on up hand preference is measured by manual preference tests, as described earlier. The child is observed performing a variety of tasks (drawing, cutting, eating with a spoon). Hand preference is then determined by the proportion of activities performed with the right hand versus the left hand. Using this form of assessment, researchers have determined that left- or right-handedness for the majority of children is present by ages 2½ to 3 and remains consistent over time (Gesell and Ames, 1947; McManus et al., 1988; Sinclair, 1971). However, this is not the case for all children. Curt and his associates (1992) found that the proportion of right hand preference increased from about 60% to over 80% between ages 2 and 4 in a sample of 765 children. (This change was not observed in left-handed children, who remained at less than 10% of the sample.)

In a longitudinal study of 199 children by Ounsted, Cockburn, and Moar (1985), children were assessed at ages 2, 4, and 7½. Of the children who were right-handed at 7½, over 70% had shown right hand preference at age 2, and 89%

at age 4. For left-handed children the numbers were similar (76% at 2 years and 86% at 4 years). They concluded that hand preference is consistent over this period.

McManus et al. (1988), in a study of 314 children ages 3, 4, 5, and 7, noted that, although the direction of hand preference appeared to be set by age 3, the degree of hand preference, or proportion of activities performed with the preferred hand, increased over time. This increase was more rapid in the left-handed children, who showed weaker hand preference than right-handers at age 3 but a similar degree at 7 years. Based on current research, Harris and Carlson (1988) have concluded that hand preference is consistent and stable in most children by ages 3 to 4, although the speed and efficiency of hand use continue to increase.

CONCLUSION

Hand preference is a complex construct that varies depending on the definition and the measures used. It does appear that the preferred use of one hand for specialized fine motor activities is determined before birth. The mechanism or mechanisms through which this occurs are subject to debate and may include genetics as well as brain damage or anomalous brain development in utero. This preference may be seen during the first year of life although it is highly variable and not seen in all children at this early age. However, a clear hand preference is usually apparent by ages 3 to 4 in normal children for tasks requiring precise fine motor movements. Although there is a higher incidence of left-handed individuals in clinical populations with various disabilities, left-handers in the general population do not appear to have more problems than do right-handers.

REFERENCES

Annett, M. (1981). The right shift theory of handedness and developmental language problems. *Bulletin of the Orton Society, 31,* 103.

Annett, M., & Kilshaw, D. (1984). Lateral preference and skill in dyslexics: Implications of the right shift theory. *Journal of Child Psychology and Psychiatry, 25,* 357-377.

Archer, L.A., Campbell, D., & Segalowitz, S.J. (1988). A prospective study of hand preference and language development in 18- to 30-month olds. II. Relations between hand preference and language development. *Developmental Neuropsychology, 4,* 93-102.

Bakan, P. (1971). Handedness and birth order. *Nature (London), 229,* 195.

Bakan, P. (1977). Handedness and birth order revisited. *Neuropsychologia, 15,* 837-839.

Bakan, P., Dibb, G., & Reid, P. (1973). Handedness and birth stress. *Neuropsychologia, 11,* 363-366.

Belmont, L., & Birch, H.G. (1963). Lateral dominance and right-left awareness in normal children. *Child Development, 34,* 257-270.

Bemporad, B., & Kinsbourne, M. (1983). Sinistrality and dyslexia: A possible relationship between subtypes. *Topics in Learning and Learning Disabilities, 3,* 48-65.

Best, C. T. (1988). The emergence of cerebral asymmetries in early human development: A literature review and a neuroembryological model. In D.L. Molfese & S.J. Segalowitz (Eds.). *Brain lateralization in children: Developmental implications.* New York: Guilford Press.

Bishop, D.V.M. (1984). Using non-preferred hand skill to investigate pathological left-handedness in an unselected population. *Developmental Medicine and Child Neurology, 26,* 214-226.

Bishop, D.V.M. (1990). Handedness, clumsiness and developmental language disorders. *Neuropsychologia, 28,* 681-690.

Blau, A. (1946). *The master hand: A study of right and left sidedness and its relation to laterality and language.* New York: American Orthopsychiatry Association.

Brown, N.A., & Wolpert, L. (1990). The development of handedness in left/right asymmetry. *Development, 109,* 1-9.

Bruner, J.S. (1969). Eye, hand, and mind. In D. Elkind & J.H. Flavell (Eds.). *Studies in cognitive development: Essays in honor of Jean Piaget.* New York: Oxford University Press.

Carlson, D.F., & Harris, L.J. (1985). Development of the infant's hand preference for visually directed reaching: Preliminary report of a longitudinal study. *Infant Mental Health Journal, 6,* 158-174.

Corballis, M.C., & Morgan, M.J. (1978). On the biological basis of human laterality. *Behavioral Brain Science, 2,* 261-336.

Cornwell, K.S., Harris, L.J., & Fitzgerald, H.E. (1991). Task effects in the development of hand preference in 9-, 13-, and 20-month-old infant girls. *Developmental Neuropsychology, 7,* 19-34.

Curt, F., Maccario, J., & Dellatolas, G. (1992). Distributions of hand preference and hand skill asymmetry in preschool children: Theoretical implications. *Neuropsychologia, 30,* 27-34.

Galaburda, A.M., LeMay, M., Kemper, T.L., & Geshwind, N. (1978). Right-left asymmetries in the brain. *Science, 199,* 852-856.

Gesell, A., & Ames, L.B. (1947). The development of handedness. *The Journal of Genetic Psychology, 70,* 155-175.

Geshwind, N. (1983). Biological associations of left-handedness. *Annals of Dyslexia, 33,* 29-44.

Geshwind, N., & Behan, P. (1982). Left-handedness: Associations with immune disease, migraine, and developmental learning disorder. *Proceedings of the National Academy of Science, 79,* 5097-5100.

Geshwind, N., & Galaburda, A.M. (1985a). Cerebral lateralization: Biological mechanisms, associations, and pathology. I. A hypothesis and a program for research. *Archives of Neurology, 42,* 428-459.

Geshwind, N., & Galaburda, A.M. (1985b). Cerebral lateralization: Biological mechanisms, associations, and pathology. II. A hypothesis and a program for research. *Archives of Neurology, 42,* 521-552.

Gillberg, C., Waldenstrom, E., & Rasmussen, P. (1984). Handedness in Swedish 10-year-olds: Some background and associated factors. *Journal of Child Psychology and Psychiatry, 25,* 421-432.

Harris, L.J., & Carlson, D.F. (1988). Pathological left-handedness: An analysis of theories and evidence. In D.L. Molfese & S.J. Segalowitz (Eds.). *Brain lateralization in children: Developmental implications.* New York: Guilford Press.

Healey, J.M., Liederman, J., & Geshwind, N. (1986). Handedness is not a unidimensional trait. *Cortex, 22,* 33-53.

Hecaen, H., & Ajuriaguerra, J. D. (1964). *Left-handedness.* New York: Grune & Stratton.

Hicks, R.E., & Barton, A.K. (1975). A note on left-handedness and severity of mental retardation. *Journal of Genetic Psychology, 127,* 323-324.

Hiscock, C.K., Hiscock, M., Benjamins, D., & Hillman, S. (1989). Motor asymmetries in hemiplegic children: Implications for the normal and pathological development of handedness. *Developmental Neuropsychology, 5,* 169-186.

Hopkins, B., Lems, Y.L., Palthe, T.V.W., Hoeksma, J., Kardaun, O., & Butterworth, G. (1990). Development of head position preference during early infancy: A longitudinal study in the daily life situation. *Developmental Psychobiology, 23,* 39-53.

Kinsbourne, M. (1988). Sinistrality, brain organization, and cognitive deficits. In D.L. Molfese & S.J. Segalowitz (Eds.). *Brain lateralization in children: Developmental implications.* New York: Guilford Press.

Levander, M., Stalling, D., & Levander, S.E. (1989). Birth stress, handedness and cognitive performance. *Cortex, 25,* 673-681.

Liederman, J. (1988). Misconceptions and new conceptions about early brain damage, functional asymmetry, and behavioral outcome. In D.L. Molfese & S.J. Segalowitz (Eds.). *Brain lateralization in children: Developmental implications.* New York: Guilford Press.

Liederman, J., & Coryell, J. (1981). How right hand preference may be facilitated by rightward turning during infancy. *Developmental Psychobiology, 14,* 439-450.

Lucas, J.A., Rosenthal, L.D., & Bigler, E.D. (1989). Handedness and language among the mentally retarded: Implications for the model of pathological left-handedness and gender differences in hemispheric specialization. *Neuropsychologia, 27,* 713-723.

McLean, J.M., & Ciurczak, F.M. (1982). Bimanual dexterity of major league baseball players: A statistical study. *New England Journal of Medicine, 2,* 1278-1279.

McManus, I.C. (1985). Right- and left-hand skill: Failure of the right shift model. *British Journal of Psychology, 76,* 1-16.

McManus, I.C., Ski, G., Cole, D.R., Mellon, A.F., Wong, J., & Kloss, J. (1988). The development of handedness in children. *British Journal of Psychology, 6,* 257-273.

Michel, G.F. (1981). Right-handedness: A consequence of infant supine head-orientation preference? *Science, 212,* 685-687.

Michel, G.F., & Harkins, D.A. (1986). Postural and lateral asymmetries in the ontogeny of handedness during infancy. *Developmental Psychobiology, 19,* 247-258.

Michel, G.F., Ovrut, M.R., & Harkins, D.A. (1986). Hand-use preference for reaching and object manipulation in 6- through 13-month-old infants. *Genetic, Social, and General Psychology Monographs, 111,* 409-427.

Morgan, M. (1977). Embryology and the inheritance of asymmetry. In S. Harnard, R. Doty, L. Goldstein, & G. Krauthamer (Eds.). *Lateralization in the nervous system.* New York: Academic Press.

Nachson, I., & Denno, D. (1986). Birth order and lateral preferences. *Cortex, 22,* 567-578.

Oldfield, R.C. (1971). The assessment and analysis of handedness: The Edinburgh Inventory. *Neuropsychologia, 9,* 97-113.

Ounsted, M., Cockburn, J., & Moar, V.A. (1985). Hand preference: Its provenance, development, and associations with intellectual ability at the age of 7.5 years. *Developmental and Behavioral Pediatrics, 6,* 76-80.

Peters, M. (1983). Lateral bias in reaching and holding at six and twelve months. In G. Young, S.J. Segalowitz, C.M. Corter, & S.E. Trehub (Eds.). *Manual specialization and the developing brain.* New York: Academic Press.

Porac, C., & Coren, S. (1981). *Lateral preferences and human behavior.* New York: Springer-Verlag.

Provins, K.A., Dalzeil, F.R., & Higginbottom, G. (1987). Asymmetrical hand usage in infancy: An ethological approach. *Infant Behavior and Development, 10,* 165-172.

Ramsay, D.S. (1980). Onset of unimanual handedness in infants. *Infant Behavior and Development, 2,* 69-76.

Ramsay, D.S. (1985). Fluctuations in unimanual hand preference in infants following the onset of duplicated syllable babbling. *Developmental Psychology, 21,* 318-324.

Ramsay, D.S., & Willis, M.P. (1984). Organization and lateralization of reaching in infants: An extension of Bresson et al. *Neuropsychologia, 22,* 639-641.

Rice, T., Plomin, R., & DeFries, J.C. (1984). Development of hand preference in the Colorado Adoption Project. *Perceptual and Motor Skills, 58,* 683-689.

Ross, G., Lipper, E.G., & Auld, P.A.M. (1987). Hand preference of four-year-old children: Its relationship to premature birth and neurodevelopmental outcome. *Developmental Medicine and Child Neurology, 29,* 615-622.

Rudel, R.G., Healey, J., & Denckla, M.B. (1984). Development of motor co-ordination by normal left-handed children. *Developmental Medicine and Child Neurology, 26,* 104-111.

Satz, P., Orsini, D.L., Saslow, E., & Henry, R. (1984). The pathological left-handedness syndrome, *Brain and Cognition, 4,* 27-46.

Satz, P., & Soper, H.V. (1986). Left-handedness, dyslexia, and autoimmune disorder: A critique. *Journal of Clinical and Experimental Neuropsychology, 8,* 453-458.

Satz, P., Soper, H.V., & Orsini, D.L. (1988). Human hand preference: Three nondextral subtypes. In D.L. Molfese & S.J. Segalowitz (Eds.). *Brain lateralization in children: Developmental implications.* New York: Guilford Press.

Sinclair, C. (1971). Dominance patterns of young children, a follow-up study. *Perceptual and Motor Skills, 32,* 142.

Soper, H.V., & Satz, P. (1984). Pathological left-handedness and ambiguous handedness: A new explanatory model. *Neuropsychologia, 22,* 511-515.

Soper, H.V., Satz, P., Orsini, D.L., Van Gorp, W.G., & Green, M.F. (1987). Handedness distribution in a residential population with severe or profound mental retardation. *American Journal of Mental Deficiency, 92,* 94-102.

Tan, L.E. (1985). Laterality and motor skills in four-year-olds. *Child Development, 56,* 119-124.

Tan, L.E., & Nettleton, L.C. (1980). Left-handedness, birth order and birth stress. *Cortex, 16,* 363-374.

Young, G., Segalowitz, S.J., Misek, P., Alp, I.E., & Boulet, R. (1983). Is early reaching left-handed? Review of manual specialization research. In G. Young, S.J. Segalowitz, C.M. Corter, & S.E. Trehub (Eds.). *Manual specialization and the developing brain.* New York: Academic Press.

10

Self-Care and Hand Skill

Anne Henderson

The performance of self-care activities is so universal that its fundamental relevance to all aspects of living is often overlooked. Eisen et al. (1980) in their Health Insurance Study (HIS) conceptualized child health to include physical, mental, and social health. Physical health was defined in terms of functional status, which in turn was defined as the "capacity to perform a variety of activities that are normal for an individual in good health" (p. 7). The categories included within functional status were self-care activities and leisure activities. Self-care activities included the basic functions of eating, dressing, bathing, and use of the toilet; they are the foci of this chapter.

The discussions of the development of self-care in this chapter include only the basic activities, although we recognize the equal importance in the health of the child of all functional status activities identified above. Furthermore, although postural control is essential for all self-care and oral-motor control is essential for feeding, this discussion is restricted to hand function. The reader must incorporate the information not covered into an overall framework of physical, mental, and social development.

The achievement of independence in basic self-care is one of the major developmental tasks of the young child since the child entering school is expected to be toilet trained and to be self-sufficient in eating, dressing, hygiene, and simple domestic tasks. These self-care activities are among the first achievements of childhood, and they provide independence, social approval, and a sense of mastery for the child.

This acquisition of self-care skills in childhood is intricately involved with the development of motor skill, particularly of the hands. The purpose of this chapter is therefore to review what is known about the development of self-care in relation to the development of hand function. We begin with comments on the importance of self-care, its measurement, and some factors that influence it. We then present a developmental review of eating, dressing, and hygiene/grooming behavior.

IMPORTANCE OF INDEPENDENCE IN SELF-CARE

Children of every society are expected to develop independence in their performance of everyday living skills. Independence is taken for granted as children reach the appropriate maturational levels. This universal expectation for competence in self-care activities is the reason for the emphasis on their acquisition in rehabilitation and education.

Importance to the Child

Independence in basic self-care is most important to the individual child. Inability to perform those activities that the child's peers have accomplished exposes the child to possible ridicule and embarrassment. The ability to feed, dress, and care for toileting needs significantly increases a child's control over both home and school environment. For example, a child who dresses himself/herself does not have to depend on the convenience of the caregiver. The child has some control of time, to be dressed without waiting or to delay dressing a bit to complete an interesting activity. A child's control over the environment comes to a large degree through mastery of daily activities (Amato and Ochiltree, 1986). The ability to meet individual needs without seeking help can result in feelings of efficacy and control (White, 1959).

The most important consideration in the development of basic self-care is in its relationship to the child's self-esteem and feelings of efficacy. Self-dependence is an important developmental task in any culture, the achievement of which wins cultural approval, and cultural pressures are such that mastery of a given task leads to satisfaction (Bernard, 1970). Teaching self-care activities provides an opportunity for caregivers to instill positive self-esteem in young children.

The observation of emerging independence in a child has been called "an early joy of parenthood" (Coley and Procter, 1989). In the United States children are encouraged and praised for self-sufficiency, with the result that most want to be independent and feel a sense of pride in their mastery (Gordon, 1992). Young children often announce achievements such as tying a bow or

buckling a shoe to family and friends, often wanting to demonstrate their new skill. When parents actively encourage and teach children to care for themselves, they are fostering the development of competence (Maccoby, 1980). Furthermore, young children demand independence: "I can do it myself." This insistence on self-sufficiency in performing activities begins during the second year (Geppert and Kuster, 1983). The desire for self-sufficiency has been related to the development of volitional behavior (Bullock and Lutkenhaus, 1988). Volition implies action in which the achievement of a goal is seen as resulting from one's own activity. This development of volitional competence begins during the toddler years.

Self-Care in Disability

The timely achievement of abilities in self-care tasks is important in the daily life of all children. Delay and inability to perform a skill are major barriers to school and home living of children with special needs. In the development of a child's potential, "acquiring daily living skills may be as important as academic qualifications" (Gordon, 1992).

The degree of disability in self-care among children with special needs varies with type and degree of impairment. A survey conducted in an Australian school district of special needs children (primarily with cerebral palsy or multiple handicaps) reported that about 65% needed help in dressing and 25% in eating. Although little attention has been given to the self-care needs of children with developmental clumsiness, descriptive studies indicate the impaired motor abilities may interfere with eating and dressing independence (Gubbay, 1975; Walton, Ellis, and Court, 1962).

The importance of self-care skills in early childhood is sometimes underestimated because infants and preschool children are naturally dependent and are easy to care for. Parents may not be too concerned about delays in activities such as dressing (Klein, 1983). However, as a child grows and siblings are born, extended dependency can add significantly to the stress within a household (Wallender, Pitt, and Mellins, 1990).

Self-dependence in everyday tasks is important to everyone, and no less so for children whose achievement is interrupted by disability. Research has demonstrated just how important it is since life outcome in social and work situations of young adults with congenital handicaps appears to be related to their independence in self-care. Wacker et al. (1983) reported that the variable most strongly related to satisfaction with life outcomes was the individuals' perception of their independence in self-care and mobility.

MEASUREMENT

Since the early years of the profession, therapists have been concerned with the assessment and treatment of dysfunctional self-care performance (Coley, 1978; Law and Usher, 1988). One of the first known checklists of self-care performance was published in 1935 (Wolf, 1969), and since that time assessment of function has been traditional in both occupational and physical therapy. Assessment forms were published from time to time in the early years, but more often treatment settings designed forms to meet the needs of their particular caseloads and treatment settings. This practice continues today.

Developmentally oriented functional assessments that incorporated information on child growth and development came into use in the 1940s. Developmental scales including basic self-care were published a few years later. For example, an upper-extremity motor development test that included age-keyed items on feeding, dressing, and grooming, as well as hand use, was developed at the New York State Rehabilitation Hospital (Miller et al., 1955). Such instruments used information on ages at which children typically master skills, and grouped the skills by the age at which achievement might be expected.

Nonstandardized Measures

Both published and nonpublished center-made nonstandardized measures are in wide use. The advantage of center-made instruments is that they can be designed for the needs of particular children in particular settings. The disadvantage is that assessment information cannot be generalized to other disabilities or settings. Furthermore, the semiformal methods of administration make it very difficult to ensure reliability among different therapists, even when a standardized method of evaluating each item has been developed. Improved skill or the lack thereof might reflect differences between therapists rather than changes in a child's performance.

One of the reasons therapists continue to construct their own instruments is because of the need for greater detail in planning treatment programs. Breakdown of self-care activities is different for a

child with an amputation, a child with cerebral palsy, a child with spina bifida, or a child with mental retardation. Published, though nonstandardized, instruments fill some of these needs (Brigance, 1978; Coley, 1978; Vulpe, 1979). These developmental scales are similar in design and purpose to center-made scales but provide a standardized administration and sometimes reliability of scoring as well. Items are often selected with disability categories in mind. For example, a comprehensive tool for evaluation of children's self-sufficiency in self-care activities was developed by the Occupational Therapy Department at Children's Hospital at Stanford, California (Bleck & Nagle, 1975) for use primarily in cerebral palsy.

Both center-made and published scales are designed for day-by-day guidance of intervention and are as detailed as available knowledge allows. The approximate ages of accomplishment are derived from multiple sources, including intelligence tests, developmental tests, and research studies. Coley (1978) described the thinking that went into the development of her center's self-care assessment. Because this tool was intended as a guide for the sequential learning of self-care skills, specifically by children with cerebral palsy, it included more steps in the achievement of skills as well as related motor abilities than are found in most developmental assessments. Coley's description (1978) of the design of the instrument exemplifies the thinking that has gone into similar instruments.

The design . . . reflects clear sequential development consistent with the maturation of the central nervous system. The arrangement of data allows the assessment to flow in concert with the appearance and integration of primitive reflexes and the evolution of more advanced patterns of movement. The plan for organizing the data collection in this handbook emerged from the analysis of each task of the activities of daily living assessment as a neuromotor developmental process. . . . As the tasks are broken down into developmental sequences, it becomes possible to define the task or activity of daily living by drawing from the description of the developmental sequence most closely associated with the level of independence being sought for the task. . . . From the numerous tasks of daily living, a basic unit of activities is selected and each activity defined. The normal sequence of behaviors is organized by using the approximate chronological age at which the child accomplishes the defined tasks. The numerical figures thus serve to maintain the order of the data, and additionally, the chronological system serves as a guide in determining the normative levels of performance (pp. 5-6).

Most other similar published self-care scales are a part of overall developmental assessments

(Brigance, 1978; Vulpe, 1979). The approximate ages at which all the tasks and subtasks are achieved were derived from many sources, which are identified in the manuals. The purpose of these assessments is to provide an ongoing inventory of a child's progress and achievements in all developmental areas. The developmental assessment published by Vulpe has a particularly detailed section on self-care.

Standardized Instruments

Derived normative age information for developmental scales is at best approximate, and the information on individual children is descriptive only. Meaningful overall scores are not obtainable because there is no way of weighing individual items. They are therefore not appropriate for use in research or the documentation of overall progress.

Recently standardized instruments that have been designed for reliable documentation of change include the Vineland Adaptive Behavior Scales (Sparrow, Balla and Cicchetti, 1984) and the Wee Functional Independence Measure (Granger, Hamilton, and Kayton 1988). These scales, however, yield only total scores within domains and are less useful in planning therapy. Two scales that can be used for both research and treatment planning are the Klein-Bell Scale (Klein and Bell, 1979) and the Pediatric Evaluation of Disability Inventory (PEDI) (Haley et al., 1992). Both these instruments were constructed with consideration for the acquisition of skills of individuals with physical disabilities.

The PEDI has several strengths as a measurement tool for children. It has been carefully standardized and yields a total score that can be used to measure the overall change in children with disabilities. Age expectations are given both for overall independence in separate domains and for individual items. The user can select the level of expectation desired, such as the age range at which 10%, 25%, 50%, 75%, or 90% of children without disabilities demonstrate mastery. The PEDI includes the evaluation of self-care, mobility, and social function.

The Klein-Bell Scale has also been shown to be reliable and valid for both use with adults (Klein and Bell, 1979) and with children (Law and Usher, 1988). Self-care items are broken down into discrete steps, each of which can be scored separately but can be combined into a total score. Because the scale was designed for adults, age norms were not needed, but Law and Usher assigned approxi-

mate age levels to each step based on developmental literature. The scale was found to discriminate between children with cerebral palsy and their age peers.

In summary, the selection of a measurement tool needs to be based upon the major purpose of the tool. Often more than one tool should be used, if multiple purposes are to be met. Possible purposes are (1) diagnostic-remedial, to provide a blueprint for selecting and sequencing treatment activities, (2) to describe self-care performance for communicating with parents and professionals, (3) to chart the acquisition of self-care skills, and (4) to evaluate the effects of treatment. Both center-made and published but not standardized evaluation instruments can be used for the first three purposes; only standardized instruments are appropriate for the fourth purpose.

FACTORS IN THE ACQUISITION OF SELF-CARE

Our knowledge of the factors that influence the development of basic self-care is based more on common knowledge derived from the experience of caregivers than on research. However, most would agree with the statement made by Key et al. (1936) about dressing—that learning is influenced by chronologic age, mental age, the child's interest, the amount of guidance given, and the type of clothing worn. Whether or not these factors are supported by research, social, psychologic, and physical factors, as well as gender and maturation, seem to play a part in when skills are acquired.

Social and Cultural Influences

Gesell and Ilg (1943) considered the development of feeding behavior in the infant to be a "story of progressive self dependence combined with cultural conformance." The broad culture and the expectations of the home and preschool all determine the degree and timing of a child's mastery of basic self-care skills (Bernard, 1970). However, there is little information on the impact of culture and society on the ages at which basic self-care skills are attained. Nevertheless, some generalizations based on common knowledge can be made.

An obvious cultural factor is in the difference in eating tools. The use of a spoon requires less motor maturation than chopsticks. The spoon is grasped in the fist and can be carried to the mouth with the forearm pronated, but chopsticks require individuation of the fingers and supination of the forearm. Another difference is the way in which knives and forks are used. In the United States, we scoop and spear with a fork and cut meat with the knife in the right hand, then switch utensils to continue eating. In some European countries the knife is used in the right hand to pile food on the back of the fork that is then carried to the mouth with the left hand. These differences may influence the sequence and timing of self-sufficiency in eating behavior.

Differences in dressing styles must certainly influence skill attainment. In some cultures children go naked until they are toilet trained. In the United States the emphasis on early self-sufficiency has led to inventions in clothing style. For example, draw-down diapers foster an earlier independence in going to the toilet, and Velcro fasteners make the preschool child self-sufficient in putting on shoes.

The development of early self-care is also determined by the philosophy of a culture. Cultures determine the appropriate time for a child to learn a skill. In the United States we generally encourage early self-sufficiency. For example, children are given finger foods and allowed to messily explore food manually. In my experience, in Mexico, many families with maids did not permit children to use spoons until they were able to do so without spilling; bibs were not used beyond early infancy. Such differences in attitudes result in differences in the timing of the child's mastery of basic skills.

Within the broad culture the performance of everyday skills is influenced by families. An example of family influence on a child's tidiness in eating was reported by Bott et al. (1928). They wondered why a child who was above average on most of their measures was so far below age expectations in eating. On questioning the parents they discovered that, because they thought the child was too young to eat well, they had made no attempt to correct him. When the expectations for the child were raised at home, his score rose to age levels within 2 weeks.

Two recent studies have investigated factors influencing competence in household tasks. A study by Zill and Peterson (cited by Amato and Ochiltree, 1986) found that the best predictor of performance on tasks such as washing dishes without help was the frequency of joint family activities. They also found that family size was related to competence in such skills. Large families may require more practical assistance from

their children in chores, and younger children are able to learn from older children. The family variables found by Amato and Ochiltree (1986) to foster the acquisition of practical skills were frequent interaction of family members and the requirement that the children take responsibility for chores.

In summary, cultural, class, and family variables influence the timing of the acquisition of independence in self-care in young children. For the most part societal expectations do not vary in respect to the need for eventual development of independence, but behavior in childhood may signify cultural and parental patterns rather than a child's intrinsic abilities.

Sex Differences

Several differences between girls and boys in the age at which self-care skills are acquired have been reported. Gesell and Ilg (1943) wrote that boys demand independence in dressing at a younger age than girls. Key et al. (1936) reported tentative sex differences in dressing ability between 2½ and 4½ years. Girls were more able than boys and tended to dress faster, and the ability of boys was generally more variable than that of girls. Sources of the differences in the ages at which dressing skills are achieved have been proposed. It has been thought that girls dress themselves earlier than boys because their wrists are more flexible, they are better coordinated, and they wear simpler clothing (Coley, 1978; Gesell et al., 1940; Key et al., 1936).

A difference has also been reported in the use of eating utensils (Gesell and Ilg, 1943). Girls shifted to an adult grasp earlier than boys, some as early as 3 years. Some boys, on the other hand, continued to use a pronated grasp at 8 years of age. Boys were also reported to sometimes demand to feed themselves before they were competent to do so.

Sex differences may be a factor in the development of individual skills, but no differences in overall functional ability were reported in recent research (Haley et al., 1992). Further study is needed to confirm the early findings.

Maturation

Although culture and family expectations play a role, it seems clear that the greatest factor in the achievement of self-care skill in childhood is maturation. Certainly Gesell and his associates thought so, and self-care items are prominent in developmental diagnosis (Gesell and Amatruda, 1965). This supposition is borne out by research. Key and her associates (1936) found the correlation between dressing ability and chronologic age to be considerably higher than that for mental age or any other factor. The composite score of self-care, mobility, and social functions of the PEDI showed high and significant correlation with age but not with demographic variables.

Personal Factors

The influence of personality factors such as volition and self-sufficiency in the performance of practical skills such as self-care has only recently begun to be studied (Bullock and Lutkenhaus, 1988; Geppert and Kuster, 1983). Most accounts are anecdotal, but they report interest, self-reliance, and perseverance to be important (Key et al., 1936; Wagoner and Armstrong, 1928). Key and her associates reported that interest in dressing develops with ability; in 2-year-old children, as mastery increased, enjoyment increased. At 3 they found interest to shift to desire for approval and achievement and found wide differences in the development of self-reliance and the perseverance needed for the performance of the more difficult tasks. These findings were based on analysis of the children's comments while dressing.

Motor Factors

Coley (1978) identified sequences of gross and fine motor development leading to independence in self-care tasks. Examples of necessary gross motor abilities needed for dressing are reaching above the head or behind the back while maintaining trunk stability. Self-feeding requires head and mouth control as well as trunk stability. Coley identified steps in the motor control leading to many individual self-care skills, and they are incorporated into the tables and discussed within each self-care domain. They include bilateral skills, finger manipulation, and tool skills.

Children learn one-handed skills before bilateral skills (see Chapter 7), and the later achievement of some skills occurs because of the need for the two hands to work together. An early example is holding the bowl with one hand while scooping with the other. Examples in dressing include pulling on boots, zipping, and buttoning, which are more difficult because they require more precision in bilateral functioning.

Children become functional in the performance of skills during their preschool years, but complete independence and adult levels of speed and precision require a long developmental period. One indication of the automatization of a skill that occurs at about 4 years of age is when children can feed themselves and dress themselves while carrying on a conversation (Klein, 1983; Hurlock, 1956).

Many self-care activities require the use of tools (Castle, 1985). Tools are defined here as a means of effecting change in other objects. The earliest self-care tools are for eating: spoons, knives, forks, and cups. Self-care in hygiene includes tools such as brushes, combs, and washcloths. Dressing fasteners, zippers, snaps, and buttons can also be considered tools. The use of most tools is complex because it involves the manipulation of one object relative to another, which results in the change of state of one or both objects (Parker and Gibson, 1977). The use of tools is goal directed by definition and requires the understanding of a means-end relationship. Even the use of a simple tool such as a spoon requires both the understanding of purpose and the motor skill to use it. However, as children mature, their understanding often moves ahead of their manipulative skill. In general, learning to use tools is acquired later than self-care without tools.

CHRONOLOGY OF SELF-CARE ACQUISITION

The following discussion presents sequences in which children learn to care for their own daily needs. The information has been compiled from different sources to provide as much detailed information as is available. The purpose of charting such information is to allow a preliminary analysis of the relationship of the acquisition of self-care skills to the development of hand skills. The child's attempts at performance are included because they show an understanding of the task, and the practicing of subskills reflects motor abilities.

The developmental information in the following discussion is organized into the domains of eating, drinking, dressing, personal hygiene, grooming, and simple household tasks. The items listed in the charts are steps in the learning of self-care that various authors have observed and reported. They are included to show some of the possible steps through which children may learn the skills. We have no definitive information as to the consistency of the sequences by which children learn, just assumptions about some overall sequences of skill development, which are based on reports of ages at which children are usually self-sufficient.

The area of research that has provided the most information on the acquisition of specific self-care skills over the years has been the area of development of evaluation tools. Two such primary sources of information were used to chart the approximate ages at which skills are achieved. The first source is the PEDI developed by Haley et al. (1992). This instrument includes extensive sections on basic self-care and provides the most reliable information available on the ages at which many skills are achieved. The ages noted in the tables indicate a group in which more than 75% of the children were reported to have achieved independence.

The works of Gesell and his associates were also a primary source. Their data on the development of self-care skills were collected by many different methods over many years. The results of most of their observations were incorporated into overviews of development (Gesell and Amatruda, 1965; Gesell and Ilg, 1943, 1946; Gesell et al., 1940). They were interested in information that would assist in the diagnosis of developmental delay and to that end selected different sorts of behaviors expected at each age level. The behaviors selected have provided developmental information on the acquisition of basic self-care skills for many years.

Several secondary sources were also used. Following the lead of the Yale Developmental Clinic, self-care items were and continue to be included in many developmental evaluation instruments. These instruments include approximate ages for the acquisition of self-care skills derived from multiple sources. The primary and secondary sources used for the tables that follow were Coley (1978), Brigance (1978), Vulpe (1979), Haley et al. (1992), Gesell and Ilg (1943, 1946), and Key et al. (1936).

It must be emphasized that the ages listed from these sources are only approximate, are not necessarily derived the same way, and reflect different levels of expectations. The data in the tables are best interpreted as ages at which many, but not all, healthy children perform under optimum circumstances. Furthermore, it must be recognized that the age at which children master self-care skills is highly variable. An important finding of the PEDI research was that there is a wide age range,

sometimes as much as 3 to 4 years, over which individual children achieve particular skills.

Eating

The progress of a child's self-feeding behavior requires both the acquisition of skill in the use of eating utensils and conformity to cultural standards. In typically picturesque speech Gesell (Gesell and Ilg, 1943) described this progression.

At 36 weeks he can usually maintain a sustained hold on the bottle. In another month he may hold it up and tilt it with the skill of a cornetist. He can feed himself a cracker. At 40 weeks, he also begins to finger feed, plucking small morsels . . . . He also handles his spoon manfully [by 15 months] and begins to feed himself in part, though not without spilling, for the spoon is a complex tool and he has not acquired the postural orientations and pre-perceptions necessary for dexterity . . . . At 2 years, he inhibits the turning of the spoon as it enters the mouth and feeds himself acceptably . . . . At 3½ years he enjoys a Sunday breakfast with the family . . . . At 5 years . . . he likes to eat away from home especially at a restaurant. He is more a man of the world!

Finger feeding and the use of a cup are early accomplishments and the basic components of self-feeding with a spoon—filling the spoon, carrying it to the mouth without spilling, and removing food—are well mastered by 3 years of age. However, self-feeding takes concentration, and it is not until after the third or fourth year that the skill is sufficiently automatic to allow eating and talking at the same time (Hurlock, 1956). The 5-year-old is skillful but slow. Skill continues to improve, for it is not until 8 or 9 years of age that the child has become deft and graceful (Gesell and Ilg, 1946), and it is not until 10 years that self-feeding is accomplished entirely independently, with good control and with attention to table manners (Hurlock, 1956).

Finger Feeding

Self-feeding with the fingers begins in the second half of the first year. Table 10-1 shows the development of the skill, which parallels the infant's acquisition of hand skills. Initial feeding is of crackers held in the hand and sometimes plastered against the mouth with the palm and with the forearm supinated. As finger skill develops, bite-size pieces of food are picked up and put into the mouth with a pincer grasp. Even when spoon use has become skillful, children prefer to use fingers for discrete pieces of food such as peas or meat (Gesell and Ilg, 1943).

Table **10-1** Eating finger foods

SKILL	AGE	SOURCE
Picks up finger foods and eats	6 mo-1 yr	Haley et al.
Feeds self cracker, whole hand grasp	6-7 mo	Coley
Feeds self spilled bits from tray	9 mo	Gesell and Ilg (1943)
Feeds self finger foods, pincer grasp	10 mo	Coley
Finger feeds part of one meal	1 yr	Gesell and Ilg (1943)
Takes bite-size pieces from plate, delicate grasp, appropriate force, with demonstrated release	1 yr	Coley

Drinking from a Cup or Bottle

Independent drinking from a cup is an early developing skill as long as safeguards are taken. The use of spout cups with lids allows a child to drink from a cup as well as a bottle in the second half of the first year of life. Table 10-2 shows the progress of skill in drinking. Cup drinking begins with the same bilateral whole hand grasp used for the bottle and progresses to the dexterous grip of one hand on the handle at 3 years of age.

Use of Utensils

Table 10-3 shows the chronology of the development of the use of spoons, forks, and knives. The many years required for learning to use utensils reflects the complexity of their use, particularly the knife and fork in cutting. The infant begins eating with a spoon held in a fisted grasp, with the arm pronated and with shoulder abduction. The adult finger grip, with forearm supination and rotation as needed, allows more fine motor control and dexterity (Haley et al., 1992) but does not develop until approximately 3 years in girls (Gesell et al., 1940); some boys continue to use a pronated pattern at 8 years (Gesell and Ilg, 1946). The fisted grasp appears again in the use of forks and knives in cutting. It appears that the force needed for holding and cutting requires the power of the whole hand. The necessary power combined with the finger dexterity for cutting is not developed until a child is about 10.

Studies of spoon use. The spoon is the first tool used by most infants (Connolly and Dalgleish, 1989). Several studies of spoon use have been reported, two involving infants and one preschool children. The earliest study, of nursery school children's eating behavior, was a part of a larger study of multiple habits (Bott et al., 1928). The eating behaviors included in the study were (1) the proper use of utensils, (2) putting the proper portion of food on a utensil, and (3) coordination, as indicated by minimal spilling. They found improvement with age in all these behaviors, but the behaviors differed as to when they improved. The use and filling of the utensils improved primarily between 2 and 3 years, but spilling decreased more between 3 and 4 years.

The cinemagraphic study of infant eating behaviors conducted by Gesell and Ilg (1937) described both prespoon activity and early spoon use. Preparation for using the spoon began when a child was being fed. Between 3 and 6 months of age the child watched the spoon, and soon mouth opening began in anticipation of the spoon

Table **10-2** Self-feeding: drinking from cup/bottle

SKILL	AGE	SOURCE
Holds and drinks from bottle/spout cup with lid	6 mo-1 yr	Haley et al.
Tips bottle to drink	10 mo	Gesell and Ilg (1943)
Lifts open cup to drink, some tipping	1½-2 yr	Haley et al.
Holds cup alone, hands pressed on side	1 yr	Gesell and Ilg (1943)
Grasps with thumb and fingertips	1 yr 3 mo	Gessell and Ilg (1943)
Holds cup and tilts by finger action	1 yr 3 mo	Gesell and Ilg (1943)
Lifts open cup securely with two hands	1½-2 yr	Haley et al.
Lifts cup to mouth, drinks well, may drop	1½ yr	Coley
Holds cup well, lifts, drinks, replaces	1 yr 9 mo	Coley
Lifts open cup to drink with one hand	3-3½ yr	Haley et al.
Holds cup or glass with one hand, free hand poised to help	2 yr	Gesell and Ilg (1943)
Cup held by handle, drinks securely, one hand	3 yr	Gesell and Ilg (1943)

Table 10-3 Self-feeding: use of utensils

SKILL	AGE	SOURCE
Spoon		
Grasps spoon in fist	10-11 mo	Gesell and Ilg (1943)
Dips spoon in food, lifts to mouth	1 yr 3 mo	Gesell and Ilg (1943)
Fisted grasp, pronated forearm, turns spoon	1 yr 3 mo	Coley
Scoops food, lifts with spilling	1½-2 yr	Haley et al.
Fills spoon, turns in mouth, spilling	1½ yr	Coley
Spoon angled slightly toward mouth	1½ yr	Gesell and Ilg (1943)
Tilts spoon handle up as removes from mouth	1½ yr	Gesell and Ilg (1943)
Uses spoon well with minimal spilling	2-2½ yr	Haley et al.
Point of spoon enters mouth	2 yr	Gesell and Ilg (1943)
Inserts spoon into mouth without turning	2 yr	Gesell and Ilg (1943)
Fills by pushing point of spoon into food	2 yr	Gesell and Ilg (1943)
Grasps spoon with fingers (girls supinate)	3 yr	Gesell and Ilg (1943)
Fills spoon by pushing point or rotating spoon	3 yr	Gesell and Ilg (1943)
Holds spoon with fingers for solid foods	4 yr	Coley
Eats liquids, spoon held with fingers, few spills	4-6 yr	Coley
Fork		
Spears and shovels food, little spilling	2-2½ yr	Haley et al.
Fork held in fingers	4½ yr	Coley
Knife		
Uses for spreading	5-5½ yr	Haley et al.
Spreads with knife	6-7 yr	Coley
Uses to cut soft foods (sandwich)	5-5½ yr	Haley et al.
Cuts meat with knife	7-8 yr	Coley
Deft and graceful in the use of utensils	8 yr	Gesell and Ilg (1946)

reaching the mouth. Later, head movements began—movement of the head toward the spoon and then away as food is removed. Whereas initially food was put in the mouth by the adult's manipulation of the spoon, the child later removed food by lip compression. These movements of the head and lips were considered to make later spoon manipulation more effective.

Gesell and Ilg noted that even as simple a tool as a spoon requires a sequence of perceptual and motor acts. One act is the discriminative grasp of the spoon handle. Infants first grasped the lower third of the handle, later the middle to upper third, and finally the end. Grasp was at first palmar, with the thumb wrapped around the spoon, but later the thumb was placed along the handle. The adult grasp was not usually seen until the age of 3.

A second perceptual and motor act is the filling of the spoon. At first the bowl of the spoon is merely dipped in the dish, often with the spoon handle perpendicular. Filling began with a rotary movement toward the body, and it was not until 16 months that children began filling the spoon by

inserting its point into the food. Lifting the spoon was at first accomplished with the arm pronated, and often with the bowl of the spoon tipping. By the end of the second year children were lifting their elbows and flexing their wrists. The insertion of the spoon into the mouth also changed from the side into the mouth to the point into the mouth.

The third study, recently reported by Connolly and Dalgleish (1989), confirmed many of the findings of Gesell and Ilg. They conducted a comprehensive videotape study on the longitudinal development of spoon use. The research procedure was more formal, and the study can serve as a model for the investigation of the learning of complex motor skills. The authors first presented an analysis of spoon use that included both intentional and operational aspects. The task was described as entailing:

. . . (a) an intention to eat, which involves the child's motivation; (b) some knowledge about the properties of the spoon as an implement with which to effect the transfer of food from dish to mouth; (c) the ability to grasp and hold the spoon in a stable configuration; (d) the loading of food onto the spoon; (e) carrying the loaded spoon from dish to mouth; (f) controlling the orientation of the spoon during this transfer to avoid spillage; and (g) emptying the spoon and extracting it (p. 897).

On the basis of on this analysis, Connolly and Dalgleish conducted a longitudinal videotape study of the development in the operation of a spoon during the second year of life. Among their descriptions was an analysis of change in the action sequences from only two actions to a complex sequence that included corrections.

The actions of putting a spoon in and out of a dish and putting the spoon in and out of the mouth were initially unconnected. The first purposeful sequence was in five steps: (1) spoon to dish, (2) remove from dish, (3) lift to mouth, (4) put in mouth, and (5) remove from mouth. Later two added actions, filling the spoon and removing food with lips, were added. The final action sequence included 11 steps that included monitoring and correction through repetition of sequences: (1) control of spoon, (2) spoon to dish, (3) steady dish with other hand, (4) remove spoon from dish, (5) check to see if there is enough food on spoon (if not, repeat 2 to 4), (6) lift spoon, (7) put spoon in mouth, (8) empty spoon with lips, (9) remove from mouth, (10) check to see if spoon is empty (if not, repeat 7 to 9), (11) pick up spilled food (repeat 6 to 8).

This change in action sequences seems to indicate that the child was learning skill both in the performance of single actions and in the use of complex movement sequences. Connolly and Dalgleish also report other changes in motor actions, such as a smoothing of the trajectory of the dish-to-mouth path, and the shifting of the angle at which the spoon was placed from side toward mouth, to point toward mouth. Children used primarily a palmar grasp; some of the wrist, shoulder, and elbow movements were also described.

Serving/Preparing Food

A part of independence in eating is serving oneself and preparing foods. Table 10-4 shows that by the time children enter school they can take care of simple preparation and self-service of food and drink. In the preschool years children also begin to help with simple household chores such as setting the table (3 to 4 years), putting away silverware (2 years), wiping up spills (3 years), and wiping dishes (3 years) (Gesell and Ilg, 1943).

One of the expectations of the nursery school children studied by Bott et al. (1928) was that their feeding area be cleaned up after they ate. At the

Table 10-4 Serving/preparing food

SKILL	AGE	SOURCE
Prepares Food		
Unwraps food	1½-2 yr	Vulpe
Opens jars	2 yr	Gesell and Ilg (1943)
Fixes dry cereal	4-5 yr	Vulpe
Makes sandwich	7 yr	Brigance
Serves self	4-5 yr	Vulpe
Prepares baked potato	8 yr	Gesell and Ilg (1946)
Prepares Drinks		
Pours from small pitcher	2-2½ yr	Vulpe
Obtains drink from tap	3-3½ yr	Gesell and Ilg (1943)
Pours from large pitcher or carton	4-4½ yr	Haley et al.
Carries glasses without spilling	6 yr	Brigance
Other Skills		
Uses napkin	4 yr	Brigance
Sets table with help	2½-3 yr	Vulpe
Wipes up spills	3 yr	Gesell and Ilg (1943)
Sets table without help	4-5 yr	Vulpe

age of 2 the children left the table, chair, and floor clean after eating in 45% of the observations. By the age of 4 years the percentage had increased to 85%. This change undoubtedly reflects the influence of nursery school expectations as well as maturation.

Dressing

The development of self-care in dressing, undressing, and managing fasteners also parallels and depends on the development of hand skills. A fisted grasp is sufficient for the tasks of removing hat and socks. Pulling up pants requires more strength and bilateral coordination than pushing them down and kicking them off. Individual finger function comes into play in loosening laces, and full independence in dressing requires complex finger manipulation of buttons and ties. It is the need for finger dexterity and planning sequences that underlies the slow acquisition of management of fasteners.

Key and her associates (1936) studied the process of learning to dress among 45 nursery school children, ages 1½ to 5½ years. Overall dressing ability was highly correlated with chronologic age. They reported the learning process to be continuous, increasingly difficult, and unstable, and that the most rapid period of learning was between 1½ years and 2½ years. Overall success rates increased over the ages studied as follows: 1½ years, 40%; 2 years, 50%; 2½ years, 80%; and 3½ years to 5½ years, 90%. Other authors have also reported that dressing skills develop rapidly between 1½ and 3½ years (Gesell et al., 1940).

Self-help in putting on and removing clothes is highly dependent on the type of clothing worn (Key et al., 1936). The variability in the age of acquisition is undoubtedly in part a result of the type of clothes selected for children by their caregivers. Characteristics of clothing that facilitate self-dressing include loose tops with large neck openings and loose pants with elastic tops and loose cuffs. The type and size of fasteners should be appropriate for children and they should be in reasonable locations (front or side). Velcro and buttons with long shanks facilitate independence (Reich and Otten, 1980). It should be noted, however, that peer fashions may be important even for young children, and compromises between independence and self-esteem may be needed.

The overall development of dressing skill proceeds from undressing to dressing without fastening to managing fasteners. Taking off an item of clothing is easier than putting it on since putting on clothing is more complex both motorically and perceptually. For example, socks slip off easily, but the coordination between the two hands and between hands and feet together are needed for putting socks on. Moreover, the sock must be rotated correctly to match its heel to the heel of the foot.

Information on the chronology of dressing is presented in four areas: antecedents of dressing skills, undressing without fasteners, dressing without fasteners, and managing fasteners.

Antecedents of Dressing Skills

Table 10-5 lists approximate ages at which children achieve abilities necessary for dressing. The earliest interaction with clothing, such as clutching and pulling at clothing, is meaningless in respect to self-care but demonstrates the ability to

Table 10-5 Antecedents of self-dressing skills

SKILL	AGE	SOURCE
Reach and Grasp		
Clutches and pulls clothing	up to 3 mo	Vulpe
Pulls off hat	6 mo	Vulpe
Pulls off booties	6-9 mo	Gesell and Ilg (1943)
Pulls off socks	9-10 mo	Vulpe
Cooperation		
Passive (lies still)	3-6 mo	Vulpe
Holds arm out	9 mo	Coley
Lifts foot for shoe or pants	1½-2 yr	Haley et al.
Attempts Skill		
Tries to put on shoes	14-18 mo	Vulpe
Tries to assist with fasteners	2-2½ yr	Haley et al.
Helps push down pants	2 yr	Coley
Interested in lacing	2½-3 yr	Vulpe
Trunk Stability		
Reaching to toes	1 yr 4 mo	Coley
Reaching above head bilaterally/ unilaterally	2-5 yr	Coley
Reaching behind back, hands together	3-6 yr	Coley
Reaching behind head, hands together	4-6 yr	Coley

grasp. The early removal of hats and socks is also hardly purposeful undressing since it is just as likely to occur during dressing as during undressing. Nevertheless, these actions demonstrate motor sequences that will later be used purposefully.

Researchers have chronicled infant beginnings of cooperation and assistance in dressing (Gesell and Ilg, 1943). These early actions of pushing with arms or legs are components of later self-dressing. Furthermore, actions such as holding arms or legs out demonstrate the child's understanding of the dressing process. Trying to assist (e.g., pulling at a zipper tab) may not be functional but is important because it demonstrates modeling behavior (Haley et al., 1992).

Table 10-6 Undressing: clothes unfastened or without fasteners

SKILL	AGE	SOURCE
Hat and Mittens		
Pulls off hat appropriately, on request	1½ yr	Gesell and Ilg (1943)
Removes mittens	12-14 mo	Coley
Socks and Shoes		
Removes socks on request	1½-2 yr	Haley et al.
Removes untied/unfastened shoes	1½-2 yr	Haley et al.
Unties and removes shoes	2-3 yr	Coley
Pants/Pull-Down Garments		
Pushes off pants if soiled	1 yr	Gesell and Ilg (1943)
Pushes down underpants/shorts	21-24 mo	Gesell and Ilg (1943)
Removes elastic top on long pants, clearing over bottom	2-2½ yr	Haley et al.
Shirt/Coat/Sweater		
Removes second arm from coat	1 yr	Brigance
Removes unbuttoned coat	1 yr	Brigance
Removes pullover garments, T-shirt, dress	2½-3 yr	Haley et al.
Assistance needed	3 yr	Coley
Little assistance	4 yr	Coley

Undressing: Clothes Unfastened or Without Fasteners

Table 10-6 identifies the sequences in which children learn to take off their clothes. Complete independence in undressing requires the release of fasteners, a skill that doesn't develop until after 3 years (Coley, 1978). However, with assistance in unfastening, the toddler can take off much clothing. Undressing requires only simple perceptual skills; knowing front from behind and left from right is unnecessary. Furthermore, fewer action sequences are needed than for dressing (Klein, 1983), and hand use requires little more than gross grasp, pulling, and pushing. Interest in taking clothes off begins in the first year; by 2½ years most children can and want to take off their clothes, and by 3 years undressing is done well and rapidly (Gesell and Ilg, 1943).

Dressing With Assistance on Fasteners

Table 10-7 lists the sequences in which dressing skills are acquired. The long 5-year developmental period is to a great extent a reflection of the perceptual skills needed. The last skills achieved are in the orientation of the heel of the sock, the front and back of garments, and, the most difficult, the distinguishing of left and right shoes.

Children know when their coat is right side out when they are 3, but they have more difficulty with other clothes. The 4- or 5-year-old gets the underclothes right side out, but it is not until 7 years that the inside and outside of all clothes are discriminated (Brigance, 1978). In addition to these perceptual skills, self-care dressing skills require complex motor planning. Gaddes (1983) described the difficulty of some children with learning disabilities in dressing as a lack of the tactile and kinesthetic awareness essential to the task of putting on one's clothes, and commented that "small children are usually unable to put on their clothes without help . . . not because they lack the physical strength but because they lack the necessary ideomotor image" (p. 109).

The hand skills needed are primarily whole-hand grasp, a power grasp for pulling clothing on, and a high level of bilateral skill. Hands must work smoothly and in unison to pull socks up to full extension, pull on boots, and pull up pants. Hands must work cooperatively in holding a shirt or coat with one hand while finding the armhole with the other.

Additional bilateral dressing skills have been identified by Thornby and Krebs (1992). Their interest was in expectations for independence for children with unilateral below-elbow amputations. The skills identified include grasping and pulling up trousers or skirt (2½-3 years), and grasping clothing while zipping a zipper (3 years 3 months to 4 years). The children with amputations achieved these skills several years later than usual.

A study of dressing. Key and her associates (1936) studied the ability of children to put on the clothing that they wore to nursery school and found wide differences in the ability to put on

Table 10-7 Self-dressing: without fasteners

SKILL	AGE	SOURCE
Hat		
Puts on, may be backward	2 yr	Gesell et al.
Socks		
Puts on with help on heel orientation	3 yr	Coley
Puts on heel correctly oriented	3-3½ yr	Haley et al.
Pulls socks to full extension	4 yr	Key et al.
Shoes		
Gets shoe on halfway	1½ yr	Gesell et al.
Puts on, may be on wrong feet	3-3½ yr	Haley et al.
If laces are loosened	2 yr	Gesell et al.
Loosens laces and puts on	2½ yr	Vulpe
Puts on correct feet	4½-5 yr	Haley et al.
Puts on boots if loose fitting	3-4 yr	Vulpe
Independent with Velcro fastenings	4½-5 yr	Haley et al.
Coat/Open-Front Shirt		
Finds large armholes	2 yr	Coley
Puts on coat with help	2 yr 9 mo	Coley
Puts on open-front shirt	3½-4 yr	Haley et al.
Adjusts collar to neck	3 yr	Key et al.
Pullover Garment/T-Shirt/Dress		
Puts on pullover garment	3-3½ yr	Haley et al.
Puts head through hole	2 yr	Key et al.
Puts arm through hole	3½ yr	Key et al.
Pulls down over trunk	3 yr	Key et al.
Distinguishes Front/Back, Inside Out	4 yr	Coley
Pants/Pull-Up Garment		
Helps pull pants up	2 yr	Gesell et al.
Tries to put on, two feet in one hole	2-2½ yr	Gesell et al.
Puts on if oriented verbally	3-3½ yr	Haley et al.
Orients correctly and puts on	4 yr	Coley
Can turn right side out	4 yr	Coley

separate garments. Overall, socks and leg garments were found to be the easiest, followed by upper body garments and dresses. Shoes, because of their fasteners, were the most difficult.

In addition to looking at the overall ability to put on the garments, the researchers recorded the success rate of separate dressing units for each garment. These data provided an index of the difficulty of the subskills needed for successful performance. An analysis of the percentage of success for each subskill at each age level shows the relative difficulties of the components of putting on shoes, socks, pull-down garments, dresses, and shirts. This list excludes fasteners, and open-front and slipover shirts were not differentiated. The order of difficulty reported here is based on the age group in which 50% or more of the children succeeded in the task.

Put one leg in hole of pants
Pulled up pants
Shoe started on foot
Opened shoe for foot
Put head in neck hole of dress
Put on dress correctly front to back
Socks started over foot
Put foot in shoe with heel down
Pulled sock up on leg
Kept tongue out of shoe while donning

Put second leg in hole of pull-down garment
Pulled sock up on foot
Put pullover garment over head
Put first arm in dress hole
Adjusted dress when on
Put second arm in sleeve hole of dress
Shirt on correctly front to back
Adjusted pants when on
Put first arm in sleeve hole of T-shirt
Adjusted shirt when on
Put second arm in sleeve hole of T-shirt
Pants on correctly front to back
Adjusted heel of sock

It can be seen that the difficulty young children have in dressing is sometimes a result of a challenging perceptual task, such as locating the front of a T-shirt or the heel of a sock, and sometimes a complex motor act, such as maneuvering an arm into a second dress hole.

Fasteners: Zippers, Snaps, Buttons, Ties

Table 10-8 shows the range of approximate ages at which children are able to fasten and unfasten their clothing. Manipulating zippers, as long as hooking and unhooking a separating zipper are not included, is the easiest form of closure while tying is the most difficult. The feature all fasteners have in common is the need for bilateral finger manipulation skills. Zippers require precision grip and pinch strength. The bilateral nature of this task is shown by the 3-year delay in skill acquisition in children with unilateral below-elbow amputations (Thornby and Krebs, 1992). Buttons require precision grip with manipulation and with both hands working cooperatively.

Another component of the management of fasteners is strength. Snaps require considerable strength in the fingers. Koch and Simenson (1992) examined functional skills in spinal muscle atrophy. Children with 1/2- to 2-lb pinch strength needed minimal help in dressing. Children with less than 1/2-lb pinch strength had trouble with tying and buttoning.

Managing fasteners is also a perceptual task, particularly buttoning and tying. For both these tasks vision is important for learning. It is only after considerable skill has been developed that back buttons and back bows can be accomplished, using touch and kinesthesia alone.

Buttoning. The ability to button has been included in developmental tests for many years, and it has been studied more than other fastenings. The ability develops in preschool over 2 to 3 years of age, and achievement depends in part on the location of

the button. Stutzman (1948) examined the ability of preschool children to button buttons on a strip on a table. Children under 2 years of age failed to button one button, but by 2 1/2 to 3 years of age 72% of the children succeeded, albeit slowly. However, Key et al. (1936) reported that only 50% of their 3-year-old children succeeded in buttoning their shirts or dresses, and only 33% their pants.

Wagoner and Armstrong (1928) reported a study of buttoning skill in 30 nursery school children between the ages of 2 and 5 years. They standardized the task by making jackets that were adjustable in size and which had front and side buttons. The major findings were: (1) children under 2 1/2 years seemed not to have the motor control needed to button; from 2 1/2 to 5 years speed of buttoning improved with age; (2) girls were better than boys, but the researchers noted that this result might have reflected an artifact of their sample; and (3) side buttons were much more difficult than front buttons; 25 children succeeded with the front buttons, but only 15 completed the side buttons (the authors noted that buttoning side buttons may require a more complex type of motor adjustment than do front buttons).

Wagoner and Armstrong also reported correlation of buttoning speed with the Stanford-Binet ($r = .33$), the Merrill-Palmer Performance Tests ($r = .62$), and the Goodenough Drawing Test ($r = .57$). Thus buttoning appeared to be more related to performance tests than to intelligence. They also found success in buttoning to be highly correlated (.83 to .91) with teacher ratings on self-reliance, perseverance, and care of details.

Learning to tie shoes. Shoe tying is an important and difficult developmental task for children. Children perceive the relationship of the loops and strings and learn the steps of looping, winding, and pulling through but still may fail. The most difficult aspect of shoe tying appears to be what Maccoby and Bee (1965) in their study of form copying termed the *perception of attributes*. Their example was that children discriminate forms such as diamonds but are unable to draw them because they do not perceive the attributes of the form, such as the relative size of lines and angles. Similarly, children do not perceive the relative sizes of loops and strings; the loop is too large and the bow fails. It is only when children perceive these attributes of the lacing process that they succeed.

Learning to tie shoes is of special importance to a child's sense of competence. The 6-year-old child has a sense of achievement and independence from adult help in the school environment.

Table 10-8 Fasteners: ties, buckles, velcro, snaps, zippers, buttons

SKILL	AGE	SOURCE
Shoes—Lace and Tie		
Unties show bow	1½ yr	Brigance
Pulls laces tight	2½-3 yr	Vulpe
Tries to lace, usually incorrect	3 yr	Coley
Laces shoes	4-5 yr	Coley
Ties overhand knot	5 yr 3 mo	Coley
Ties bow on shoes	6-6½ yr	Haley et al.
Sashes, Necktie		
Unties back sash of apron or dress	5 yr	Coley
Ties front sash of apron or dress	6 yr	Coley
Ties back sash of apron or dress	8 yr	Coley
Ties necktie	10 yr	Coley
Buckles		
Unbuckles belt or shoe	3 yr 9 mo	Coley
Buckles belt or shoe	4 yr	Coley
Inserts belt in loops	4½ yr	Coley
Velcro Fasteners		
Manages shoes with Velcro	4½-5 yr	Haley et al.
Snaps		
Unsnaps front snaps	1 yr	Brigance
Unsnaps back snaps	3 yr	Brigance
Snaps most snaps, front/side	3½-4 yr	Haley et al.
Snaps back snaps	6 yr	Coley
Zippers		
Zips and unzips, lock tab	2-2½ yr	Haley et al.
Opens front separating zipper	3½ yr	Coley
Zips front separating zipper	4½ yr	Coley
Opens back zipper	4 yr 9 mo	Coley
Closes back zipper	5½ yr	Coley
Zips, unzips, hooks, unhooks, separating zipper	5½-6 yr	Haley et al.
Buttons		
Unbuttons most front and side buttons	3 yr	Coley
Buttons one large front button	2½ yr	Coley
Buttons series of three buttons	3½ yr	Coley
Buttons/unbuttons most buttons	4-4½ yr	Haley et al.
Buttons back buttons	6 yr 3 mo	Coley

Hygiene and Grooming

Tables 10-9 and 10-10 present the sequences in which hygiene and grooming skills are acquired by children. The development of parts of the skills begins in early childhood, but independence in most hygiene and grooming skills is a middle childhood achievement.

Many hygiene and grooming tasks are bilateral. Hands are rubbed together in washing; in drying, towels are held alternately while drying each hand. Applying toothpaste on a brush is a skilled bilateral activity. This was shown by the delay in which children with unilateral amputations were found to achieve this task (Thornby and Krebs, 1992). The toothbrush is a tool that requires a high

Table 10-9 Hygiene

SKILL	AGE	SOURCE
Washing/Drying Hands		
Holds out hands to be washed	1½-2 yr	Haley et al.
Dries with help	1½ yr	Coley
Rubs hands together to clean	1½-2 yr	Haley et al.
Turns faucet on/off	2½-3 yr	Haley et al.
Dries hands thoroughly	3½-4 yr	Haley et al.
Without supervision	3½ yr	Coley
Washes hands thoroughly	3½-4 yr	Haley et al.
Without supervision	3 yr 9 mo	Coley
Disposes of paper towel or replaces towel	4 yr	Coley
Washes hands at appropriate time before meals	6 yr	Coley
Washing Face		
Washes/dries face thoroughly	5½-6 yr	Haley et al.
Without supervision	4 yr 9 mo	Haley et al.
Washes ears	8-9 yr	Haley et al.
Bathing Body		
Tries to wash body	1½-2 yr	Haley et al.
Bathes down front of body	3 yr	Coley
Washes body well	3½-4 yr	Haley et al.
Soaps cloth and washes	4½ yr	Coley
Teeth Brushing		
Opens mouth for teeth to be brushed	1-2 yr	Haley et al.
Holds brush, approximates brushing	1½-2 yr	Haley et al.
Brushes teeth, not thoroughly	2-2½ yr	Haley et al.
Thoroughly brushes teeth	4½-5 yr	Haley et al.
Prepares brush, wets and applies paste	4½-5 yr	Haley et al.
Brushes routinely after meals	7 yr	Coley
Nose Care		
Allows wiping of nose	1½-2 yr	Haley et al.
Wipes on request	2-2½ yr	Haley et al.
Wipes without request	3-3½ yr	Haley et al.
Attempts to blow nose	1½-2 yr	Haley et al.
Blows and wipes alone	6-6½ yr	Haley et al.
Toileting		
Assists with clothing management	2-2½ yr	Haley et al.
Manages clothes before and after toileting	3-3½ yr	Haley et al.
Tries to wipe self after toileting	3-3½ yr	Haley et al.
Manages toilet seat, toilet paper, flushes	3-3½ yr	Haley et al.
Wipes self thoroughly	5½-6 yr	Haley et al.
Completely cares for self at toilet	5 yr	Coley

level of skill, as wrist and hand movements are complex in placing the brush and brushing all the teeth. It is also a skill accomplished without vision.

Independence in hair care is greatly influenced by social factors, especially for girls. At about the time when hair becomes manageable by the 4-to 7-year-old child, independence is often delayed in girls by choice of hairstyles (e.g., braids are usually a teenage accomplishment). Hair styling requires a complex manipulation of many tools—brush, comb, pins, dryers—all of which must be used without vision or with mirror vision.

Table 10-10 Grooming

SKILL	AGE	SOURCE
Hair		
Holds head in position for combing	1-1½ yr	Haley et al.
Brings comb to hair	1-1½ yr	Haley et al.
Brushes or combs hair; combs with supervision	2½-3 yr	Haley et al.
Manages tangles/ parts hair	7 yr	Haley et al.
Combs using mirror to check style	7½	Coley
Uses rollers, hairspray	12 yr	Coley
Shoes		
Shines shoes	7 yr	Brigance
Deodorant		
Uses daily	12 yr	Coley
Nail Care		
Scrubs fingernails with brush	5½ yr	Coley
Maintains clean nails, files, clips both hands	8 yr	Coley

The ability to perform grooming and hygiene skills develops far earlier than the acceptance of responsibility for performing them. Grooming and hygiene skills are particularly likely to be neglected by school-age children. Note that the performance ages in the tables reflect when a child can do a skill and not whether it is done without supervision.

DISCUSSION

Independence in the performance of the daily activities of basic self-care requires the mastery of complex hand skills that children learn over many years. The skills have varying degrees of manipulative, perceptual, and cognitive components. The action sequences are learned through extensive practice until they become automatic and efficient. We have some knowledge of the usual ages at which the skills are mastered, but very little knowledge of what Connolly and Dalgleish (1989)

called the general patterns of behavioral change, which occur as children acquire specific self-care skills.

Most of the studies of the development of self-care skills cited in this chapter were conducted before 1940 and are few. Recent studies are even more scarce: as noted by Amato and Ochiltree (1986), despite an increasing interest in the development of competence in childhood during the last decade, practical life skills have been virtually ignored. Interest in the study of children's self-care skills over the years has been largely limited to their use in identifying developmental milestones, and most of our knowledge is of that kind. This information has been presented in this chapter as a summary of what is currently known about the chronology of skill acquisition that can function as a possible source for finding clues to the understanding of the process by which skills are acquired.

Although the ages identified are approximate and represent an unspecified average behavior, they provide a tentative chronologic order in which skills develop. However, the sequences of skill development that are suggested by the information in the tables may be an artifact of the use of average ages. Of course, some of the steps in learning are clearly acceptable, that is, a partial skill would precede a complete skill. Many of the sequences have been repeatedly observed and verified by teachers, parents, and therapists. Furthermore, these overall sequences have value in that they provide information that could be used in planning longitudinal studies since they identify the age span in which skills usually develop. However, individual differences among children could result in different routes to competence in an overall skill, and the differences in the process of skill acquisition may be obscured by the use of group data. Nevertheless, some generalizations can be made about some of the factors affecting the general patterns of change in the acquisition of self-care.

Hand Skills in Self-Care

The examination of the chronology of self-care acquisition allows a preliminary, although fragmentary, analysis of the relationship of the development of hand use to the development of self-care. We do not know when these self-care skills reach adult levels of efficiency and precision, but clearly skill acquisition is a gradual process that requires many years. It appears that aspects of skill acquisition over the years include (1) abilities in grip, (2) the use of two hands in a complementary fashion, (3) the ability to use the hands in varied positions with and without vision, (4) the execution of increasingly complex action sequences, and (5) the development of automaticity.

Grip Abilities

Infants have developed whole hand and pincer grips before they begin to acquire self-care skills. However, the whole hand to pincer grip sequence occurs repeatedly as skills develop. Examples in the young child include progression from a whole hand to a finger grip on a spoon and from a whole hand grip pulling up pants to a thumb and finger grip on socks. This progression can be observed again in older children when power grips are needed. A child lifts a cup or glass with one hand before he/she has the finger grip power needed to lift a cup by the handle. In cutting with a knife and fork, a child first uses a fisted grip on both utensils to exert the pressure needed. The power finger grips used by adults for cutting are not achieved until the preteen years.

Bilateral Hand Use

Most self-care skills are bilateral. The challenge posed by these skills depends on their complexity. The simple act of drinking from a cup held in two hands is one of the first achievements of an infant, and an infant is soon able to hold a dish while spooning food. The order in which further bilateral dressing skills develop seems to depend on the added need for power, whether hands work in unison or cooperate in different functions, and the extent of the motor sequencing involved. Undressing is easier with two hands but requires less coordination of the two hands than does dressing. Intermediate bilateral skills include holding a shoe open with the tongue out and manipulating buttons. The greatest difficulty comes when the two hands must perform different sequences, as in tying bows.

Position of the Hands

Two factors appear to influence a child's ability to perform a task with the hands someplace other than in front of the body. Young children seem unable to perform tasks such as buttoning without seeing their hands, and performing with the hands in awkward positions such as at the side of the body is difficult. These two factors probably combine in the delay in learning to manipulate back buttons and bows.

Executing Motor Sequences

Even the early-developing task of self-feeding with a spoon requires the learning of a multiple sequence of actions. Through analysis, therapists have identified the steps involved in many dressing skills, but the sequences followed by healthy children in learning particular dressing skills have not been studied. However, it is to be expected that the ease of learning a skill is related to the number of action sequences involved.

Automaticity

Self-care literature provides a clue to the development of automaticity in skill performance. There appears to be a delay following a child's ability to perform a skill in eating and dressing before the skill can be performed while carrying on a conversation. This suggests that an automatic level of skill execution does not develop until several years after a skill is first mastered.

Combined Motor Abilities

Examples of skills involving different facets of hand manipulation have been given for illustrative purposes. Nevertheless, clearly most of these facets occur in combination. The highest level of self-care skill appears to require some combination of bilateral sequencing and complementary hand use, the combination of power and precision in grip, the ability to perform hand tasks with the hands behind the back or head, and the ability to visualize what the hands are doing.

Perceptual Factors

The sequences of self-care acquisition also clearly demonstrate the need for development of perceptual skills. Perceptual skills are required for tool use, ranging in difficulty for spoons, toothbrushes, and combs. Perceptual factors are particularly evident in dressing. Children often have the motor skills to dress before they can dress correctly. Over several years they learn, in this order, whether clothes are inside or outside out, the difference between front and back, and which is left or right. Their ability to respond first to more obvious cues is shown by this sequence as well as by their ability to locate a dress front by its decoration before the front of pants or T-shirts for which labels must be noted.

Cognitive and Personality Factors

We have little data on the importance of cognitive and personality factors in self-care acquisition, but the few studies suggest that, for children whose intelligence is within normal limits, the level of intelligence is less important than the personality characteristics of persistence and self-reliance. There is good reason to believe that the role of personal and social characteristics is as important as perceptual and motor maturation. Children are highly variable in the chronologic ages at which they acquire skills. The finding that a 3- to 4-year span may separate the earliest and latest age at which healthy children master a particular skill is a powerful indication that there are large personal and situational differences among children. We know very little about the sources of these individual differences, but we can hypothesize that they are multiple and include differences in problem-solving abilities as well as in personality characteristics such as persistence and self-reliance. We also know virtually nothing about the extent to which and in what combinations these intrinsic factors influence the maturation of self-care skills or how much is a function of family and cultural variables. Many studies are needed to understand the variables that have an impact on the learning of self-care skills. The PEDI promises to provide a rich resource for the determination of which cultural, cognitive, motor, and personality factors have an impact on the acquisition of self-care skills. The interest in the development of competence and volition will also hopefully include more attention to basic practical skills.

CONCLUSION

This chapter has focused on how and when healthy children learn the separate skills and subskills of self-care. Knowledge of the sequences in which healthy children acquire self-sufficiency in daily activities can be valuable in understanding the roadblocks of children with physical or mental disability. Sequences of skill acquisition can provide guidance in selecting levels of skills at which to introduce training.

The acquisition of self-care in healthy children provides only a part of the picture needed for treatment planning. We need to know how skills are learned in the presence of different disabilities. Therapists work with children with disabilities, each of which influences learning capacity in different ways. Part of the art of therapy is to identify the individual differences in ability as well as the impact of disability. It would be helpful to know more about the factors affecting the learning process, the differences and similarities in the

ways in which children with disabilities learn complex skills, and whether or not an alternate method or adapted equipment is facilitating. We particularly need to know more about the limitations and learning of self-care skills by children who have motor dysfunctions that may accompany a learning disability.

The importance of self-care skill acquisition in a healthy child's sense of efficacy and the parent-child interaction around self-care issues should be investigated. Furthermore, although we know that independence in self-care is important to an individual's quality of life, disability is sometimes so severe that independence cannot be achieved, and we know little about the importance of partial independence to the individual or of its meaning to an individual's sense of mastery and control. Research in self-care with both healthy children and children with disabilities has the potential for discovering information that will be applicable to designing rehabilitation programs.

Parents should be helped to understand the importance of the mastery of self-care skills to the child and to give the child a sense of pride in this most mundane of accomplishments. Time in the daily schedule is needed for practice of self-care for all children. The child with a disability will have a different timetable for mastery, but the same rules should apply. Time must be scheduled for the child to acquire skills, and self-reliance and self-confidence must be engendered.

REFERENCES

Amato, P.R., & Ochiltree, G. (1986). Children becoming independent: An investigation of children's performance of practical life-skills. *Australian Journal of Psychology, 38*(1), 3, 13, 59-68.

Bernard, H. (1970). *Human development in western culture* (2nd ed.). Boston: Allyn & Bacon.

Bleck, E.E., & Nagel, D.A. (1975). *Physically handicapped children—A medical atlas for teachers.* New York: Grune & Stratton.

Bott, E.A., Blatz, W.E., Chant, N., & Bott, H. (1928). Observation and training of fundamental habits in young children. *Genetic Psychology Monograph, 4,* 1-161.

Brigance, A.H. (1978). *Diagnostic inventory of early development.* North Billerica, MA: Curriculum Associates.

Bullock, M., & Lutkenhaus, P. (1988). The development of volitional behavior in the toddler years. *Child Development, 59,* 4, 15, 664-674.

Castle, K. (1985, May/June). Toddlers and tools. *Childhood Education, 16,* 352-355.

Coley, I.L. (1978). *Pediatric assessment of self-care activities*. St. Louis: Mosby.

Coley, I., & Procter, S. (1989). Self maintenance activities. In P. Pratt & A. Allen (Eds.), *Occupational therapy for children*. St. Louis: Mosby.

Connolly, K., & Dalgleish, M. (1989). The emergence of a tool-using skill in infancy. *Developmental Psychology, 25*(6), 894-912.

Eisen, M., Donald, C.A., Ware, J.E., & Brook, R.H. (1980). *Conceptualization and measurement of health for children in the health insurance study*. Santa Monica, CA: RAND.

Gaddes, W.H. (1980). *Learning disabilities and brain function*. New York: Springer-Verlag.

Geppert, U., & Kuster, U. (1983). The emergence of "Wanting to do it oneself": A precursor of achievement motivation. *International Journal of Behavioral Development, 6*, 355-369.

Gesell, A., & Amatruda, C.S. (1965). *Developmental diagnosis (2nd ed.)*. New York: Harper & Row.

Gesell, A., Halverson, H.M., Thompson, H., Ilg, F.L., Castner, B.M., Ames, L.B., & Amatruda, C.S. (1940). *The first five years of life: A guide to the study of the preschool child*. New York: Harper & Row.

Gesell, A., & Ilg, F. (1937). *Feeding behavior of infants*. Philadelphia: J.B. Lippincott.

Gesell, A., & Ilg, F. (1943). *Infant and child in the culture of today*. New York: Harper & Row.

Gesell, A.L., & Ilg, F. (1946). *The child from five to ten*. New York: Harper & Row.

Gordon, N. (1992). Independence for the physically disabled. *Child: Care, Health and Development, 18*, 97-105.

Granger, C.V., Hamilton, B.B., & Kayton, R. (1988). *Guide for the use of the functional independence measure for children (Wee-FIM)*. Buffalo, NY: State University of New York Research Foundation.

Gubbay, S.S. (1975). *The clumsy child: A study of developmental apraxia and agnostic ataxia*. Philadelphia: Saunders.

Haley, S.M., Coster, W.L., Ludlow, L.H., Haltiwanger, J.T., & Andrellos, P.J. (1992). *Pediatric evaluation of disability inventory*. Boston: New England Medical Center Hospital Inc., and PEDI Research Group.

Hurlock, E.B. (1964). *Child development (4 ed.)*. New York: McGraw-Hill.

Key, C.B., White, M.R., Honzik, W.P., Heiney, A.B., & Erwin, D. (1936). The process of learning to dress among nursery-school children. *Genetic Psychology Monographs, 18*, 67-163.

Klein, M. (1983). *Pre-dressing skills*. Tucson: Community Skill Builders.

Klein, R.M., & Bell, B. (1979). *The Klein-Bell ADL Scale manual*. Seattle: University of Washington Medical School, Health Sciences Resource Center, SB-56.

Koch, B.M., & Simenson, R.L. (1992). Upper extremity strength and function in children with spinal muscular atrophy type II. *Archives of Physical Medicine and Rehabilitation, 73*, 241-245.

Law, M., & Usher, P. (1988). Validation of the Klein-Bell Activities of Daily Living Scale for Children. *Canadian Journal of Occupation Therapy, 55*, 63-68.

Maccoby, E.M. (1980). *Social development: Psychological growth and the parent-child relationship*. New York: Harcourt, Brace, Jovanovich.

Maccoby, E.M., & Bee, H.L. (1965) Some speculations concerning the gap between perceiving and performing. *Child Development, 36*, 367-378.

Miller, A., Stewart, M., Murphy, M.A., & Jantzen, A. (1955). An evaluation method for cerebral palsy. *American Journal of Occupational Therapy, 9*, 105-111.

Parker, S.T., & Gibson, K.R. (1977). Object manipulation, tool use and sensorimotor intelligence as feeding adaptations in cebus monkeys and great apes. *Journal of Human Evolution, 6*, 623-641.

Reich, N., & Otten, P. (1980). Are buttons and zippers confidence trippers? *Accent on Living, 25*, 98-99.

Sparrow, S.S., Balla, D.A., & Cicchetti, D.V. (1984). *Vineland Adaptive Behavior Scales*. Circle Pines, MN: American Guidance Service.

Stutzman, R. (1948). *Guide for administering the Merrill Palmer Scales of Mental Tests*. New York: Harcourt, Brace & World.

Thornby, M.A., & Krebs, D.E. (1992). Bimanual skill development in pediatric below-elbow amputation: A multicenter, cross-sectional study. *Archives of Physical Medicine and Rehabilitation, 73*, 697-702.

Vulpe, S.G. (1979). *Vulpe Assessment Battery for the atypical child*. Toronto: NI on Mental Retardation.

Wacker, D.P., Harper, D.C., Powel, W.J., & Healy, A. (1983). Life outcomes and satisfaction ratings of multi-handicapped adults. *Developmental Medicine and Child Neurology, 25*, 625-631.

Wagoner, L.C., & Armstrong, E.M. (1928). The motor control of children as involved in the dressing process. *Journal of Genetic Psychology, 35*, 84-97.

Wallander, J.L., Pitt, L.C., & Mellins, C.A. (1990). Child functional independence and maternal psychosocial stress as risk factors threatening adaptation in mothers of physically or sensorially handicapped children. *Journal of Consulting and Clinical Psychology, 58*(6), 818-824.

Walton, J.N., Ellis, E., & Court, S.D.M. (1962). Clumsy children: A study of developmental apraxia and agnosia. *Brain, 85*, 603-612.

White, R.N. (1959). Motivation reconsidered: The concept of competence. *Psychological Review, 66*, 297-333.

Wolf, J. (1969). *The results of treatment in cerebral palsy*. Springfield, IL: Charles C Thomas.

11

The Development of Graphomotor Skills

Jenny Ziviani

GENERAL GRAPHOMOTOR COMPETENCY
Processes of Acquisition
Implement Grasp and Manipulation

DRAWING
The Nature of Drawing
Drawing and Developmental Evaluation

WRITING
The Nature of Writing
Writing and Developmental Expectations

CONCLUSION

Graphomotor skills comprise those conceptual and perceptual-motor abilities involved in drawing and writing. Drawing is defined as the art of producing a picture or plan with implements such as pencils, pens, or crayons. Writing is the process of forming letters, figures, or other significant symbols, especially on paper (*Webster,* 1988).

At the conceptual level, graphomotor skills in drawing consist of the formulation of the way in which forms and objects are to be produced so as to represent the perceptions of the individual; in writing they consist of the formulation of letters in such a way as to produce meaningful words and sentences. At the perceptual-motor level, graphomotor skills comprise the interplay between envi-

ronmental conditions and individual sensory, perceptual, and motor abilities in the process of executing a drawing or a piece of written work.

Graphomotor skills offer one method of nonverbal communication and are hence important in the attainment of developmental maturity. The usual developmental sequence is that drawing (with at least some level of proficiency) precedes writing, and it has been argued that drawing in fact acts as an apprenticeship for writing (Willats, 1985).

However, although there are descriptive data about what children can be expected to achieve in drawing and writing at different ages, our knowledge of the underlying, facilitating processes remains ill defined. This chapter addresses some of the gaps according to the following plan.

Because both drawing and writing involve inscription with a tool or implement, it is possible to present a generic overview of graphomotor skills. Therefore the first section of the chapter analyzes the processes involved when a child begins basic inscription, with foci on the acquisition of the necessary graphomotor skills and on methods of grasp and manipulation of appropriate tools.

This introduction paves the way for two subsequent reviews, the first of drawing and the latter of writing. In each the nature of the task is assessed and developmental considerations outlined.

The chapter concludes with a statement on research needs, both in the general domain of graphomotor skill acquisition including grasp and manipulation and in the more specialized fields of drawing and writing.

GENERAL GRAPHOMOTOR COMPETENCY

Processes of Acquisition

Children, when presented with tools for inscription, regularly smear paint, scribble with crayons, or draw (Phelps, Stempel, and Speck, 1984). The execution varies depending on the developmental status of individuals and their prior exposure to graphic experiences. In its most basic form simple inscription with an implement onto a page can be conceived of as a perceptual-motor act (Sovik, 1981). The learning of a skilled task such as writing or drawing, however, is more dependent on the cognitive-perceptual-motor skills of the performer (Laszlo and Broderick, 1985).

Most theories of motor learning now acknowledge the interplay between individual and environment in the acquisition of skills (Schmidt, 1988). Factors internal to the performer include affective state, motivation, cognition, sensory perception, motor planning, and biomechanical considerations. External considerations relate to the spatial and temporal requirements of the task, prior learning, and the types of tools and equipment available for use.

Motor learning theorists have postulated that the acquisition of drawing and writing skills can be best understood within the framework of a closed loop theory (Sovik, 1981). Once learned, however, handwriting moves into the domain of an open loop skill (van der Meulen et al., 1991). This means that, instead of remaining dependent on vision, the skilled writer is able to write so quickly that there is no time to modify performance on the basis of visual feedback.

Laszlo and Bairstow (1985a) have argued that kinesthetic memory, more than kinesthetic acuity, is primarily responsible for the skilled performance of writers. These researchers based their observations on the performance of children on an assessment they developed—The Kinaesthetic Sensitivity Test (KST) (1985b). The psychometric properties of the KST, however, continue to be debated in the literature (Hoare and Larkin, 1991; Lord and Hulme, 1987). Furthermore, Copley and Ziviani (1990) demonstrated that the Kinesthesia Test (Ayres 1972), which assesses both kinesthesis and motor planning, was a better predictor of children with poor handwriting than the KST alone. The relative importance, therefore, of the role of kinesthesis in acquisition of proficient handwriting remains unclear. There is, however, evidence from animal experimentation to support the reliance upon kinesthetic information once skill has been acquired (Leonard et al., 1992).

The visual sense, however, has been thought to remain active in children who are experiencing difficulties in mastering handwriting. Wann (1987) found that good and poor writers used different movement patterns when asked to reproduce letters and words. Performance was recorded using an xy digitizer, and movement patterns were identified as (1) ballistic (high peak velocity, high acceleration and deceleration, with peak duration occupying a low percentage of series length); (2) step (one primary peak, medium velocity acceleration and deceleration); and (3) ramp (several velocity maxima, low velocity, very little acceleration). Step and ramp patterns are both atypical of programmed movement and more in line with the feedback model of control. Because visual cues are seen as the major source of environmental information during handwriting, the increased incidence of ramp patterns in poor quality writers was seen as indicating their continued reliance on visual feedback. Although not suggesting that the more proficient writers were not using visual feedback during letter production, Wann (1987) postulated that they were probably less dependent on it as a means of control. He went on to point out that deprivation of visual feedback would result in the deterioration of performance of even the most proficient writer. He did, nevertheless, postulate that a skilled writer could maintain performance of chunks of script (a few words) by only occasional visual checks. Other researchers (van der Muelin et al., 1991) have supported the view of Wann and suggest that children with difficulty in visual-motor control compensate by adopting a greater reliance on visual monitoring and that this in turn results in slower performance. These issues warrant greater attention because they can influence the adoption of appropriate remedial strategies.

Implement Grasp and Manipulation

Brushes, crayons, pencils, and pens are the primary tools used by children in their graphic endeavors. These implements form an extension of the hand, and their control and manipulation are important in the attainment of skilled copying, drawing, and writing. Only through experimentation do children become skilled in adapting to implements of differing weight, length, and graphic quality (Schwartz and Reilly, 1980).

After progressing through a range of precursor grips—palmar, incomplete tripod, and static tripod—most children generally acquire the dynamic tripod grip as their means of implement manipulation for drawing and writing (Rosenbloom and Horton, 1971; Saida and Miyashita, 1979). The dynamic tripod grip is efficient for the execution of precision control and is therefore well suited to graphic tasks (Napier, 1956). Not all children, however, use this grip. Variations include those in which a developmentally less mature grip is used (palmar grasp) and those in which an unusual version of the dynamic tripod is evident.

However, aberrant grips can be found in the population at large among people who do and do not experience graphomotor difficulties (Sassoon, Nimmon-Smith, and Wing, 1986; Schneck and Henderson, 1990; Ziviani and Elkins, 1986). The frequency with which a lateral tripod grip was found in the adult population led Bergmann (1990) to conclude that it was such a common variant that it could be considered normal. Opinions vary, nevertheless, pertaining to children (Levine et al., 1981).

Handwriting speed and legibility have not been found to be adversely affected by pencil hold alone (Sassoon et al., 1986; Ziviani and Elkins 1986). Diverse ways of categorizing variations in the dynamic tripod grip have been used. Ziviani and Elkins (1986) used a series of four nonexclusive categories that described grips on the basis of the number of fingers held on the shaft of the writing implement, the degree of forearm supination, the hyperextension of the distal interphalangeal joint of the index finger, and the thumb/ index finger opposition. On the basis of these variations no significant relationship could be attributed to the grips employed and the speed and legibility of handwriting achieved.

Sassoon et al. (1986) used a classification of penholds that examined the position of digits on the pencil shaft, their proximity to the writing tip, and the shape of the digits. Furthermore, grips were described in relation to the shaping of the hand, the positioning of the upper body, as well as the specific orientation of the writing paper. This study also found writing speed was not compromised by unconventional pencil holds. However, both of the previous studies have examined only static grips; the dynamic quality of grip usage is still to be explored, as is the impact of extensive writing tasks and consequent fatigue.

Developmentally immature grips have been linked to poorly established lateral preference (Rosenbloom and Horton, 1971; Schneck, 1989) but can also result when insufficient prerequisite experience has been obtained. Poor hand preference is thought to impede the refinement of the manipulative skills needed for good pencil control. This view is consistent with the development of in-hand manipulation skills outlined by Exner (1990).

In research by Schneck (1991), the presence of proprioceptive/kinesthetic finger awareness was found to be an important determinant in children with unusual grips. In other words, unusual grips may not of themselves lead to poor writing but, in conjunction with poor proprioceptive/kinesthic perception, they might contribute to poor writing performance. Increased pencil grip pressure may also be associated with limited proprioceptive feedback (Levine et al., 1981).

In a practical and clinical sense, therapists will be confronted by the issue of whether to assist children to modify the grip they are using as part of an overall strategy to facilitate an improvement in handwriting performance. A number of points may be worth considering when this situation arises:

- Mechanically the dynamic tripod grip offers a high level of precision and control. If the child is young enough, therefore, and has not developed a fixed writing posture, then the dynamic tripod grip should be encouraged.
- Variations of the dynamic tripod grip do not, of themselves, contribute to handwriting difficulties. If the grip adopted allows for intrinsic muscle action and some opposition, then it may be acceptable for the task.
- Differentiation should be made, however, between a modified version of the dynamic tripod grip and a grip that is developmentally immature. The latter requires intervention because it may indicate that the child has not developed the necessary prerequisites to progress to a more mature hold.

DRAWING
The Nature of Drawing

When considering drawing, it is important to differentiate the simple copying of shapes and figures from the creation of pictures from memory or imagination. It is with the copying skills (the perceptual-motor elements of drawing) that the present discussion is primarily concerned. It is not the purpose here to review the many investigations that have dealt with the symbolic nature of drawing or those that view drawing as a way of probing a child's thought processes or knowledge of the world (Moore, 1987). For those interested in drawing as an indicator of symbolic intent, the research of Koppitz (1968) and DiLeo (1983) may be of help. Equally, Thomas and Silk (1990) provide an interesting review of findings in the field along with some cautionary considerations for those interpreting children's drawings.

Research into copying has tended to be experimental and has focused on the perceptual-motor nature of the skill, primarily when examining errors in reproduction (Freeman, 1980). In explaining outcomes and end products, difficulties in the processing of sensory information and modification of performance on the basis of feedback have been highlighted (Laszlo and Broderick, 1985).

Certain general characteristics are thought to distinguish children's drawings from those of adults. Children's drawings have been described as being formula-like, segregating elements into non-overlapping spatial bounds, inappropriate with respect to relative positioning of elements within a scene, and depicting subjects as they are perceived to be rather than how they look (Freeman, 1980). Apart from exceptional children, such as a few with autism (Selfe, 1985), most subjects in their preschool and early school years construct their drawings from simple geometric forms and do not compose broad outlines that are then detailed. Fenson (1985), in a detailed longitudinal study of one child, found that a fundamental shift occurred between 3 and 7 years of age in the structure of drawing. The child moved from a constructional style to the use of contoured forms.

The term *constructional* in this context relates to the assembling of simple geometric forms into a pictorial representation (such as the use of a circle for a face and a rectangle for a body when drawing a person). The term *contoured,* on the other hand, refers to the sketching of an outline, which is subsequently detailed to achieve the desired representation. Although no attempt is made to explain why a shift might occur from the former to the latter, it is postulated that the motivation is a quest for realism. This quest, in conjunction with greater skill in visually controlling actions and the ability to plan spatially and execute actions, constitutes the move from a juvenile to a more adult approach. Obviously, such assumptions require further investigation.

A number of writers have recorded the ontogenetic transition of children's drawings (Kellogg, 1969; Luquet, 1927). There is general agreement that between ages 2 and 3 children are thought only to make scribbling marks on paper with no representational intent. When, between the ages of 3 and 4 years, a child begins to interpret a drawing, the interpretation occurs only *after* he/she has produced it. The representational intent is not there at the outset. In the next stage (4 to 5 years) the nature of the drawing is announced before its commencement, but the coordination of individual elements remains difficult. Subsequently (6 to 7 years) the child is able to include all the characteristics of objects being drawn as they are known to him/her. This is not always consistent with the way they are in an adult reality. Finally, from around 8 years of age the child begins to take into account visual persepective, and object position and orientation also become more important.

Graphic perspective has also received considerable attention (Freeman, Eiser, and Sayers, 1977; Light and MacIntosh, 1980). Whereas some see its onset as evidencing cognitive maturation (Reid and Sheffield, 1990), Hagen (1985) highlights the necessity to learn the rules governing the ability to represent something in true perspective. His outlook proceeds from a series of studies that found little difference between the way in which children handle the three-dimensional plane and the methods adopted by adults. In both populations, if individuals have no special artistic talent or training, they will reproduce the visual structures that they see in natural perspective along a continuum from orthogonal (no diminishing projected size with increasing distance) to projective (image size decreases as distance increases).

The research of van Sommers (1984) has detailed a number of characteristics of the way in which individuals approach specific drawing tasks. For example, right-handed subjects tend to commence the drawing of a free-standing circle at around the 12 o'clock position and invariably rotate counterclockwise, whereas a little over 60% of left-handers continue in a clockwise manner. Van Sommers (1984) also notes that a developmental change in children occurs between 3 and 6 years of age. During these years right-handed children's circle production changes from clockwise to counterclockwise. Another feature is the direction in which profiles are facing. Most profiles of faces are turned to the left, as are most cars. Glasses have lenses to the left, pencils have points to the left, spoons and pipes have bowls to the left. On the other hand, most flags fly right, and cups and buckets have their handles to the right. The impact of hand preference and convention is implicated in these findings.

Developmentally, although children may have constant access to other children's drawings, they maintain variety in even the most common objects. Even when they do adopt stereotyped formulas, they not infrequently include their own versions alongside. The drawings of one child over time may be very repetitious in the treatment of individual motifs (van Sommers, 1984). The logic is that flexibility is lost due to the repetition of early drawing strategies. However, this is not to say that their drawings never change but rather that they often evolve by modulation or amendment of existing devices, rather than through a revolutionary rethinking of the basic representational strategy. By this reasoning, innovation in drawing is thought to occur late in the sequence of reproduction and not in the initial strokes (van Sommers, 1984).

Drawing and Developmental Evaluation

Both the spatial (Beery, 1982) and representational (Goodenough, 1926) aspects of drawing have been used in the measurement of developmental levels. The ability to reproduce a cross and a circle is, for example, required in the Griffith Mental Measurement Scales (Griffith, 1970). Notwithstanding variations in the ages at which children are expected to complete these tasks (Hanson and Smith, 1987; Moore and Law, 1990), ability continues to condition our interpretations of children's developmental status.

One of the most widely used tests of visual-motor integration (Beery, 1982) evaluates children's accuracy in the reproduction of shapes to determine their visual-motor maturity. Some researchers have determined ability in this assessment as being directly associated with subsequent handwriting skill (Oliver, 1990).

Cognitive and intellectual developments have also been associated with children's drawing performance. A number of studies have found positive correlations between scores on the Goodenough Draw-A-Man Test and scores on individual items in other psychologic tests. Harris (1963) summarized these studies. Although the nature of this association remains unclear, one group of authors (Lark-Horovitz, Lewis, and Luca, 1967) has as-

sumed that children who can draw well are invariably bright and that, although they progress through the same stages in the development of drawing skills, their progress is at an accelerated rate. Little substantive research is available to support this assumption.

Obviously, for those children with impairment of effector mechanisms (as in cerebral palsy and spina bifida) the quality of drawn productions may be affected. How their works differ from the drawings of children without disability needs to be considered within the context of the child's perceptual-motor limitations, cognitive impairment, and possible environmental restrictions. Determining the relative contribution of each factor is not easy. Unfortunately many assessments of developmental and cognitive abilities rely, in part, on copying abilities, especially for preschool children (Moore and Law, 1990).

An attempt has been made by Reid and Sheffield (1990) to accommodate perceptual-motor limitations when examining children's drawings. These authors adopted a cognitive-developmental basis for the analysis of drawings in children with myelomeningocele. The structure of children's thought is said to progress through four stages: sensorimotor, relational, dimensional, and vectorial. It is the dimensional stage (thought to occur between the ages of 4 and 10 years) on which the authors concentrate in an alternative approach to analyzing children's drawings. Instead of attending to the quality of drawings, Reid and Sheffield (1990) argue that the subject matter and its depiction should become the focus for determining developmental maturity. They propose the following four dimensional substages:

- Operational consolidation, in which the drawing of a recognizable unit (human figure or object) is assembled from previously acquired circles and lines
- Unifocal coordination, which occurs when two units are placed together to create a scenelike quality
- Bifocal coordination, at which stage an element of depth is introduced into drawings by the use of foreground and background
- Elaborate bifocal coordination, in which the use of perspective becomes more elaborate and less rigid

Preliminary observations suggest that this is a useful analytic scheme for children with myelomeningocele. Yet, since other experimenters argue against the developmental significance of perspective (Bremner and Batten, 1991; Hagen, 1985), further research is warranted to examine the potential clinical utility of Reid and Sheffield's (1990) findings.

WRITING
The Nature of Writing

The acquisition of writing proceeds hand in hand with children's confidence and understanding of language. Berninger and Rutberg (1992) currently suggest that different kinds of constraints operate on the writing acquisition process at different developmental stages. During the primary school grades neurodevelopmental constraints in orthographic coding, fine motor function, and orthographic-motor integration are likely to interfere with the rapid automatic production of written language. Later, when most children can automatically write the alphabet and spell a set of functional words, the writing process is more probably constrained by verbal working memory and ability to generate the major units of written language—the word, the sentence, or text-level structures. Once proficiency in generating units of language is achieved, writing can be constrained by cognitive processes such as planning, translating, and revising when composing larger pieces of text.

For older children constraints may still be operating at the neurodevelopmental and/or linguistic, as well as the cognitive, levels. Inefficiencies in the low-level neurodevelopmental processes early in writing acquisition can contribute to future higher-level writing disabilities, both directly (because production of written material continues to be a problem) or indirectly (because of an aversion to writing arising from early frustration and failure).

Writing and Developmental Expectations

Historically and cross-culturally several factors seem to operate in the continuing production of written script: the writing may become abbreviated; the size of the writing diminishes; form becomes simplified and standardized; and cursive forms evolve with curves replacing angles and ligatures joining letters (van Sommers, 1991). Disregarding personalization of writing style, many of these features can be identified as individual children acquire graphic proficiency (e.g.,

writing becomes smaller and more economical with the cursive form being preferred for speed).

As children master the skill of handwriting, their performance changes both qualitatively and quantitatively. How do we judge if either or both of these aspects are appropriate for the child's chronologic or developmental level? Handwriting is heavily influenced by the nature of the instruction received and the extent of practice undertaken by the individual. We suspect that handwriting receives little emphasis in school curricula (Rubin and Henderson, 1982). Therefore, to exercise a semblance of experimental control, an individual's performance needs to be compared with that of peers who have been exposed to the same degree of instruction and the same model script. In this sense teachers are often the best judge and provide extensive referrals (Alston and Taylor, 1987; Oliver, 1990).

Although children with handwriting difficulty need to be seen within their social and educational context, general developmental expectations do exist for these populations. Handwriting quality and quantity translate respectively into legibility and speed. Handwriting quality appears an elusive concept. Years of work have produced a wide variety of handwriting scales (Phelps, Stempel, and Speck, 1984; Stott, Moyes, and Henderson 1985; Ziviani and Elkins, 1984) and checklists (Alston, 1985). Most of these efforts have identified characteristics considered to contribute to handwriting legibility. In general, these characteristics can be classified as either giving form (formation, size) or as creating space division (space between letters, words, and lines). There are also other factors, arguably overlooked, that relate to movement (pressure while writing, frequency of pen lifts). Of all the elements mentioned, formation and letter shaping have been considered the most important (Mojet, 1991).

Handwriting legibility has been examined either globally or in detail via its various components. When a global measure is used, the individual's performance is compared with a series of model specimens. Increasingly, researchers have sought to break down handwriting samples into their component parts. This provides a better way of understanding legibility difficulties and offers a basis for designing appropriate remedial interventions. One study documents the grade level expectations of children between 7 and 14 years of age in terms of writing size, horizontal alignment, spacing consistency, and letter formation (Ziviani and Elkins, 1984). Drawn from a population of

Table 11-1. Reported mean handwriting speeds (letters per minute) by school grade, various authors (1961–1990)

AUTHOR	SCHOOL GRADE				
	3	4	5	6	7
Groff (1961)		35.1	40.6	49.6	
Hamstra-Bletz and Blotz (1990)	25	37	47	57	62
Phelps et al. (1985)	35	46	54	66	
Sassoon et al. (1986)		64			
Ziviani and Elkins (1984)	32.6	34.2	38.4	46.1	52.1

Australian schoolchildren, these data support the assumption that children's writing speed increases with age and that girls write more quickly than boys. In terms of the legibility characteristics, letters become more accurately formed, spacing becomes more consistent, size diminishes (more particularly in girls), and writing attains better horizontal alignment.

Findings such as these provide a useful baseline measure for children exposed to similar educational instruction. Children with spina bifida myelomeningocele, for example, are at risk for developing difficulties in the acquisition of proficient handwriting (Anderson and Spain, 1977). Ziviani, Hayes, and Chant (1990) used the normative data discussed previously to help specify the nature of difficulties experienced by children with spina bifida who were able to attend regular schools. Their findings indicated that speed, horizontal alignment, and letter formation were the handwriting characteristics most detrimentally affected. Writing size, meanwhile, fell within two standard deviations of the normative means, and spacing consistency was often better than in the normative sample. Such findings are useful in delineating handwriting dysfunction and not just accepting a global disability.

Handwriting speeds, although not necessarily related to legibility (Wann, 1987), indicate an individual's confidence in written production. Since most examination papers remain handwritten, a certain level of proficiency is still seen as an educational goal. Authorities differ in terms of expected handwriting speeds for children at various ages. A summary is presented in Table 11-1. Most variation can be attributed to differing instructions to children ("write normally" vs. "write fast"). In assessing past research, additional consideration needs to be given to the nature of the material being copied or written, the date of data collection, and variation in teaching practices. Further work is required to update and validate findings. When deciding if a child's performance

is within developmental expectations, therefore, attention to a teacher's observations within a peer-appropriate context is necessary. Also, if standardized data are available, they should reflect the child's cultural and educational environment.

CONCLUSION

This review of graphomotor skills shows a field dotted with light and shade. The 'light' of more thorough and extensive research falls on the following aspects of general graphomotor competency, drawing, and writing:

- General graphomotor competency has been the subject of research effort in relatively recent times and, at the present, demonstrates no particular or major thrusts. By its very nature it is open to experimental manipulation through the control of stimuli presented to subjects and the measurement of output. The introduction of computer technology has greatly assisted the measurement of output and has provided information on the timing and spatial aspects of graphic actions (see Wann, Wing, and Sovik [1991] for details of some of these experiments).

- After many years of comparative neglect, children's drawings have received renewed attention in the late 1980s and early 1990s (Thomas and Silk, 1990; van Sommers, 1984). Now the main research foci are on the use of perspective in drawings and the processes that influence children in their graphic representation of the visible world. These findings link up with research in other fields and disciplines on the interpretative aspects of drawings.

- Handwriting as a functional outcome of the cognitive-perceptual-motor ability of children has come under closer scrutiny by both educators and therapists alike. In the process greater attention has been given to handwriting instruction and remediation.

As a result practitioners have been alerted to the need for greater research in the area, and, although such research is still scant, there is evidence of activity (Laszlo and Bairstow, 1985; Oliver, 1990).

The areas of shade in graphomotor research remain extensive and are of potentially wider concern in childhood skill acquistion. This chapter concludes by pointing to some of the major gaps in knowledge regarding general graphomotor competency, drawing, and writing, with suggestions, where appropriate, for research initiatives and interventions.

- Why some children demonstrate difficulty in the attainment of graphomotor abilities is still not clear. Wann (1987) suggests that a reliance on visual feedback may hinder some endeavors. The importance of kinesthesis in the proficient execution of both drawing and writing warrants further investigation (Laszlo and Bairstow, 1985; Lord and Hulme, 1987). This may indeed shed light on both acquistion and remediation strategies in the future.

- Research in the area of implement grasp and manipulation suggests that the type of grip being used need not impede graphomotor production (Bergmann, 1990; Sassoon et al., 1986; Ziviani and Elkins, 1986). As yet unanswered is the issue of long-term fatigue and resulting variations in both grips used and quality of written work. This has practical implications for examination situations, which apply time constraints to students.

- Children's drawing abilities in the reproduction of shapes and in the way they represent their environment continue to be used as test items in developmental assessments. The relative impact of innate ability and the amount of instruction to which the child has been exposed remain unclear and beg further investigation.

- Handwriting requires the child to learn and apply a number of rules as well as to develop motor programs for the efficient execution of script. To this end the nature and extent of instruction are highly influential as are a prerequisite linguistic base and a knowledge of the way in which to form individual letters and join them to manufacture words. One area that has not

received much attention in the literature is the influence of different scripts in the attainment of proficient handwriting. The relative merits of learning print (ball and stick) and then moving on to learn cursive writing, as opposed to starting with a simple modified cursive script, also requires further investigation. Both approaches are, in fact, currently used in school systems throughout the world. We simply do not know which is better.

- The neuromuscular and biomechanical subskills necessary for the execution of a fine motor skill such as handwriting need to be ascertained. Penso (1991) provides a practical guide to some of these factors in relation to children with motor disabilities. Determining their relative impact on performance is essential if appropriate intervention is to be designed.

- In remediation of writing, decisions as to whether to skill train (a behavioral approach) or process intervene (using sensory-perceptual-motor methods) can currently draw little on the research literature. Scant evidence about the success of either method exists (Laszlo and Bairstow 1985; Oliver, 1990). Current practices, therefore, need to be further researched, and the selection of both teaching and remediation approaches needs to be related more to properly conducted research than to tradition.

REFERENCES

Alston, J. (1985). The handwriting of 7- to 9-year-olds. *British Journal of Special Education, 12,* 68-72.

Alston, J., & Taylor, J. (1987). *Handwriting.* London: Croom Helm.

Anderson, E. M., & Spain, B. (1977). *The child with spina bifida.* London: Methuen.

Ayres, A. J. (1972). *Southern California Sensory Integration Tests.* Los Angeles: Western Psychological Services.

Beery, K. E. (1982). *Revised administration, scoring and teaching manual for the developmental test of visual-motor integration.* Chicago: Follett.

Bergmann, K. P. (1990). Incidence of atypical pencil grasps among nondysfunctional adults. *American Journal of Occupational Therapy, 44,* 736-740.

Berninger, V. W., & Rutberg, J. (1992). Relationship of finger function to beginning writing: Application to diagnosis of writing disabilities. *Developmental Medicine and Child Neurology, 34,* 198-215.

Bremner, J. G., & Batten, A. (1991). Sensitivity to viewpoint in children's drawings of objects and relations between objects. *Journal of Experimental Child Psychology, 52,* 375-394.

Copely, J., & Ziviani, J. (1990). Kinaesthetic sensitivity and handwriting in grade one children. *Australian Journal of Occupational Therapy, 37,* 39-43.

DiLeo, J. H. (1983). *Interpreting children's drawings.* New York: Brunner/Mazel.

Exner, C. E. (1990). The zone of proximal development in in-hand manipulation skills of non-dysfunctional 3- and 4-year-old children. *American Journal of Occupational Therapy, 44,* 884-891.

Fenson, L. (1985). The transition from construction to sketching in children's drawings. In N. H. Freeman & M. V. Cox (Eds.). *Visual order: The nature and development of pictorial representation.* Cambridge: Cambridge University Press.

Freeman, N. H. (1980). *Strategies of representation in young children.* London: Academic Press.

Freeman, N. H., Eiser, D., & Sayers, T. (1977). Children's strategies in producing three-dimensional relationships on a two-dimensional surface. *Journal of Experimental Child Psychology, 23,* 305-314.

Goodenough, F. (1926). *Measurement of intelligence in drawings.* New York: World.

Groff, P. J. (1961). New speeds in handwriting. *Elementary English, 38,* 564-565.

Griffith, R. (1970). *The abilities of young children: A comprehensive system of mental measurement for the first eight years of life.* London: Child Development Research Centre.

Hamstra-Bletz, L., & Blote, A. W. (1990). Development of handwriting in primary school: A longitudinal study. *Perceptual and Motor Skills, 70,* 759-770.

Hanson, R., & Smith, J. A. (1987). Achievements of young children on items of the Griffith Scales: 1980 compared with 1960. *Child: Care, Health and Development, 13,* 181-195.

Hagen, M. A. (1985). There is no development in art. In N. H. Freeman & M. V. Cox (Eds.). *Visual order: The nature and development of pictorial representation.* Cambridge: Cambridge University Press.

Harris, D. B. (1963). *Children's drawings as measures of intellectual maturity.* New York: Harcourt, Brace & World.

Hoare, D., & Larkin, D. (1991). Kinaesthetic abilities of clumsy children. *Developmental Medicine and Child Neurology, 33,* 671-678.

Kellogg, R. (1969). *Analyzing children's art.* Palo Alto: National Press Book.

Koppitz, E. M. (1968). *Psychological evaluation of children's human figure drawings.* New York: Grune & Stratton.

Lark-Harovitz, B., Lewis, H., & Luca, M. (1967). *Understanding children's art for better teaching.* Columbus, OH: Charles Merrill.

Laszlo, J. I., & Bairstow, P. J. (1985a). *Perceptual motor behaviour: Developmental assessment and therapy.* London: Holt, Rinehart & Winston.

Laszlo, J. I., & Bairstow, P. J. (1985b). *Kinaesthetic sensitivity test.* Perth, Australia: Senkit Pty. Ltd.

Laszlo, J. I., & Broderick, P. A. (1985). The perceptual-motor skill of drawing. In N. H. Freeman & M. V. Cox (Eds.). *Visual order: The nature and development of pictorial representation.* Cambridge: Cambridge University Press.

Leonard, C. M., Glendinning, D. S., Wilfong, T., Cooper, B. Y., & Vierck, C. J. (1992). Alterations of natural hand movements after interruption of fasciculus cuneatus in the macaque. *Somatosensory and Motor Research, 9,* 75-89.

Levine, M. D., Oberklaid, F., & Meltzer, L. (1981). Developmental output failure: A study of low productivity in school-aged children. *Pediatrics, 67,* 18-25.

Light, P. H., & MacIntosh, E. (1980). Depth relationships in young children's drawings. *Journal of Experimental Child Psychology, 30,* 79-87.

Lord, R., & Hulme, C. (1987). Kinaesthetic sensitivity of normal and clumsy children. *Developmental Medicine and Child Neurology, 29,* 720-725.

Luquet, G. H. (1927). *Les dessin enfantin.* Paris: Alcan.

Mojet, J. (1991). Characteristics of the developing skill in elementary education. In J. Wann, A. M. Wing, & N. Sovik (Eds.). *Development of graphic skills: Research, perspectives and educational implications.* London: Academic Press.

Moore, V. (1987). The influence of experience on children's drawings of a familiar and unfamiliar object. *British Journal of Developmental Psychology, 5,* 221-229.

Moore, V., & Law, J. (1990). Copying ability of preschool children with delayed language development. *Developmental Medicine and Child Neurology, 32,* 249-257.

Napier, J. P. (1956). The prehensile movements of the human hand. *The Journal of Bone and Joint Surgery, 38,* 902-913.

Oliver, C. E. (1990). A sensorimotor program for improving writing readiness skills in elementary age children. *American Journal of Occupational Therapy, 44,* 111-116.

Penso, D. E. (1991). *Keyboard, graphic and handwriting skills: Helping people with motor disabilities.* London: Chapman & Hall.

Phelps, J., Stempel, L., & Speck, G. (1984). *Children's handwriting evaluation scale.* Dallas: CHES.

Phelps, J., Stempel, L., & Speck, G. (1985). The children's handwriting scale: A new diagnostic tool. *Journal of Educational Research, 79,* 46-50.

Reid, D. T. & Sheffield, B. (1990). A cognitive-developmental analysis of drawing abilities in children with and without myelomeningocele. *Physical and Occupational Therapy in Pediatrics, 10,* 33-57.

Rosenbloom, L., & Horton, M. E. (1971). The maturation of fine prehension in young children. *Developmental Medicine and Child Neurology, 13,* 3-8.

Rubin, N, & Henderson, S. E. (1982). Two sides of the same coin: Variations in teaching methods and failure to learn to write. *Special Education: Forward Trends, 9,* 17-24.

Saida, Y., & Miyashita, M. (1979). Development of fine motor skill in children: Manipulation of a pencil in young children 2-6 years old. *Journal of Human Movement Studies, 5,* 104-113.

Sasson, R., Nimmo-Smith, J., & Wing, A. M. (1986). An analysis of children's penholds. In H. S. R. Kao, G. P. van Galen, & R. Hoosain (Eds.). *Graphonomics: Contemporary research in handwriting.* Amsterdam: North Holland Press.

Schmidt, R. A. (1988). *Motor control and learning: A behavioral emphasis.* Champaign IL: Human Kinetics.

Schneck, C. M. (1989). *Developmental changes in the grasp of writing tools in normal 3- to 6.11-year-old children in first grade with handwriting problems.* Unpublished doctoral dissertation, Boston University.

Schneck, C. M., & Henderson, A. (1990). Descriptive analysis of the developmental progression of grip position for pencil and crayon control in nondysfunctional children. *American Journal of Occupational Therapy, 44,* 893-900.

Schneck, C. M. (1991). Comparison of pencil grip patterns in first graders with good and poor writing skills. *American Journal of Occupational Therapy, 45,* 701-706.

Schwartz, R. K., & Reilly, M. A. (1980). Learning tool use: Body scheme recalibration and the development of hand skill. *The Occupational Therapy Journal of Research, 1,* 13-29.

Selfe, L. (1985). Anomalous drawing development: Some clinical studies. In N. H. Freeman & M. V. Cox (Eds.). *Visual order: The nature and development of pictorial representation.* Cambridge: Cambridge University Press.

Sovik, N. (1981). An experimental study of individualized learning/instruction in copying, tracking, and handwriting, based on feedback principles. *Perceptual and Motor Skills, 53,* 195-215.

Stott, D. H., Moyes, F. A., & Henderson, S. E. (1985). *Diagnosis and remediation of handwriting problems.* Guelph, Ontario: Brook Educational.

Thomas, G. V., & Silk, A. M. J. (1990). *An introduction to the psychology of children's drawings.* New York: Harvester Wheatsheaf.

van der Meulen J. H. P., Denier van der Gon, J. J., Gielem, C. C. A. M., Goosken, R. H. J. M., & Willemse, J. (1991). Visuomotor performance of normal and clumsy children. 1. Fast goal-directed arm movements with and without visual feedback. *Developmental Medicine and Child Neurology, 33,* 40-54.

van Sommers, P. (1984). *Drawing and cognition: Descriptive and experimental studies of graphic production processes.* Cambridge: Cambridge University Press.

van Sommers, P. (1991). Where writing starts: The analysis of action applied to the historical development of writing. In J. Wann, A. M. Wing, & N. Sovik (Eds.). *Development of graphic skills: Research, perspectives and educational implications.* London: Academic Press.

Wann, J. P. (1987). Trends in the refinement and optimization of fine-motor trajectories: Observations from an analysis of the handwriting of primary school children. *Journal of Motor Behavior, 19,* 13-37.

Wann, J. P., Wing, A. M., & Sovik, N. (1991). *Development of graphic skills: Research, perspectives and educational implications.* London: Academic Press.

Webster's encyclopedic dictionary of the English language. 1988. New York: Lexicon Publications.

Willats, J. (1985). Drawing systems revisited: The role of denotation systems in children's figure drawings. In N. H. Freeman & M. V. Cox (Eds.). *Visual order: The nature and development of pictorial representation.* Cambridge: Cambridge University Press.

Ziviani, J., & Elkins, J. (1984). An evaluation of handwriting performance. *Educational Review, 36,* 251-261.

Ziviani, J., & Elkins, J. (1986). Effect of pencil grip on handwriting speed and legibility. *Educational Review, 38,* 247-257.

Ziviani, J., Hayes, A., & Chant, D. (1990). Handwriting: A perceptual motor disturbance in children with myelomeningocele. *The Occupational Therapy Journal of Research, 10,* 12-26.

Therapeutic Intervention

12

Remediation of Hand Skill Problems in Children

Charlotte E. Exner

HISTORY OF INTERVENTION IN HAND SKILL PROBLEMS

Addressing fine motor problems in children who have motor control difficulties is of substantial interest to occupational therapists. However, fine motor skills have not always been a strong area of focus in these children's treatment. Several theoretic and legal movements have affected how this area of treatment was and is now addressed.

In the 1960s behavioral theory and perceptual-motor approaches were being applied to treatment of children, particularly children with mental retardation. Both approaches used the strategy of analyzing tasks or activities for their component parts so that these parts could be taught to children. In behavioral intervention, shaping and chaining of subskills were used in teaching skills, and children were rewarded for their accomplishment of incremental improvements in these skills. The fine motor activities selected for these children to learn via either approach consisted primarily of activities on developmental checklists, such as stacking blocks, putting pegs into holes, and stringing beads. Although it was found that children could be taught these skills, the value of such skills to the children's daily life functioning or as a basis for acquiring higher-level skills was not addressed or was only inferred. Generalization of skills to other tasks or situations received little attention.

For children with motor impairment in the 1960s, two main approaches were also being used: a neurodevelopmental approach and a functional-compensatory approach. The neurodevelopmental approach consisted of emphasis on reflex-inhibiting postures, but these postures did not address fine motor control. The functional-compensatory approach did focus on fine motor control but typically did so by attempting to circumvent the fine motor problem through adaptations, such as typewriters, eating utensils, and clothing, and by providing children with splints to wear during functional activities. The splints were designed to increase range of motion at the wrist and fingers.

In the early 1970s, theory became a much stronger force in treatment, and neurophysiologic concepts about central nervous system functions and muscle functions began to be applied to treatment of children and adults with motor control problems. These principles addressed improving motor control by facilitation and inhibition of specific muscles or muscle groups through either localized application of stimuli (such as tapping and vibration), which was believed to influence neural control at the level of the muscle spindle or golgi tendon organ, or through generalized tone or arousal/inhibition techniques (such as use of neutral warmth and facilitation of extension through use of an inverted position). The application of these principles in treatment strongly influenced the use of splinting for children and adults with spasticity. Traditional splinting was believed to have a negative effect on spasticity although the empirical studies did not necessarily show this to be true. However, new types of splints, which were designed using neurophysiologic principles, were proposed in an attempt to affect hand posturing and function (MacKinnon, Sanderson, and Buchanan, 1975). Yet no empirical studies of these splints' effectiveness on children's hand function were conducted until the early 1980s (Exner and Bonder, 1983).

By the middle 1970s neurodevelopmental treatment was changing focus from a more passive type of intervention to a more dynamic approach; the focus on reflex-inhibiting postures was replaced with the concept of active treatment as seen in handling of the child by the therapist. Emphasis was placed on facilitation and inhibition of tone (normalization of tone) and development of trunk control. Treatment of problems with the trunk was believed to be crucial before addressing other motor problems of the child. Upper extremity weight bearing in a variety of positions became a commonly used treatment technique for normalizing the tone throughout the upper extremities, facilitating scapulohumeral stability, and developing trunk control. Attention to fine motor problems, beyond preparing the hand for weight bearing, was minimal. The difficulty with this focus on shoulder and trunk control was that for many children those areas were long-standing problems. To wait to address fine motor problems until trunk and scapulohumeral control were fully developed meant that some children would never receive attention to fine motor problems. Also, improvement in scapulohumeral and trunk control did not necessarily translate into improved use of the hands.

Another theory that came into prominence in the early to middle 1970s was sensory integration. At that time sensory integration theory focused almost exclusively on factors felt to underlie the functional problems of the child. Emphasis was placed on enhancing functioning of the vestibular, proprioceptive, and tactile systems and the integration of these systems with one another. This theory proposed that, with improved integration of these systems, improved functioning would occur. Again attention to fine motor problems was minimal since these problems were expected to resolve when the underlying problems were addressed. The difficulty was that waiting for these problems to resolve with treatment could take a year or more, and not all children showed an improvement in fine motor control with this treatment.

However, passage of Public Law (P.L.) 94-142 affected the role of the occupational therapist in addressing fine motor problems in the treatment of children. Teachers in the classroom were responsible for teaching children with severe involvement and multiple handicaps. They had to focus on more basic life skills as well as academic skills, so fine motor skills became one of the goal areas for children. Teachers were skilled in task analysis and reinforced learning of tasks in increments; the behaviorist approach to working with fine motor problems fit well within the teachers' framework for teaching. It lent itself to addressing skills in a focused time period and the documentation of progress as required by the educational system. In addition, using behaviorist techniques did not require understanding of neurophysiologic principles or theories typically used by therapists. Occupational therapists, who were in more limited supply in the school systems than were teachers, assumed the role of consultants to teachers about fine motor skills and became direct service providers for hands-on treatment using neurodevelopmental or sensory integration approaches with children. Therapists usually did not consider addressing fine motor problems directly to be of high interest or high priority relative to the higher priority of treating children using a neurodevelopmental treatment or sensory integration approach. The latter approaches were seen as more "medical" because of their theoretic bases and were considered more appropriate for therapists to use because of their focus on the child's underlying problem. In general, therapists were less interested in any approach that seemed to promote a child's development of splinter skills.

Gradually, however, by the early 1980s a shift back toward function began occurring in the therapeutic community and with that shift came an increasing interest in children's hand function. Therapists who used neurodevelopmental treatment or sensory integration treatment approaches began to focus more on how the child functioned in his/her environment. Attention was still given to children's underlying problems, but, with limited therapy time available to children in school systems and limited reimbursement for treatment privately, therapists had less time to address all of the underlying problems. The importance of carry-over into the child's daily activities began receiving more attention, and increasing emphasis began to be placed on the occupational therapist's role as a consultant to others who spent more time with children, especially teachers. Parents, teachers, and school administrators began placing greater emphasis on educational relevance, which caused therapists to address the particular concerns that related to the child's academic performance and his/her ability to manage in the school environment (e.g., in the bathroom, in the cafeteria, and in getting to and from classes).

Because of the direct and obvious importance of hand function for independent task accomplishment, fine motor skills began receiving more attention. Many children were recognized as having fine motor difficulties. McHale and Cermak (1992) concluded that approximately 10% of children in the early school years have significant fine motor problems, yet the demands in schools for fine motor performance are high. Preschool children must be able to manage the manipulatives that are in the classroom environment, including puzzles, scissors, crayons, blocks, pegs, and beads. Elementary school–age children must be able to manage the entire writing process, which includes handling a pencil or pen effectively, using an eraser, tearing and folding paper, putting paper into notebooks and folders, and doing art projects. McHale and Cermak (1992) found that "all the classrooms observed [in the study] had a high level of fine motor demands," with fine motor tasks being carried out for 30% to 60% of the classroom day and the majority of these tasks involving writing activities.

As children reach middle school and high school age, they not only have a high volume of written work, but they also take courses that have labs (science, industrial arts, home economics) that require the ability to handle small materials with dexterity. Children of all ages need effective hand function to manage eating, dressing, toileting, and hygiene care independently in school as well as at home and in the community.

Recent theory development and empirical study of theories that have been used as a basis for treatment have also influenced a trend toward a focus on hand function in the therapeutic process. Whereas therapists were taught that proximal development precedes distal development (and this principle influenced therapists for many years to focus primarily on proximal control issues with children who had upper extremity and fine motor problems), current research suggests that the relationship is more functional than causal (Case-Smith, Fisher, and Bauer, 1989). Different neurologic tracts control proximal and distal functions (Lawrence and Kuypers, 1968a, b); the corticospinal tracts are responsible for distal functions, including well-controlled forearm movements (Paillard, 1990) but do not regulate proximal functions. Therefore treatment of proximal control problems will not necessarily cause distal control to improve, unless the distal control problem is due solely to difficulty placing and holding the hand in space. As Pehoski (1992) notes, distal control problems need to be treated specifically.

Another factor influencing the return to emphasis on fine motor treatment was the development and refinement of motor learning theory. This theory emphasizes that skills are acquired using specific strategies and are refined through a great deal of repetition and the transfer of skills to other tasks (Croce and DePaepe, 1989).

Finally, a major factor influencing therapists to specifically address fine motor problems with their children is that they can help the child to immediately use these skills in activities that are meaningful to the child. Furthermore, most therapists observe that children improve in their fine motor skills with intervention. However, very little was written describing fine motor treatment of children in the 1980s; only Erhardt (1982) specifically focused on hand function in assessment and intervention. More recent literature has discussed fine motor treatment (Boehme, 1988; Exner, 1989; Case-Smith and Pehoski, 1992).

However, as yet few studies have focused on treatment of fine motor problems. In keeping with the theoretic focus on underlying problems, almost all empirical studies conducted that address the improvement of fine motor skills are those that use treatment techniques designed to influence tone or proximal control. For example, in Embry's (1993) annotated bibliography of efficacy studies conducted within the last 10 years that focused on improving upper extremity function, the categories of body position, weight bearing, neurodevelopmental treatment, and orthoses/splints were included. Some studies have addressed the influence of body positioning on hand function in children with cerebral palsy (Noronha, Bundy, and Groll, 1989; Seeger, Caudrey, and O'Mara, 1984; Nwaobi, 1987). Barnes (1986, 1989a, b) studied the effectiveness of upper extremity weight bearing on hand function. MacKinnon, Sanderson, and Buchanan (1975) and Exner and Bonder (1983) studied the effectiveness of splinting in improving hand function in children with cerebral palsy. Smelt (1989) combined use of an orthotic device with weight bearing in her study. More recently the effectiveness of upper extremity casting for decreasing tone and improving hand function has been discussed by Yasukawa (1992), and a single-subject study of upper extremity casting conducted by Tona and Schneck (1993) showed some empirical support for this approach. Although the effectiveness of neurodevelopmental treatment has received some study, only Law et al. (1991) considered its effect specifically on hand function. In this research study some children also received casting so the effects of casting could be assessed separately and in conjunction with neurodevelopmental treatment. Again, casting was shown to be an effective adjunct to other treatment.

Carmick (1993) discussed the use of neuromuscular electrical stimulation to improve upper extremity/fine motor control in children with cerebral palsy. The electrical stimulation was used to increase muscle activity in muscle groups opposing those with spasticity. The treatment appeared to be effective with the two children discussed in the study.

Visual-motor skills as demonstrated in standardized tests in which children are asked to draw increasingly complex designs are often used as part of a fine motor evaluation. Many standardized fine motor tests (such as the Bruininks-Oseretsky Test of Motor Proficiency and the Peabody Fine Motor Scales) include drawing of shapes and designs within their subtests. Kleinman and Stalcup (1991) studied the effectiveness of using crafts that involved manipulation of objects within increasingly complex activities to improve visual-motor integration in children with psychosocial problems. They established a sequence of craft activities based on complexity in terms of sensorimotor skills, visual-perceptual skills, and cog-

nitive skills. More of the children who participated in the graded sequence of craft activities improved significantly in their performance on the Developmental Test of Visual-Motor Integration than did children who completed craft activities but not in a specifically graded sequence. The degree of improvement that may have resulted from improved fine motor coordination or from improved visual perception is not known. However, the children's ability to integrate visual perceptual information with fine motor output did seem to improve.

In contrast to the previously mentioned studies, DeGangi et al. (1993) empirically studied the use of fine motor activities (and other activities) to improve fine motor skills. They compared child-centered intervention, in which the adult facilitates the child's activities but the child selects the activities from among those provided in a therapeutic environment, with structured sensorimotor intervention in which the adult directs the child's activities. The child-centered intervention seemed to result in more change in the children's fine motor skills, as measured by the Peabody Fine Motor Scales, than the sensorimotor program did, but the difference in gains between the two approaches was not significant. DeGangi et al. (1993) concluded that "in practice, the therapy approaches used in this study may be blended or sequenced one after the other for best results" and that "this study provides preliminary evidence that children with sensorimotor dysfunction benefit from approaches that elicit adaptations to environmental and task demands through the use of play and structured learning techniques as therapeutic mediums" (pp. 782-783). The remainder of this chapter addresses structured approaches that may be used through playful activities. The importance of the environment is also stressed.

GOAL SETTING FOR HAND SKILL INTERVENTION
Functional and Developmental Considerations

Interventions for fine motor problems, whether they are compensatory strategies or interventions to improve the child's actual fine motor abilities, need to be linked to a functional problem that the child is experiencing. Typical childhood functional problems that are likely to have a fine motor component (and are likely to have other components as well) include the following:

- Poor handwriting
- Difficulty managing materials in the classroom
- Difficulty with artwork, including scissor use
- Limited constructive play skills
- Avoidance of play with peers
- "Messy" eating
- Slow dressing, with avoidance of fasteners
- Lack of independence in getting ready for school

Once it is determined that the child's functional problem has a fine motor component, the therapist must delineate the specific aspects of the fine motor problem and identify the child's areas of strength. This process should yield an understanding of both the child's deficits and the potential for change. At this point the therapist can determine the focus of the intervention program for the child. Gilfoyle, Grady, and Moore (1990) present five overall goals of intervention programs; one or more of these goals may be used. They include:

- Prevention: The potential of primary or secondary problems is minimized
- Modification: The child changes based upon self-participation in activities
- Remediation: Another individual facilitates change to modify or enhance skills
- Compensation: Actions are modified or the task is modified
- Maintenance: Ongoing use of the skills is encouraged

One strategy that can be useful in determining if intervention should focus on remediation or compensation is to consider the child's zone of proximal development, a concept introduced by Vygotsky (1978). The zone of proximal development describes skills the child can demonstrate but only with adult or peer collaboration or assistance. This concept can be useful in designing a treatment plan with goals that are realistic and achievable. Using this concept, the therapist is interested in determining those skills that are close or within reach, not the skills for which the child is still missing many prerequisites. Those skills not within reach may be those which the child needs; if so, adaptations or compensations may be needed to reach these goals. When attempting to improve fine motor skills, however, the child needs to have the prerequisite skills or be able to be facilitated in using a particular fine motor skill before that skill is established as a goal. Setting goals for fine motor treatment involves prioritizing the areas that need to be addressed as well as determining those

areas most likely to be responsive to direct intervention and those that may need adaptation.

Another important consideration in planning intervention for fine motor skills is the child's cognitive functioning. The child's understanding of objects and their relationships and potential for other relationships affects the desire to use the hands to make objects move and interact with one another. Although children acquire some aspects of understanding objects and their actual and potential relationships through manipulating them, the child's cognitive functioning seems to drive (or at least set the stage for) the acquisition of increasingly complex fine motor skills. Therefore it seems important for the child to understand activities that use the fine motor skills that will be addressed in treatment before the therapist sets goals for these skills. Otherwise, the child will have no context for the use of the skills. For example, the child who cannot attend to two objects simultaneously will not be able to bang two objects together or stabilize materials with one hand while manipulating with the other. Erhardt (1992) also makes the point that, in planning intervention for eye-hand coordination, the therapist must take into account the child's intrinsic desire to play and the child's cognitive development since these are the impetus for "purposeful, goal-directed, eye-hand coordination behaviors" (p. 23).

Sample Short-Term Goals

The following represent examples of short-term goals or objectives for remediation programs. They may be quantified for a particular child so documentation of progress or lack of progress can be measurable. They can also be modified so that the focus is on the task that the child will be able to accomplish, rather than specifically on the fine motor skill used to accomplish the task. For example, adding tasks or additional information to one of the following statements, such as "the child will be able to handle money to pay for items in a store by using effective in-hand manipulation skills of translation and shift" places emphasis on the functional outcome rather than the type of fine motor skill.

Sample Short-Term Goals for Grasp

The child will:
- Use a power grasp on tools such as eating utensils, toothbrush, hammer
- Modify use of a radial finger grasp according to pressure requirements for small objects

- Supinate the forearm slightly during approach and maintain this during a radial finger grasp
- Use a full palmer grasp with wrist extension and varying degrees of elbow flexion-extension

Sample Short-Term Goals for Voluntary Release

The child will:
- Release objects that are stabilized by a supporting surface (such as a pegboard)
- Voluntarily release lightweight objects onto a flat surface
- Place an object within 1 inch of other objects without disturbing these by using minimal finger extension
- Release objects while maintaining the forearm in midposition

Sample Short-Term Goals for In-Hand Manipulation

The child will:
- Use shift skills in handling fasteners on clothing
- Use shift skills in managing paper for cutting
- Use translation and shift skills in handling money
- Use simple rotation (or complex rotation) to position a crayon or pencil appropriately in the hand
- Use simple rotation to open and close bottles
- Use translation skills (with or without stabilization) to finger feed in a socially acceptable manner

Sample Short-Term Goals for Bilateral Skills

The child will:
- Stabilize small containers by grasping with one hand while the other hand places objects into the container
- Stabilize paper effectively with one hand during a brief coloring activity
- Manipulate paper by shifting with the non-preferred hand, while using scissors to cut with the other hand

In selecting fine motor areas to address in treatment, the therapist must always keep in mind the importance of assisting the child in improving functionally, not just in a particular fine motor skill or set of fine motor skills. We often assume that our intervention for grasp problems, for example, will have a positive effect on many of the child's functional skills. To determine the validity of this assumption we need to assess the child's performance on standardized tests of fine motor skills (when possible and appropriate) and in particular fine motor activities *and* functional life tasks. The latter is, however, the most important assessment. As Bundy (1990) stressed, we need to be clear in our articulation of the functional changes we expect as a result of our treatment.

INTERVENTION STRATEGIES FOR FINE MOTOR PROBLEMS

To address any particular fine motor skill, the therapist may need to address a variety of subcomponents that contribute to that skill. For example, when the goal is the ability to modify pressure and finger position in a radial digital grasp pattern, emphasis may be placed on radial-ulnar dissociation within the hand, wrist stability, ability to extend the fingers with the wrist in a neutral position, ability to grade finger opening for an object, ability to use a small range of finger flexion (rather than full flexion), or ability to sustain interphalangeal (IP) extension so as to grasp a flat object. The therapist may need to prepare the child to work on these skills by addressing tone, strength, cocontraction, range of motion, and sensory factors.

When planning fine motor treatment for a child, the therapist must also give substantial consideration to the child's interest in the fine motor materials and activities presented. Upper extremity weight bearing and intervention to improve the child's postural control may be done without the child being interested in these activities yet with the child benefiting from the intervention. In contrast, fine motor treatment cannot be done *to* a child. It must be done with the child's involvement in the activities and with the child's belief that he/she can be successful in accomplishing the activities presented. Just having the child do the activity, with little or no attention to the task and no intrinsic investment in the activity, is likely to be of little value with regard to assisting the child in improving fine motor skills. Therefore each treatment session's activities must be suited to the particular child; activities that are particularly good for one child may hold little interest for another.

Within a treatment session the therapist may focus on a variety of fine motor skills or may address only one key area. The following 10 areas may be addressed when the therapist can treat the child directly for 45 to 60 minutes; the order of the suggested interventions is such that skills can build on one another. Obviously some areas will be omitted or addressed only very briefly when a shorter treatment session is used or when intervention is being provided in a classroom setting or through consultation. However, to address even one area the therapist always needs to consider some aspects of the environment being used for treatment and preparation of the child for that intervention. A typical sequence of activities that may be included in a treatment session that focuses on fine motor problems follows:

1. Positioning of the child and the therapist
2. Inhibition/facilitation of tone
3. Postural control
4. Proximal upper extremity control
5. Isolated arm and hand movements
6. Grasp
7. Voluntary release
8. In-hand manipulation
9. Bilateral skills
10. Integration of skills into functional activities

Although all of these areas may not be addressed in every treatment session, the therapist must always address positioning of the child and the therapist and integration of skills into functional activities. These areas and the others are discussed in detail following.

Positioning of the Child and the Therapist

Positioning should be selected to present the type of postural support or challenge that the therapist believes is most desirable for the fine motor skills that will be addressed. In a treatment session it may be appropriate to work on a particular skill first with the child in a relatively nondemanding position, then to work on the same skill in a somewhat more posturally demanding position. For other children it seems most appropriate to work with them in the position in which they will be using the fine motor skill(s) being emphasized. The most commonly used position for treatment and functional use of fine motor skills is sitting, but supine, side-lying, prone, and standing positions may also be used.

For the child with very limited motor skills, the most appropriate position for working on hand function may be supported supine or supported side-lying. In these positions the focus is likely to be on visually regarding the hand(s), using a palmer grasp pattern, sustaining grasp during arm movements, sustaining grasp with the wrist in neutral extension, reaching followed by gross/palmar grasp, and using crude voluntary release.

The prone position can be useful for assisting children in developing a variety of hand skills, but the complexity of the hand skills that can be elicited depends on the child's ability to stabilize effectively at the shoulders in this position. If the child has some difficulty with stability, the emphasis may be on the child being able to sustain the elbows at 90 degrees of flexion, without pulling into more flexion. Sustaining a position of 90 degrees of elbow flexion is very important for both upper extremities because effective hand use in most table-top activities and some standing activities requires that the forearm remain on or near the work surface. Stabilizing materials with the non-preferred hand requires that pressure be exerted into elbow extension while maintaining 90 degrees of elbow flexion. Other typical skills that can be addressed with the child prone on forearms are supination, grasp with the wrist in neutral or slight extension, in-hand manipulation without stabilization of other materials in the hand, bilateral activities in which one hand is stabilizing while the other is manipulating, and bilateral simultaneous in-hand manipulation. For these fine skills to be carried out in the prone position, activities that require a relatively small range of movement must be used. Children can usually use a wider range of movement in sitting or standing positions.

Sitting at a table is often preferred over other positions for carrying out fine motor treatment. When a table is used, it should be at or very slightly above elbow height. Use of a lower table tends to facilitate upper trunk flexion, which is accompanied by humeral internal rotation. Use of a higher table places the child's arms in abduction and internal rotation. Both of these positions are counter to the desired position of humeral adduction and slight external rotation; the humeral position of internal rotation makes it difficult for the child to use slight supination. Without slight supination the child does not have freedom to use thumb and radial finger movements easily.

Sitting in a chair but with no table (or for some children sitting on the floor or on another surface) may also be useful, particularly if the goal is to improve skill in moving objects in space while maintaining a good-quality grasp. When a table is not in front of the child, the therapist often has more opportunity to do both proximal and distal handling to facilitate the child's movements into external rotation, elbow extension, supination, wrist extension, and finger flexion or extension.

Standing is an important position to use when working on some fine motor tasks if the child has the postural control to manage standing and hand use. Generally children find it easier to develop a degree of proficiency when carrying out the skills in sitting, then begin using these skills in standing. Examples of skills that may benefit from a sitting to standing progression are buttoning, engaging the bottom of zippers, brushing teeth, and handling money. For many of these skills the child may initially find it easier to accomplish the fine motor tasks while standing by leaning against a surface to obtain some stability. Gradually the use of this support surface may be faded.

Inhibition/Facilitation of Tone

Inhibition and/or facilitation of tone may be addressed for the child's entire body or for only a particular area of the body. For intervention suggestions to address problems with tone see Boehme (1988) and Danella and Vogtle (1992).

Postural Control

Postural control is a significant consideration in the treatment of many children who have fine motor difficulties. Head control, trunk control, prone skills, and sitting skills are often problem areas for these children. If the therapist has specific goals or the child needs proximal intervention to allow for more effective hand placement in space, postural control needs to be addressed next. Boehme (1988) provides treatment suggestions for this area.

Proximal Control

For strategies that may be useful in dealing with some of the underlying problems and for strategies designed to address more proximal (scapulohumeral) problems in the upper extremities (particularly reach) see Boehme (1988) and Danella and Vogtle (1992). Barnes' studies (1986, 1989a, b) have provided some empirical data supporting the effectiveness of upper extremity weight bearing in improving hand function in children with spastic cerebral palsy. In her single-subject studies she found that extended-arm weight bearing increased the children's use of wrist extension in initiation of grasp and during voluntary release. In her first study (1986) she found that reach with an

extended elbow increased also. In a later study (1989a) she did not find an increase in elbow extension but did find an increase in index finger extension during initiation of grasp. Supination and the quality of grasp did not improve as a result of the weight-bearing intervention. Thus the components that changed as a result of the weight-bearing intervention were those inherent in the weight bearing itself. These components are important for good-quality hand function and need to be emphasized. However, intervention that specifically focuses on supination and hand function is needed also. The focus of the remainder of this chapter is primarily on using structured activities and some degree of handling to address children's difficulties with hand function.

Isolated Arm and Hand Movements

Children often find it easier to work on a new movement component in isolation from other movement components, or when not handling objects, or when handling well-stabilized objects as compared to using that movement component within an activity using unstabilized objects. For example, supination and pronation, wrist flexion/extension, and metacarpophalangeal (MP) flexion/extension with IP extension may be addressed by playing a game with the child in which the child is tapping the table, or his/her leg, or a drum and is only using the desired upper extremity motion. The therapist may assist the child in stabilizing a more proximal body part (e.g., stabilizing the humerus if using supination/pronation, the forearm if using wrist extension/flexion, the dorsum of the hand if using MP flexion/extension). The therapist also may assist the child with using internal rotation, pronation, and wrist flexion, since even children who posture in these patterns have functional difficulty using these movements. They need assistance in developing control over the movements as well as assistance in posturing/holding differently.

Supination is a particularly difficult movement component for children with abnormal tone to use; even children with only slightly low tone will tend to stabilize in full pronation when engaging in fine motor tasks. Yet being able to move into and hold various degrees of supination is critical for hand function. Full pronation interferes significantly with thumb mobility and distal finger control. The ability to use full supination is helpful in performing activities, but for functional hand use the most important range of supination seems to be from full pronation to midposition. The ability to hold in any degree of this range is also important. During most fine motor skills that involve controlled use of the radial fingers and thumb, the forearm is in approximately 30 to 45 degrees of supination.

Treatment to enhance use of supination can take into account the positions and activities in which supination is easiest to use vs. those in which it is more difficult to use. Use of supination is easiest when the humerus is adducted (close to the side of the trunk) and the elbow is flexed. It is much more difficult to use supination when the humerus is in 90 degrees of flexion and the elbow is fully extended, or when the humerus is in full horizontal adduction and the elbow is extended (as in crossing midline).

The process that normal babies seem to use in developing control with supination may also be considered in planning treatment. In normal development babies appear to work first on using supination when the elbow is in a great deal of flexion. Supination can be observed as babies bring their hands and toys to their mouths when in supine, supported sitting, and prone on forearms positions. In the latter position they also begin to move the forearms from full pronation into varying degrees of supination while weight shifting. Gradually babies appear to use more supination in sitting with the elbows in about 90 degrees of flexion. For example, by about 8 or 9 months of age the normally developing baby can bang two objects together; this occurs as a result of two aspects of motor development (and other areas of development as well): the ability to use a finger surface grasp and the ability to hold at least one forearm in midposition so that the surfaces of the

two blocks can come together. In another month or so the baby is able to clap the hands together, thus demonstrating the ability to sustain full finger extension with supination to midposition in both hands. Babies also begin to use this range of supination (0 to 90 degrees) to carry out simple activities such as holding a cup, finger feeding, and visually inspecting objects they are holding. The baby now can reach with supination to midposition. When the baby is reaching laterally (using abduction), a greater degree of supination may be observed as compared with forward reaching (using shoulder flexion).

Specific treatment suggestions for enhancing supination, in approximate order from least to most difficult, include the following:

1. *Encourage mouthing of toys (if age appropriate) and finger feeding.*
2. *Facilitate supination with the forearm on a surface,* such as in weight bearing on the floor or on a mat or while seated at a table. While the child is sitting, the therapist may find it helpful to place an object in the child's hand with the child's forearm pronated, then use his/her hand to stabilize the ulnar border of the child's forearm so the child has a surface to work against for the rotation (and so that the child can see the object placed in the hand) (Figure 12-1). This strategy may also be helpful if the child attempts to compensate for difficulty with supination by using wrist hyperextension.
3. *Encourage the use of 45 to 90 degrees of supination followed by grasp of an object*

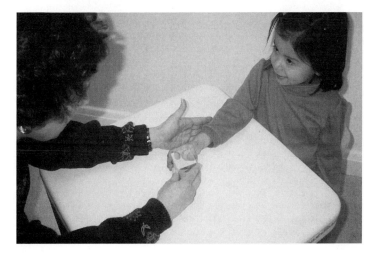

Figure 12-1. Therapist facilitates the child's use of supination by providing stability at the ulnar border of the child's forearm and cues the child to look at the object in the hand.

with the elbow in 90 degrees of flexion, with at least the elbow supported on a surface. The object should be presented in a vertical orientation to facilitate the use of forearm rotation. Some children respond well to the verbal cue "keep your thumb up" since this provides them with visual information about the desired arm/hand position. The child may be encouraged to sustain this position if he/she must transport the object a short distance before placing it into a container or board that requires the forearm to be held in supination. An example of this sequence is reaching and grasping large birthday candles, then putting them into a pretend cake. If the child can accomplish supination to midposition with both hands, banging objects together may be possible. He/she may also be encouraged to hold large blocks or nesting cans by putting one hand on either lateral side of the block or can and stacking these. In this activity the child is being asked to supinate, then initiate grasp and maintain the supination while engaging in a simple activity.

4. *Encourage lateral reach followed by grasp.* Most children with limited use of supination will find it easier to combine humeral abduction with external rotation and supination than to use humeral flexion with external rotation and supination. Objects may initially need to be presented laterally to the child's body to allow the child to continue using abduction but to move out of internal rotation (and into external rotation), which will allow for the use of supination. Objects may be presented low (relative to the child's body) initially and gradually raised higher (Figure 12-2). The therapist may find it possible to gradually present objects diagonally to the child's body (in 60 degrees of horizontal abduction, then 45 degrees, then 30 degrees) to assist the child in moving toward a more anterior reaching pattern.

5. *Encourage forward reach using shoulder flexion and some degree of external rotation.* The object is positioned in front of the child's shoulder, *not* at midline. The object may be placed anywhere between the child's leg (in sitting) and the shoulder, depending on the child's ability to control external rotation and supination while completing the reach. With increasing height of the object in front of the child's body, the child will have a greater tendency to substitute with shoulder elevation, humeral abduction, and internal rotation. Positioning of the object at the optimal height for the child and using slight facilitation at the child's elbow to

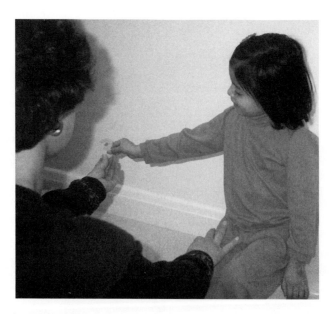

Figure 12-2. An object is presented lateral to the child's body and lower than shoulder height to facilitate the use of external rotation and supination during reaching.

help the child initiate and complete the external rotation during the reach may help the child to achieve the supination needed.

6. *Encourage reach to midline,* following the strategies suggested for reaching in front of the shoulder.

7. *Facilitate reach across midline,* following the strategies suggested for reaching in front of the shoulder.

The therapist who is working with a child on supination, as with any other skill, needs to be sensitive to the child's zone of proximal development in determining the most appropriate level or levels for use in intervention. In a treatment session the therapist may find it possible to begin at one level, then to move up one or even two levels for a few object presentations. When the child has difficulty maintaining skill at the higher level, the therapist should move back down to a lower-level skill. Most sessions consist of using two or more levels, with the therapist helping the child to develop greater competence at the lower level and to explore a level that is slightly more challenging.

Grasp

In clinical practice, treatment for problems with grasp is interwoven with treatment for voluntary release problems and in-hand manipulation problems. However, in this section of the chapter strategies for each of these skills are addressed separately.

In preparation for working on grasp skill with a child, the therapist should assess the child's current use of a wide variety of grasp patterns and determine the problem(s) most interfering with one or more functional grasp patterns. The more careful the analysis of the problems affecting the child's hand function, the more specific the intervention can be. The therapist needs to determine if an opposed grasp pattern is possible for the child, and, if so, the sizes of objects with which it can be used, that is, larger ones, medium-size ones, or small and tiny ones. Some children can functionally use an opposed grasp pattern on larger objects but not on small or tiny ones due to the lesser degree of stability that these objects provide and the index finger control that is necessary. Some children are able to use grasp patterns that rely on the use of the long finger flexors and extensors (e.g., a palmer grasp or a hook grasp) but are unable to effectively use the intrinsic muscles of

the hand to allow for more variety and function in grasp. This may be particularly obvious in a child's difficulty with holding a ball using a spheric grasp (which requires the combination of long flexor activity with dorsal interrossei and lumbrical activity) or with holding a piece of paper (which requires use of the palmar interrossei and lumbricals). Many children lack adequate thumb stability for opposition and substitute with thumb adduction, whereas others are pulled into thumb adduction by an overactive adductor pollicis.

The child's functional needs should be considered in determining the types of grasp patterns to be emphasized in treatment. Some children have an adequate grasp with the finger pads but lack the effective full palmar grasp pattern necessary for many dressing activities. Some children have only a palmar grasp pattern with the thumb adducted into the palm, so they cannot pick up small or tiny objects in a functional manner. Thus activities such as finger feeding, cup drinking, and fastener use are negatively affected. Therefore use of grasp within functional activities, not only in performance on standardized test items, should be assessed as a basis for treatment planning.

General Intervention Principles for Grasp Problems

The following general principles are suggested for structuring intervention for grasp problems.

If fisting is a problem, address voluntary hand opening before setting any other goals for grasp. In children who have limited ability to voluntarily open their hands, the priority is voluntary hand opening and being able to sustain some degree of finger extension with arm movement, if this seems to be within their zone of proximal development. For children who have tonic fisting and need maximal assistance in obtaining and even briefly maintaining hand opening, the goal of intervention for grasp is to have them be able to open their hands more readily and perhaps to initiate and sustain a palmar grasp pattern with changing arm positions.

Upper extremity weight bearing may be used to facilitate finger extension with wrist extension, but, in children who have marked fisting, weight bearing with open hands may need to be used cautiously. Most of the children with marked fisting do not have sufficient length in their finger flexors to tolerate this position without compromise in the finger positions used. In this type of weight bearing the therapist must control both the thumb, which is typically pulled into adduction, and the fingers, which may pull up into a boutonnière deformity position. Weight bearing on a curved surface may be more effective than on a flat surface, or the therapist may wish to consider use of a weight-bearing splint or other device (Smelt, 1989). Weight-bearing activities that do not ask the child to assume full body weight, such as having the child sit and place the hand on a surface with the humerus in approximately 90 degrees of flexion or abduction, may be effective and minimize the abnormal positioning of the fingers and thumb that may occur in a weight-bearing position in which the child takes the weight of his/her body.

Encouraging a greater range of arm movements without the use of tonic patterns may be used to help the child open the hands and maintain them open. Tactile/proprioceptive input to the child's arms and hands can be used directly with this technique. Emphasis on arm movements often is most easily accomplished with the child supine. In this position the child can be provided with opportunities to see his/her hands and to bring both hands together—simple activities that these children have had little opportunity to do. As the child brings the hands together, the therapist can encourage the use of supination with elbow flexion. The child may be assisted with touching stuffed animals with fisted hands, an activity that does not require that the hands be open. Activities that encourage the child to dissociate the two sides of the body may be incorporated, such as having the child touch the stuffed animal's ear with one hand and his/her own ear with the other hand. In this way one elbow is more extended and the other is more flexed. The child may be encouraged to assist with rubbing lotion on one arm with the other hand to facilitate crossing midline and hand contact on the body while the elbow position is changing.

During these activities to promote active arm movement, the child's hand often becomes open or at least less fisted, and the therapist can begin activities to encourage a full palmar grasp pattern and to facilitate changing arm positions while maintaining this grasp. If the child's fingers and thumb remain somewhat flexed, techniques recommended by Boehme (1988) for facilitating hand opening may be used.

Once the child has some degree of hand opening in a supine position, it may be possible to change the child to a sitting position and carry out similar activities. The change in body positions often presents the next level of challenge to the child. Partial or full weight bearing may be added to reinforce the hand opening, if tolerated by the child.

Address supination and wrist stability if these are problems. Problems with supination tend to be evident when the child needs to use grasp patterns that require more precision, such as a three-jaw chuck (see Glossary), a pincer, or a lateral pinch. These problems may be addressed through use of the strategies suggested earlier. Problems with wrist stability must be addressed before or in conjunction with specific intervention for grasp. Wrist stability may be addressed through use of weight-bearing techniques and through emphasis on developing a palmar grip (Boehme, 1988). Wrist extension will tend to be used more with holding objects in a full palmar grip than in patterns in which only the finger surfaces or pads are involved. The size of the object to be used for a palmar grip may need to be explored with the child; some children use more wrist extension with small-diameter objects, whereas others use more with somewhat larger-diameter objects.

Expect inconsistency in performance. Another consideration in planning and carrying out treatment is that inconsistency in performance, not consistency, is to be expected as skills are emerging. This clinical observation is supported by empirical data on development of grasp patterns in nondysfunctional infants. Hirschell, Pehoski, and Coryell (1990) found that normal 13- to 14-month-olds were consistent in the pincer grasp pattern they used. However, 7- to 8-month-olds and 10- to 11-month-olds tended to use a variety of grasp patterns when attempting to obtain the object.

Consider the stability of the child and of the object. The stability of the child, the surface on which the object is presented, and the object itself are considerations in planning treatment. This principle is supported by findings of Hirschell et al. (1990). In their study babies who were beginning to develop control of a particular grasp pattern were most successful when grasping from a very firm surface and less successful on an unstable surface.

Consider object characteristics and orientation of objects that are presented. The size, shape, weight, texture, and slipperiness of the objects selected for use in treatment must be given careful consideration. Round objects, such as dowels, will tend to be held in a palmar grasp unless the child has good stability in the fingers and thumb and can maintain a grasp by opposing the thumb to several finger pads. Therefore many children can handle blocks and other objects with straight sides more effectively than round objects. Children who do not have good internal stability within their hands should not be expected to hold unstable objects (round, squishy, or lightweight ones) with control in any pattern other than a palmar grasp.

Grasp of small or tiny objects should not be the priority for all children. An opposed grasp can be introduced to the child with larger objects, particularly if the child has sufficient hand expansion to accommodate the object. People use an opposed pattern to grasp items such as a cup (a cylindric grasp), a ball (a spheric grasp), a telephone receiver, and a large block. In many of these opposed grasp patterns the thumb is opposed to two, three, or all four fingers. Some children with disabilities can be assisted in developing skilled use of all types of opposed grasp patterns as well as the power grasp and the lateral pinch. Therefore the pincer grasp need not be considered the best grasp. For many children less attention should be paid to the pincer grasp and more attention to developing a variety of functional grasp patterns.

Consider initially emphasizing grasp without reach. Grasp can be addressed in treatment without asking the child to first reach, then grasp. To reach and grasp, the child is required to preposition the arm and the hand, often against gravity. Initially, in treatment for grasp, children respond better to intervention in which they only have to preposition the hand.

Assist the child in developing skill in carrying objects while maintaining quality of grasp, before actually using that grasp within an activity. Many children have difficulty transporting an object while sustaining a good-quality grasp pattern. It is often useful to have the child maintain a stable grasp pattern, transport the object in space, and release it before expecting that the child be able to maintain this pattern within a more challenging activity.

Developing Radial Finger Grasp Patterns

Children with whom the following strategies are used are those who can voluntarily grasp and release objects but lack good quality in one or more grasp patterns or are not able to use grasp patterns involving distal finger control. These grasp patterns include a lateral pinch or an opposed grasp with one or more fingers contacting the object and thumb opposition. Further preparation of the hand may be needed before using these strategies. Objects selected should be appropriate for the grasp pattern being addressed but should also be presented within the context of an activity that the child finds interesting. In this sequence the

emphasis is on first assisting the child with grasping while not asking the child to reach. Objects are initially stabilized well when presented, then gradually presented with less external stability, in response to the child's development of internal stability. Gradually reach and grasp are combined.

The therapist should explore the grasps used by the child at each of the levels to determine the best place to begin therapeutic intervention. Not all children need to begin at the first level described in the following. In a treatment session the therapist may find it useful to move back and forth between two or three levels. For example, the therapist may give three object presentations at level 2, then, finding that the child's performance has deteriorated slightly, give two or three presentations at level 1, then give a few at level 2 again. It may then be possible to give a few presentations at level 3 before finishing that aspect of the treatment session with other object presentations at level 2.

Level 1: Grasp from therapist's fingers. The child is in a sitting position (usually in a chair) with humerus adducted and the forearm stabilized on his/her leg or on the table surface. The child's hand is in front of the shoulder, not at midline. The therapist holds the object in his/her fingers and places the object just at the child's fingers (Figure 12-3). The child positions the hand for grasp, then grasps the object and carries it a short distance before

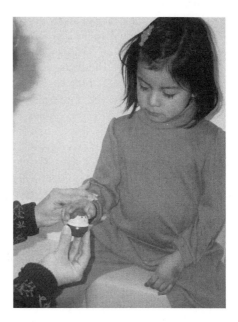

Figure 12-3. To promote use of an opposed grasp pattern, the therapist stabilizes the dorsum of the child's forearm and presents an object held with her finger pads directly to the child's fingers.

voluntary release. The therapist notes the degree and quality of wrist extension and finger and thumb positioning in the grasp. If the child does not use sufficient wrist extension, the therapist may find it helpful to stabilize the dorsum of the child's forearm and to hold the object just slightly higher for the next object presentation. If the fingers are too flexed, other preparation of the hand to decrease tone may be needed before the next object presentation. If the quality of the pattern appears good, the therapist will probably find it helpful to give several other presentations in this manner to ensure that the child can consistently maintain this quality before moving to the next level.

Level 2: Grasp from palm of therapist's hand. The child's arm and hand are positioned as in the first level. The therapist positions the object in the palm of his/her hand with the hand sufficiently cupped to stabilize the object. Then he/she places this hand just under the child's hand. In this way the child is required to position the hand for grasp and grasp the object that is just slightly less stabilized than when it was in the therapist's fingers. Again the therapist notes the quality of the pattern used and determines if other handling would be useful, if the child would benefit more from greater repetitions at the preceding level before trying this level again, or if this type of presentation should be used again.

Level 3: Grasp from surface, near body with object in front of shoulder, not midline. Now the object is placed on the table surface, which provides it with less stability than the therapist's hand does. The child's arm position is similar to that used in the previous two levels. The therapist may find it helpful to place the object on a nonskid surface or to stabilize the object slightly with the fingers. The child needs to control the positioning of the hand more in preparation for grasp at this level.

Level 4: Grasp from surface, further from body with the object in front of shoulder. At this level the child begins to combine supported reaching with preparation of the hand for grasp. The hand preparation is often better with the object in front of the shoulder since this position allows slight supination to be more easily used.

Level 5: Grasp from surface, near midline. The child now begins to work on grasping at midline while controlling the hand, forearm, and elbow position. The child is still not expected to control the humerus against gravity while initiating the grasp pattern. The therapist needs to explore the best position for the object in terms of its distance from the child's body. Typically a distance that incorporates greater than 90 degrees

of elbow extension is helpful initially. Then this distance can be varied as the child develops increasing skill.

Level 6: Grasp with object off surface. At this level the child needs to control the humerus against gravity and control the degree of external rotation used. At the previously described levels, external rotation could be assisted by the surface. Positioning of the object by the therapist can be used to help the child orient the arm into slight external rotation and the forearm into slight supination (as described in the section on supination). Again, distance from the child's body can be varied, as can positioning of the object in front of the child's shoulder or at midline.

The previous strategies can be used when assisting a child to develop a variety of grasp patterns. However, some children need additional focus on development of intrinsic muscle control so that they are able to hold flat objects by using MP flexion and IP extension of the fingers with the thumb in opposition/adduction. Activities that involve finger adduction with extension, such as rolling out clay while keeping all fingers together and straight, finger games that involve finger abduction and adduction, squeezing balls of clay until they are flat by using the thumb pad against the entire pad of the index and middle fingers, shaking dice in the palm of the hand by cupping the hand (curving the transverse metacarpal arch and the carpal arch), and games or activities that involve holding thick flat objects may be helpful (Figure 12-4). Additional activities for enhancing

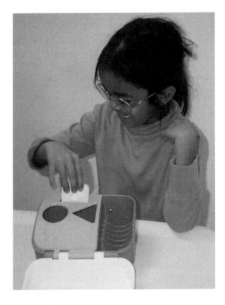

Figure 12-4. Use of a thick, flat object may assist the child in developing grasp with MP flexion and IP extension.

refined grasp patterns have been suggested by Myers (1992). Verbal cues regarding the desired pattern may also be useful in helping the child to perform the desired pattern.

Developing a Power Grasp Pattern

The strategies that have been discussed tend to be less helpful in facilitating a power grasp than they are in facilitating opposed grasp patterns. Children with poor stability in their hands tend to use a palmar grasp on tools (such as knives, toothbrushes, hairbrushes, and hammers) rather than a power grasp in which the ulnar fingers provide stability for the handle and the radial fingers are more extended so that they can reorient the tool as necessary (Figures 12-5 and 12-6). Not all children with motor disabilities are able to

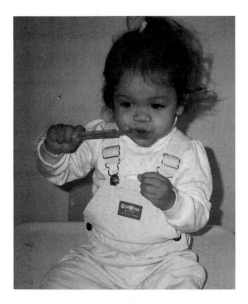

Figure 12-5. Young child demonstrates use of a palmer grasp on a "tool."

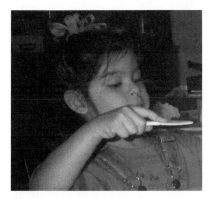

Figure 12-6. An older child demonstrates use of a power grasp on a "tool."

develop a power grasp, just as not all children will develop a pincer grasp. However, for those children who are able but do not use a power grasp, development of this skill enhances their ability to be more effective and efficient with many daily life tasks. Usually the children who can develop a power grasp are those who have some degree of instability in their hands but have reasonable thumb opposition and finger control in grasping stable objects.

A strategy that may be used in working toward a power grasp with the child is to encourage the child to use radial-ulnar dissociation within the hand. The child can be assisted in developing skill in retaining one or more objects in the middle to ulnar side of the palm with flexed ulnar fingers, while using the radial finger(s) and thumb to grasp and release objects. Initially the object held in the ulnar side of the hand might be medium sized so that the degree of finger flexion required (and the degree of differentiation in radial-ulnar finger positions) is less; gradually the size of this object may be reduced. Similarly, the size of the objects grasped with the radial fingers and thumb may be decreased as the child's proficiency increases.

The therapist who is working with a child on developing or improving a power grasp may also consider carefully selecting or modifying the diameter and shape of the object to be held with a power grasp. Tools with thin or rounded handles are more difficult for the child to grasp well; handles that are slightly larger in diameter or have ridges or indentations may be more effectively grasped by a child with instability. Also the degree of power needed within the activity should be graded because with increased demands for power the child tends to move from the more refined power grasp pattern to a palmar grasp pattern.

Following grasp of any object, the child may use the object to complete a task (e.g., use a hammer to pound a nail), use in-hand manipulation to adjust the object after grasp (e.g., turn a key to fit it into a lock), or voluntarily release the object (e.g., put coins into a machine to buy a candy bar). Because voluntary release quality depends so much on grasp quality and the two skills can often be worked on effectively within the same activity, voluntary release is discussed next.

Voluntary Release

Motor control problems with voluntary release typically result from three key areas of difficulty: (1) poor arm stability, (2) increased flexor tone, which causes fisting or difficulty with grasp using the finger surface, and (3) lack of effective use of the intrinsics. In the latter case, problems are seen in poor IP joint extension or poor MP joint control. A typical pattern seen in poor-quality voluntary release is MP joint extension with or without IP joint extension. These problems with stability and lack of extensor activity appropriately balanced with flexor activity interfere with the effectiveness and efficiency of voluntary release. Some children with these problems resort to using tenodesis action by flexing at the wrist to initiate the voluntary release (and may use the same pattern in reverse to initiate grasp).

Interference with voluntary release due to arm instability is often a key problem for children with involuntary movement or tremors. However, instability may also negatively affect voluntary release in children with low tone or high tone who do not have excess movement. For effective voluntary release the child needs to release where and when he/she wants to release. The arm is important in transporting the hand to where the child wants to release, and holding the arm in position during hand opening contributes to when he/she wants to release.

Several strategies may be used with children who have stability problems that affect voluntary release. Upper extremity weight bearing, particularly on extended arms, may help the child to develop improved cocontraction at the scapulohumeral area, the elbow, and the wrist. Reaching activities that involve touching a desired target and holding that position for a few seconds may also be helpful, particularly if the reaching is done in a variety of planes of movement. For the child who has marked instability or needs to function despite some instability, teaching the child to stabilize the arm against the body or on a surface prior to opening the hand may be a helpful compensatory strategy.

With most children who have stability problems, achieving wrist stability with finger extension is a primary area of intervention so they can release without the need for tenodesis action. Some children use the wrist flexion pattern when they are in elbow flexion, but they are able to voluntarily release with the wrist in extension if the elbow is extended. For these children, and even those who have significant flexor tone at the wrist and fingers when the elbow is flexed, an effective treatment strategy can be to facilitate releasing objects away from midline and with the elbow extended. As with the strategy discussed for facilitating supination, humeral abduction and ex-

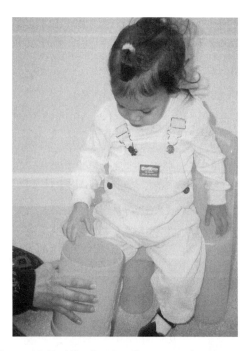

Figure 12-7. Allowing for elbow extension by placing a container on or near the floor may encourage use of wrist and finger extension for voluntary release.

ternal rotation may make it easier for the child to use elbow extension and slight supination, which may in turn allow voluntary release with wrist extension to occur. Releasing into a container placed on the floor, or at least lower than the seat of the child's chair, may also allow the child with high tone or little voluntary control to learn to take advantage of gravity or at least relax the finger flexors (Figure 12-7). Gradually the container used for release can be brought onto a table surface (if it was down low), closer to the child's body (if release was being worked on away from the body), and closer to midline (if release was being worked on in front of the shoulder or lateral to the child's body). These strategies are, however, unlikely to be beneficial for the child who can release with adequate control at the shoulder, elbow, and wrist but has difficulty grading finger extension.

In addressing problems of voluntary release as seen in poorly graded finger extension, it is important to consider the role that quality of the child's grasp plays in the problem. *The quality of voluntary release can be no better than the quality of the grasp.* However, the quality of voluntary release can be poorer than the quality of grasp. Therefore, if the child holds an object in a palmar grasp, voluntary release is initiated with full extension (or almost full extension) of the fingers. If, on the other hand, the child holds an object with the finger pads, he/she may release with just slight finger extension or much more finger extension may be seen. Because grasp and release are associated with one another, the therapist must address the quality of the child's grasp in intervention for voluntary release problems. For some children the focus is on decreasing wrist and finger flexor tone to allow for grasp on the finger surface rather than in the palm. For other children the emphasis is on enhancing the use of intrinsic muscle activity to allow for more control in the grading of both the grasp and release patterns. For children who have mild problems, attention to stabilization of the forearm in a slight degree of supination during voluntary release may help them place objects with more accuracy and without bumping other objects with their hands.

As children develop more control with voluntary release, the therapist can gradually decrease object weight, stability, and/or size, and the size of the area used for object placement. With mildly involved children, emphasis may be placed on using smaller size objects, objects that are less solid (paper balls rather than solid rubber balls, cotton balls rather than paper balls), and inexpensive toys that tend to be lighter in weight than sturdy, high-quality toys. Games in which the importance of accuracy of placement is obvious to the child can be selected or developed. For example, some children's game boards have large areas for the game pieces, whereas others have small areas. Activities that involve the child holding tweezers and using these to grasp and release objects may help the child focus on graded pressure and graded release with a steady arm position. When using the tweezers and other small materials, the therapist also can address precise grasp with the child.

In-Hand Manipulation

Skill Types

In-hand manipulation skills seem to be the most complex of all fine motor skills. In-hand manipulation involves the adjustment of objects by movements of the fingers so that the objects are more appropriately placed within the hand for the task to be accomplished (Exner, 1989, 1990, 1992). In-hand manipulation occurs within one hand. Five basic types of in-hand manipulation skills have been described (Exner, 1992):

- *Finger-to-palm translation*: Movement of an object from the fingers to the palm
- *Palm-to-finger translation*: Movement of an object from the palm to the finger pads

- *Shift*: Slight adjustment of the object on or by the finger pads
- *Simple rotation*: Turning or rolling the object 90 degrees or less, with the fingers acting as a unit
- *Complex rotation*: Turning an object over (turning it 90 to 360 degrees) using isolated finger and thumb movements

Each of the in-hand manipulation skills may occur with no other object in the hand at the time of the manipulation or while the ulnar fingers are holding one or more objects in the center or ulnar side of the palm (Exner, 1989, 1990, 1992). When other objects are held in the hand during manipulation, the skill has the term added: "with stabilization."

Although almost all children with fine motor problems have difficulty with these skills, not all of these children are candidates for intervention for their in-hand manipulation problems. To be considered for intervention specifically for in-hand manipulation problems, the child needs to have good skills in basic grasp and release patterns. He/she needs to be able to grasp a variety of objects and to accommodate the hands to these objects effectively. The child needs to be able to grasp objects at least on the finger surface (not only show use of a palmar grasp) and preferrably with the pads of the fingers. In terms of finger isolation the child needs to be able to isolate the index finger at least. If the child can use some degree of supination and thumb opposition, in-hand manipulation skills are more functional. Evidence of radial-ulnar dissociation is important, particularly when considering use of in-hand manipulation with stabilization of other objects within the child's hand. In general, in-hand manipulation activities are realistic only for children who have mild motor disabilities; most children with moderate disabilities lack the ability to use adequate grasp patterns (and lack the associated intrinsic muscle control) to make in-hand manipulation skills possible.

General Principles for Developing In-Hand Manipulation Skills

The following principles are useful to consider in planning and implementing treatment for children who have difficulty with in-hand manipulation.

Provide somatosensory stimuli. Many children with fine motor problems have difficulty with tactile perception. Case-Smith (1991) found that children with both tactile discrimination problems and tactile defensiveness had significantly poorer performance on in-hand manipulation tasks than did other children. Some children seem to have little awareness that they have five digits on each hand and instead use all four fingers as a unit. They also seem to have little awareness that they have different areas on the palms of the hand. Therefore, with children who have in-hand manipulation problems, intervention that addresses increasing their sensory awareness and discrimination and deals with any tactile defensiveness may need to be carried out before working on in-hand manipulation. If these problems are significant, intervention for them may take the major focus of the treatment session. If they are milder, some amount of time may be spent on these areas before working specifically on in-hand manipulation within the treatment session. In some cases the activities used for sensory awareness may be the same as those used for in-hand manipulation. Typical activities used for sensory awareness and discrimination may include finding objects in beans, rice, or sand (graded finger movements are used to get the grains of rice or sand off the objects), pulling pieces of clay off a ball of clay, pushing fingers into therapy putty or clay, stretching rubber bands around the fingers, and rubbing lotion on the fingers one at a time.

Facilitate the use of the intrinsic muscles in grasp and other hand functions. Many of the sensory activities (such as pulling clay) can be done to facilitate use of the intrinsic muscles. It seems helpful to stress development of the grasp pattern that uses MP flexion with IP extension because this pattern requires use of the intrinsic muscles, as does in-hand manipulation, and also because this is often the ending pattern after the child has completed the manipulation. This grasp pattern indicates the child's degree of stability with the intrinsics; in-hand manipulation relies on both mobility and stability of joints controlled by the intrinsics. Therefore we need to ensure that the child has the ability to use stability before expecting mobility with stability. Emphasis on a spheric grasp that uses a combination of long flexor activity and intrinsic activity and requires cupping of the palm may also be useful (see section on grasp for strategies to facilitate grasp patterns and use of the intrinsics).

Encourage use of bilateral manipulation and skills that substitute for in-hand manipulation. Infants manipulate objects *between* the two hands (Ruff, 1984). Young children often turn objects over between the two hands as well. They also spontaneously use any supporting surface to stabilize materials as they are attempting to manipulate them. For example, young children use a surface on which to turn a puzzle piece, rather than picking up the puzzle piece and turning it within

the hand. These substitutions may not be abnormal patterns in older children; however, they do seem to be developmentally less mature. Case-Smith (1993) noted the frequent use of stabilization on a surface by preschoolers with developmental delays, in contrast to the preschoolers without developmental delays. These substitution patterns can be effective for handling many objects, but they are not efficient, particularly when handling small or tiny objects or when both hands need to be manipulating simultaneously.

Use small objects first with a new skill. Objects that are small in relation to the child's hand size are typically easier for them to manipulate than are tiny or medium size objects. For example, children typically find nickels easier to manipulate than dimes or silver dollars. Pegs that are larger in diameter or length are more difficult to handle than are pegs that are 1 to 1½ inches long and ½ inch in diameter. Children who are ready to use in-hand manipulation skills can grasp tiny pegs well, but manipulating them is very difficult. Another example is that, whereas 1-inch beads are easy to grasp, they are usually more difficult for the child to manipulate than are ½-inch beads. Therefore, when introducing a new skill, the therapist will often find it helpful to carefully select objects that are small so that the child can have sufficient finger contact on the object during manipulation but does not need to use all fingers to stabilize the object during manipulation. As the child develops a particular skill, the therapist can begin to vary the size of the objects used.

Use cues to facilitate the child's use of in-hand manipulation skills. Exner (1990) studied the effectiveness of cues in increasing 3- and 4-year-old children's in-hand manipulation skills. She found that, as a group, the children improved significantly when given either verbal cues or demonstrations. Although some skills improved more with verbal cues and some improved more with demonstrations, the use of palm-to-finger translation with stabilization and rotation with stabilization improved with both types of cues. However, it should be noted that not all children showed improved performance with cues. As with other aspects of children's fine motor skills, their zone of proximal development for in-hand manipulation should be considered in setting goals. In addition, the therapist needs to determine the best mode for cues for each child. During testing in this study (Exner, 1990) it was observed that some children who were provided with demonstrations (but not verbal cues) seemed unsure of the aspect of the skill that they should imitate. Therefore demonstration cues alone may not be as helpful to the child as demonstration cues with verbal cues. Some children may need only verbal cues to remind them to try the skill with one hand.

Consider the tentative sequence of skill difficulty. Children appear to use finger-to-palm translation earlier than other in-hand manipulation skills. Simple rotation and palm-to-finger translation skills appear to be somewhat more difficult. Shift and complex rotation seem to be the most difficult of the in-hand manipulation skills. Therefore, in determining the type of in-hand manipulation skills that will be the focus of intervention for a child who has no skills in this area, the therapist will probably find finger-to-palm translation the easiest to help the child develop. Verbal cuing to the child to "hide the object in your hand" may be helpful in working on this skill. Small pieces of cereal or coins are good objects for the child to hide.

If the child is able to use finger-to-palm translation with a variety of objects, the therapist may begin to work on palm-to-finger translation and simple rotation. For palm-to-finger translation the intervention strategy that tends to be most effective is to use a backward shaping approach. This is done by the therapist initially placing the object on the volar surface of the child's fingers at approximately the crease for the distal IP (DIP) joint and (if possible) asking the child to bring the object out

to the pads or tips of the fingers (Figure 12-8, *A*). If verbal cuing is unlikely to be understood by the child, the therapist needs to rely even more heavily on the structuring of the activity, for example using a bank with a narrow slot or a small container or a small surface that requires the child to use a precision grasp (one on the finger pads or tips) to be successful with placement. For example, a game piece may be placed on the child's finger surface, and the child is asked to place the game piece on a particular color square on the board.

After the child is able to move objects well from the DIP creases on the fingers, the object may be moved closer to the proximal IP (PIP) crease but still kept on the index or index and middle fingers (Figure 12-8, *B*). Eventually it can be placed on the MP crease, at which time placement should be between the index and middle fingers. Finally, objects may be placed in the center of the palm (Figure 12-8, *C*). Some children are able to work on bringing objects from the ulnar side of the hand to the radial fingers and thumb. Objects that may be useful when working on palm-to-finger translation are small pieces of food or cereal, small cookies, coins, game pieces, small puzzle pieces, beads for stringing, paper clips, caps for markers and pens, pegs, and small blocks.

Simple rotation skills can often be addressed early in a treatment program designed to facilitate in-hand manipulation skills. Simple rotation tends

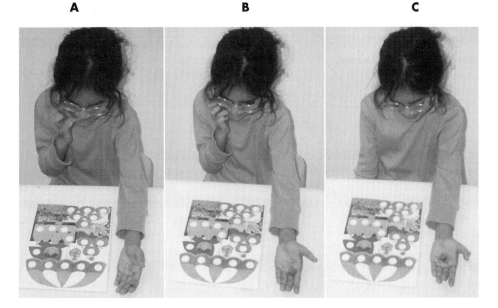

Figure 12-8. A, Use of palm-to-finger translation may be encouraged by grading the activity. Initially the object is placed on the distal surface of the child's radial fingers. **B,** Gradually the object is placed more proximally on the child's finger surface. **C,** After success with more proximal placement, the child may be able to use palm-to-finger translation when the therapist places the object in the palm of the child's hand.

to be "simple" because the fingers move as a unit to turn the object for a partial turn only. These skills may be encouraged by placing an object in the child's fingers (with appropriate finger contact and forearm pronated) and asking the child to make the object upright. It may be helpful to slightly stabilize the child's arm to help prevent the use of forearm rotation as a substitution for manipulation by the fingers. Although some supination is to be expected, the child should not be allowed to complete the entire motion with forearm rotation and without use of individual finger movements. Activities that may be useful for encouraging simple rotation skills include unscrewing a bottle top, picking up a pen, pencil, or marker that has been placed horizontally on the surface with the writing end oriented toward the ulnar side of the child's preferred hand, picking up pegs (or a similar object) from a surface and putting them into a pegboard, and rolling clay or a toy person between the thumb and radial fingers. Again, the therapist may find that demonstrations and visual cues are helpful to the child in understanding what to do with the materials; in addition, it is possible to physically assist children with simple rotation skill more readily than it is to physically assist them with the translation skills. This may be done by the therapist placing his/her fingers over the child's fingers to facilitate the finger movements for rotation.

Shift skills often require the child to have more sustained control of the fingers in IP extension; therefore shift skills are more difficult for children who have particular trouble with this pattern. In working on shift skills, use of one shift movement (such as moving a coin from the finger pads to the fingertips for placement) is easier than repetitive shifts (moving fingers around paper to allow for cutting with scissors). In treatment, children may be encouraged to use single shift movements, then gradually to increase the number of shift movements used. For example, the child who is holding the fingers on a marker approximately 1½ inches from the writing end may be asked to stretch the fingers down toward the tip and then to move the thumb so that he/she is holding the marker more effectively for writing or coloring.

When the child can use a single shift movement, the therapist should facilitate the use of shift skills in adjusting paper during cutting. To initiate this, the therapist will need to ensure that the child can hold the paper with the thumb on top of the paper and the fingers in a relatively extended position on the underneath surface. Use of index cards may make this easier than paper would be,

since the cards are slightly thicker and more sturdy than paper (but are still easy to cut) and are smaller to handle. As the child's skill in shifting the card improves, larger and larger sizes of index cards may be used for cutting. Eventually regular paper may be used.

In facilitating the use of complex rotation the therapist needs to rely on selection of materials that readily facilitate the use of complex rotation and cues to the child. Children need to have the cognitive skills to attend and to focus well on verbal and demonstration cues when complex rotation skills are addressed in treatment. This ability to respond to cues is important because it is very difficult for the therapist to physically assist the child with these skills. Games and imaginative play activities can be used for working on these skills, thus allowing for attention to other goals as well, particularly those having to do with cognitive concepts and visual perception. Materials that work well for enhancing complex rotation include pegs that can be placed upside down for the child to turn over, cubes that have pictures on one or more sides and can be turned to find the appropriate picture for a category of pictures or a puzzle, a pencil with an eraser that can be turned over to allow for its use and turned back for writing again, markers with caps so the cap can be placed in the child's hand upside down before the child places it on the marker, and toy people or figures that can be inverted on a surface or in the child's hand and that need to be rotated before placement.

When children are first working on complex rotation, they tend to need a surface for support, both for their arms and for the objects. Therefore it is easier for the child if the therapist places the object on a table surface. Soon, however, it is usually possible to place the object in the child's hand and encourage the child to at least start the rotation before using a surface for support. Later the child can be asked to use the skill without depending on a supporting surface at all and to completely finish the rotation before putting the object down. Once the child can do one complex rotation with an object, the child may be encouraged to attempt repetitive rotations by turning the object over two times, then three times, and so on. This emphasis in treatment encourages use of sustained stability with sustained mobility, which is difficult for many of the children with low tone.

Fully develop each skill before asking the child to combine skills within an activity. Children seem to find that using palm-to-finger translation immediately before using either simple or

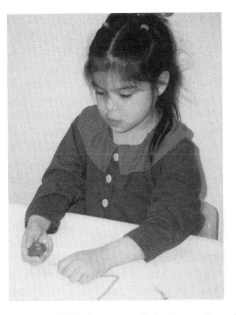

Figure 12-9. Child shows use of simple rotation with stabilization by holding two objects in the hand. One object is stabilized by the ulnar fingers, while the other object is rotated slightly before stringing.

complex rotation (e.g., moving a key from the palm to the fingers, then turning it for placement) is much more difficult than using simple or complex rotation alone. Therefore children should be assisted with developing palm-to-finger translation that does not involve rotation of the object for placement and simple and complex rotation without palm-to-finger translation before asking for the combination of these skills.

Fully develop a skill before asking the child to use that skill with stabilization. Stabilizing other materials in the hand while manipulating an object is quite difficult because it relies on good radial-ulnar dissociation of movements and the ability to carry out the manipulation without use of the ring or little fingers (Figure 12-9). Therefore the therapist should ensure that the child can use the skill easily before asking the child to hold even one object in the hand while manipulating. Children find it easier to hold one other object in the hand than to hold two or more. Usually they also find it easier at first if the objects to be held are placed in the ulnar side of the hand by the therapist. Later they may be asked to pick up and move an object into the hand and hold it there while manipulating another object with the radial fingers.

The easiest in-hand manipulation skill to use with stabilization is finger-to-palm translation, since this is only slightly more difficult than using this pattern without stabilization. It requires the

child to keep the ulnar fingers flexed while grasping with the radial fingers, and storing another object in the hand only requires movement into finger flexion (which is easier than moving into finger extension). It also seems to be a skill that many young children develop spontaneously as they try to hold several pieces of cereal or candy or small crackers in their hands at one time.

After mastering finger-to-palm translation with stabilization, most children seem to find it easier to work on palm-to-finger translation with stabilization than simple rotation with stabilization. However, the therapist should explore these with the child, then select the easier skill to work on next. The size of the object being held in the hand can be a factor in making the skill seem easier or more difficult. If it is too small, a great deal of ulnar flexion will be needed, thus increasing the requirement for radial-ulnar dissociation. If the object is too large, the child may need to use the middle finger to assist in the stabilization and then will not have this finger available for manipulation.

Children with very mild disabilities may find it possible to learn to use shift and complex rotation with stabilization, but many children find these skills too difficult. If these skills look possible for the child, the therapist may find that one skill is easier than the other for the child to develop. For complex rotation the size of the object being stabilized is particularly critical, since complex rotation often is carried out by the index, middle, and ring fingers. When stabilization of objects is required, the ring finger typically is not available to assist in the rotation. Therefore smaller objects are easier to use for manipulation than are larger ones.

Bilateral Hand Skills

In the normal development process babies initially develop gross symmetric bilateral skills (such as holding objects with two hands, clapping, banging objects together), then begin to stabilize objects with one hand while the other is manipulating (holding paper while coloring, holding a container while putting objects in), then manipulate objects with both hands simultaneously (stringing beads, tying a knot). Children with motor control problems all have difficulty with bilateral simultaneous manipulation; they often cannot use in-hand manipulation with one hand at a time, and certainly not with two hands at one time. Many children with motor control problems, even subtle problems, also have difficulty stabilizing an object with one hand while manipulating

with the other, since this skill requires good dissociation of the two sides of the body. Within this
category of bilateral skills the therapist can find it
helpful to determine if the child has greater difficulty
stabilizing while grasping an object (e.g., holding a
jar while putting the lid on) or stabilizing without
grasp (holding paper with an open hand while writing). Children with marked asymmetry in their upper
extremity functions also find gross symmetric skills
to be very difficult, whereas children with milder
problems can typically use the more basic skills in
this category. However, these children usually have
difficulty catching a ball with two hands.

As with other fine motor skills, the therapist
will find a thorough knowledge of normal fine
motor development to be very helpful in understanding the child's problem areas, in determining
goals that are appropriate, and in selecting and
modifying treatment activities. However, this information should be viewed as only a guide. In
bilateral skills, as in other areas of fine motor
performance, the therapist should be guided by
judgment about the most important functional
skills for the child now and in the future.

Children with Moderate-to-Severe Motor Involvement

The child who has significant asymmetry or significant involvement bilaterally has difficulty with
all three categories of bilateral skills. Even most
gross symmetric skills require that the child spontaneously open both hands and use supination to midposition. Although gross bilateral skills may be
done in therapy to help prepare the child for other activities, goals in the gross bilateral skill area may not
be the most appropriate, particularly when the child
has cognitive skills for performing functional tasks.

Often the focus for these children needs to be on
developing their skills for stabilizing with one hand
(the more involved hand) while the other hand is
manipulating. Initially the therapist may address
either stabilizing objects with grasp or stabilizing
objects without grasp. Consideration needs to be
given to the type of stabilizing that seems to be
within the child's zone of proximal development
and the most frequent needs that the child has. For
example, when stabilizing with grasp, the ability to
hold the forearm of the stabilizing hand in supination to midposition is important.

Stabilizing materials without grasp but with an
open hand may not be feasible for many children;
however, they may achieve sufficient dissociation
between the two sides of the body to be able to
hold materials down with a fisted hand. An impor-

tant component to address with these children is
maintaining the elbow in approximately 90 degrees
of flexion so that stabilization with the hand on a
surface is possible. In stabilizing materials without
grasp, some children can extend their fingers initially, but as they persist with the activity the fingers
and wrist flex more. Ultimately the wrist flexion
becomes a greater problem to them than the finger
flexion and interferes more with the effectiveness
of the stabilization. Therefore, at least initially in
treatment for stabilizing without grasp, emphasis is
on holding the wrist in neutral extension rather than
on finger extension. Activities in prone on forearms
weight bearing and in less stressful tabletop activities that involve stabilizing materials are often introduced early in treatment. At times the therapist
may ask the child to hold materials down while the
therapist does the manipulation. For example, the
child may hold his/her hand on the paper while the
therapist draws a picture and asks the child to guess
what is being drawn. Gradually the child is asked
to do more with the manipulating hand while using
the stabilizing hand to maintain materials on the
surface or in the grasp.

In treatment of children with marked asymmetry, giving as much attention to the *less* involved
hand as to the more involved hand is important.
Even though the side with the greater degree of
disability is a more obvious area of treatment, the
hand with a mild disability also needs to be
addressed specifically in treatment. A child with
significant asymmetry needs a very skilled hand to
accomplish tasks unilaterally that other children
may do bilaterally. The less involved arm and hand
have a greater degree of potential for improvement
in skill than do the more involved arm and hand.
Thus treatment needs to focus on this hand as well
as the more involved hand.

Bilateral simultaneous manipulation can rarely
be a therapeutic goal for children with moderate-to-
severe motor involvement. Therefore for these
children focus needs to be on developing or improving in-hand manipulation in the hand with less
involvement (if possible) and adaptations or compensatory strategies for dealing with other skills if
independence in these areas seems possible. The
child's cognitive and perceptual skills influence
decisions about the motor skills that seem reasonable for the child.

Children with Mild or Minor Motor Involvement

Children with low tone and those with milder
degrees of asymmetry may be able to work on

gross symmetric skills and become functional with them. Therefore setting goals in the area of gross symmetric bilateral skills may be reasonable. Treatment for these problems typically uses a graded approach for decreasing the size of the objects used for the bilateral tasks (such as the size of the ball to be caught) or increasing precision or timing in the activity (such as holding a stick with both hands to hit a stationary target, then a slowly moving ball, then a quickly moving ball).

Although children with mild involvement typically need some intervention for gross symmetric bilateral skills, they need more attention to skills involving stabilizing with one hand while manipulating with the other. Many times these children tend to avoid stabilizing materials with one hand, yet appear to have the potential to do this task effectively. At times these children show good skills in stabilizing materials when given verbal cues to do so, but do not in spontaneous situations. Intervention for this type of problem depends, in part, on the therapist's assessment of the child's reason(s) for not consistently stabilizing materials. Such reasons may include poor sensory awareness of one upper extremity, poor ability to dissociate the two sides of the body so that the hands can assume different functions, and the need to adduct or hyperextend one upper extremity to assist with maintaining good postural control. Intervention typically is directed, at least in part, on the underlying problem. However, intervention may also address the specific skill of holding materials with one hand while the other is manipulating.

In intervention specifically to facilitate spontaneous stabilization of materials, the therapist may try (and suggest to others) activities that *require* the use of one hand to stabilize. A highchair tray or a slightly wobbly table may be useful, since materials tend to be less stable on these surfaces than on others. Less expensive toys that are less sturdy than more expensive ones may be helpful in encouraging the child to use one hand to hold materials down. Simple toys that can be put together without requiring manipulation of objects in both hands can be appropriate, such as a padlock that a key can be put into, markers with caps to put on, and a box with a lid and objects to put inside the box. Children who have good sitting balance may be asked to sit in a chair, but not have a table in front of them, and hold a cup or other small container with one hand while putting objects in with the other hand. This type of activity may be done while standing if the child has good standing balance.

Children with mild or minimal motor involvement may be able to work toward accomplishing bilateral simultaneous manipulative tasks, such as buttoning with both hands, tying a bow, and doing craft projects. To do so, they need refined grasp patterns and ability to sustain these patterns, in-hand manipulation skills with at least one hand and preferably both, and skill in dissociating the movements on each side of the body. For these children a graded progression of activities that require stabilizing materials with a refined grasp while using manipulation with the other hand, and activities that require changing the hand that is doing in-hand manipulation, may be useful. In these activities children are usually more successful with more stable materials such as blocks that fit together and other building construction sets before having success with unstable materials such as fabric with buttons and shoelaces. Once the child is ready to try bilateral manipulation with unstable materials, grading may also be used. Large, then medium, then small buttons may be tried; most children find it easier to button when the buttons are low (in their visual field) and on their own body or on another person's body so the fabric is well stabilized. Initially it is important for the fabric to overlap in the correct direction for the child (right over left for girls, left over right for boys) regardless of the placement of the item of clothing. Later this may be varied as well. For lacing and tying, thicker (but not inflexible) shoelaces that are just the right length need to be used at first; then the thickness of the laces and their length can gradually be decreased.

Integration of Skills into Functional Activities

The child's ability to generalize the skills emphasized in the treatment session to other times of the day and other settings is a crucial consideration in planning and implementing intervention. At least some amount of each treatment session needs to be spent in engaging the child in activities that will be done in other situations. Unique ways of modifying materials and object presentations may work well in treatment settings, but parents and teachers often have difficulty presenting materials in the same way. Thus typical ways of presenting materials should also be used, as well as materials that the child has in the home or school setting. Asking a child to generalize a new skill to a new setting with new materials when the materials are not being presented as they were in therapy is a great deal to ask. Ultimately therapists expect skills to be generalized, but first we need to support this generalizability, not only with instructions and suggestions to the other key adults who will be with the child, but also in the materials and activities being used. Therapy sessions need to include the specific materials that we expect children to practice with when they are in other settings. These activities must be presented in ways that are reasonable for children to do on their own or with adults who are not therapists. Standard pegboard sets are an example of typical therapy or classroom materials that children are unlikely to have at home, are unlikely to have someone structure the presentation of to facilitate a finger pad grasp on the pegs (which are unstable because they are round), and are typically uninteresting to children. Therefore it is suggested that although pegs (and other such materials) may be a reasonable activity for the motor skill element of therapy, they may not be a good activity for engaging the child's interest or for carryover into real life situations.

Integrating new skills into functional performance also requires the involvement of parents or caretakers and teachers. Working with these individuals in the child's program involves more than asking the individuals to carry out specific skills with the child. They "may need to modify their expectations of the child's performance abilities" (Gilfoyle et al., 1990, p. 259) so the child is able to accomplish activities that are appropriate. To support the child's performance of skills, the therapist must address the child's environment, as well as the child's ability to perform specific skills (Gilfoyle et al., 1990).

CONCLUSION

The treatment of children with fine motor problems is guided by the prevailing theory used by the therapist, a careful assessment of the problems that the child has and how fine motor difficulties play a role in these problems, delineation of factors that contribute to the child's fine motor difficulties, and judgment about the child's current needs and future potential and needs. Therapists need to consider what the child and parents needs are today and what the child's needs will be in 5 years or in 10 or more years. These judgments are made based on information from the child whenever possible, the parent(s) or caregivers, and teacher, as well as test results. Needs for fine motor intervention must be balanced with other types of interventions and the child's other life needs and

interests, such as academic skills, social skills, and play. The therapist must balance the child's need for direct intervention designed to improve fine motor skills and the child's need for any adaptations or compensatory strategies to assist in accomplishing daily life tasks. The child's perceptual and cognitive functioning affect this planning, since fine motor skills are intimately related to the child's perception of objects and space and his/her desire to accomplish a meaningful end goal.

To assist in determining the child's potential for improvement from direct intervention for specific fine motor skills, the therapist needs information that typically cannot be derived solely from standardized tests of fine motor skills. For realistic intervention designed to improve the child's fine motor skills the therapist must consider the child's zone of proximal development, those skills that are within reach for the child.

Fine motor treatment typically integrates a variety of strategies, which depend upon the child's overall motor problems as well as the child's particular problems in hand function. Tactile-proprioceptive input may be an important aspect of treatment. Physical handling to enhance the child's performance may be used with many of the fine motor intervention strategies. Verbal cuing for the type of motor action desired and verbal reinforcement for performance of particular motor skills is appropriate for almost all children. Repetition of actions is necessary for building skill in new motor patterns, so games and imaginative activities to engage the child's interest and sustain the child's performance of the activities are important. The therapist must keep in mind that fine motor activities cannot be done *to* the child; they must be done *with* the child's active participation. Although children often respond well to initially trying out new skills in a one-on-one situation with a therapist, after gaining initial skill they must practice these skills in more settings than therapy and with more materials than are used in the therapy environment. Therefore collaboration with the child, the parents or caregivers, and teachers is crucial in helping the child develop fine motor skills that can be spontaneously used to enhance the child's performance in a variety of daily life skills.

REFERENCES

Barnes, K. J. (1986). Improving prehension skills of children with cerebral palsy: A clinical study. *Occupational Therapy Journal of Research, 6,* 227-240.

Barnes, K. J. (1989a). Relationship of upper extremity weight bearing to hand skills of boys with cerebral palsy. *Occupational Therapy Journal of Research, 9*, 143-154.

Barnes, K. J. (1989b). Direct replication: Relationship of upper extremity weight bearing to hand skills of boys with cerebral palsy. *Occupational Therapy Journal of Research, 9*, 235-242.

Boehme, R. (1988). *Improving upper body control: An approach to assessment and treatment of tonal dysfunction.* Tucson, AZ: Therapy Skill Builders.

Bundy, A. (1990, July). The challenge of functional outcomes: Framing the problem. *NDTA Newsletter, 1*, 21-22.

Carmick, J. (1993). Clinical use of neuromuscular electrical stimulation for children with cerebral palsy. Part 2. Upper extremity. *Physical Therapy, 73*, 514-522.

Case-Smith, J. (1991). The effects of tactile defensiveness and tactile discrimination on in-hand manipulation. *The American Journal of Occupational Therapy, 45*, 811-818.

Case-Smith, J. (1993). Comparison of in-hand manipulation skills in children with and without fine motor delays. *Occupational Therapy Journal of Research, 13*, 87-100.

Case-Smith, J., Fisher, A. G., & Bauer, D. (1989). An analysis of the relationship between proximal and distal motor control. *The American Journal of Occupational Therapy, 43*, 657-662.

Case-Smith, J., & Pehoski, C. (1992). *Development of hand skills in the child.* Rockville, MD: The American Occupational Therapy Association.

Croce, R., & DePaepe, J. (1989). A critique of therapeutic intervention programming with reference to an alternative approach based on motor learning theory. *Physical and Occupational Therapy in Pediatrics, 9* (3), 5-33.

Danella, E., & Vogtle, L. (1992). Neurodevelopmental treatment for the young child with cerebral palsy. In J. Case-Smith & C. Pehoski (Eds.) *Development of hand skills in the child.* Rockville, MD: The American Occupational Therapy Association.

DeGangi, G. A., Wietlisbach, S., Goodin, M., & Scheiner, N. (1993). A comparison of structured sensorimotor therapy and child-centered activity in the treatment of preschool children with sensorimotor problems. *The American Journal of Occupational Therapy, 47*, 777-786.

Embry, D. G. (1993). Efficacy studies in children with cerebral palsy: Focus on upper extremity function. *Physical and Occupational Therapy in Pediatrics, 12* (4), 89-95.

Erhardt, R. (1982). *Erhardt Developmental Prehension Assessment.* Laurel, MD: Ramsco Publishing.

Erhardt, R. (1992). Eye-hand coordination. In J. Case-Smith & C. Pehoski (Eds.). *Development of hand skills in the child.* Rockville, MD: The American Occupational Therapy Association.

Exner, C. E. (1989). Development of hand functions. In P. N. Pratt & A. S. Allen (Eds.). *Occupational therapy for children* (2nd ed.). St. Louis: Mosby.

Exner, C. E. (1990a). In-hand manipulation skills in normal young children: A pilot study. *Occupational Therapy Practice, 1* (4), 63-72.

Exner, C. E. (1990b). The zone of proximal development in in-hand manipulation skills of nondysfunctional 3- and 4-year-old children. *The American Journal of Occupational Therapy, 44*, 884-891.

Exner, C. E. (1992). In-hand manipulation skills. In J. Case-Smith & C. Pehoski (Eds.). *Development of hand skills in the child.* Rockville, MD: The American Occupational Therapy Association.

Exner, C. E., & Bonder, B. R. (1983). Comparative effects of three hand splints on the bilateral hand use, grasp, and arm-hand posture in hemiplegic children: A pilot study. *Occupational Therapy Journal of Research, 3*, 75-92.

Gilfoyle, E. M., Grady, A. P., & Moore, J. C. (1990). *Children adapt* (2nd ed.). Thorofare, NJ: Slack.

Goodman, G., & Bazyk, S. (1991). The effects of a short thumb opponens splint on hand function in cerebral palsy: A single-subject study. *The American Journal of Occupational Therapy, 45*, 726-731.

Hirschel, A., Pehoski, C., & Coryell, J. (1990). Environmental support and the development of grasp in infants. *The American Journal of Occupational Therapy,* 721-727.

Kleinman, B. L., & Stalcup, A. (1991). The effect of graded craft activities on visuomotor integration in an inpatient child psychiatry population. *The American Journal of Occupational Therapy, 45*, 324-330.

Law, M., Cadman D., Rosenbaum, P., Walter, S., Russell, D., & DeMatteo, C. (1991). Neurodevelopmental therapy and upper-extremity inhibitive casting for children with cerebral palsy. *Developmental Medicine and Child Neurology, 33*, 379-387.

Lawrence, D. G., & Kuypers, H. G. (1968a). The functional organization of the motor system in monkey. I. The effects of bilateral pyramidal lesions. *Brain, 91*, 1-14.

Lawrence, D. G., & Kuypers, H. G. (1968b). The functional organization of the motor system in monkey. II. The effect of lesions of the descending brainstem pathways. *Brain, 91*, 15-36.

MacKinnon, J., Sanderson, E., & Buchanan, J. (1975). The MacKinnon splint—A functional hand splint. *Canadian Journal of Occupational Therapy, 42*, 157-158.

McHale, K., & Cermak, S. A. (1992). Fine motor activities in elementary school: Preliminary findings and provisional implications for children with fine motor problems. *The American Journal of Occupational Therapy, 46*, 898-903.

Myers, C. A. (1992). Therapeutic fine-motor activities for preschoolers. In J. Case-Smith & C. Pehoski

(Eds.). *Development of hand skills in the child.* Rockville, MD: The American Occupational Therapy Association.

Noronha, J., Bundy, A., & Groll, J. (1989). The effect of positioning on the hand function of boys with cerebral palsy. *The American Journal of Occupational Therapy, 43,* 501-512.

Nwaobi, O. M. (1987). Seating orientations and upper extremity function in children with cerebral palsy. *Physical Therapy, 67,* 1209-1212.

Paillard, J. (1990). Basic neurophysiological structures of eye-hand coordination. In C. Bard, M. Fleury, & L. Hay (Eds.). *Development of eye-hand coordination across the life span.* Columbia, S.C.: University of South Carolina Press.

Pehoski, C. (1992). Central nervous system control of precision movements of the hand. In J. Case-Smith & C. Pehoski (Eds.). *Development of hand skills in the child.* Rockville, MD: The American Occupational Therapy Association.

Ruff, H. A. (1984). Infants' manipulative exploration of objects: Effects of age and object characteristics. *Developmental Psychology, 20,* 9-20.

Seeger, B. R., Caudrey, D. J., & O'Mara, N. A. (1984). Hand function in cerebral palsy: The effect of hip-flexion angle. *Developmental Medicine and Child Neurology, 26,* 601-606.

Smelt, H. R. (1989). Effect of an inhibitive weight-bearing mitt on tone reduction and functional performance in a child with cerebral palsy. *Physical and Occupational Therapy in Pediatrics, 9* (2), 53-80.

Tona, J. L., & Schneck, C. M. (1993). The efficacy of upper extremity inhibitive casting: A single-subject pilot study. *The American Journal of Occupational Therapy, 47,* 901-910.

Vygotsky, L. S. (1978). *Mind in society: The development of higher psychological processes.* Cambridge, MA: Harvard University Press.

Yasukawa, A. (1992). Upper-extremity casting: Adjunct treatment for the child with cerebral palsy. In J. Case-Smith and C. Pehoski (Eds.). *Development of hand skills in the child.* Rockville, MD: The American Occupational Therapy Association.

CHAPTER

13

Toys and Games: Their Role in Hand Development

Michelle V. Tobias   Ilene M. Goldkopf

Why a chapter on toys and games in a book addressing the development of the hand and hand skills? Pediatric occupational therapy's emphasis on (1) the use of purposeful activity and (2) the principles of normal development has naturally led to the use of play and toys in the intervention process. Children and adults automatically view toys and games as play and therefore fun, motivating, and nonthreatening. For these reasons they are ideal tools for use in therapy to facilitate motor development.

This chapter reviews concepts and theories of play and describes toys and the ways in which they can be used in the development of hand skills. Methods of analyzing toys for different purposes are presented as well as descriptions of specific toys and games.

THERAPY, PLAY, AND PLAY ACTIVITIES

Play in therapy, therapy in play: as pediatric therapists we know how well they fit together, but they are not synonymous. In the therapeutic setting play often becomes a tool used to work toward a goal. Therefore a differentiation is suggested between the terms *play* and *play activities*. Rast (1986) begins to clarify the difference. She believes that "play is an intrinsically motivating activity done voluntarily and for its own sake. Therapy proceeds according to the therapist's plan to achieve definite treatment objectives." When working with children, these treatment objectives may be as diverse as improving hand skills, dressing skills, or play skills.

Characteristics of Play

Play must be intrinsically motivating, spontaneous, voluntary, and for its own sake (Rast, 1986; Pratt, 1989; Florey, 1971; Schaaf, 1992). The idea is that the activity itself is enticing to the child. It appears to be fun and enjoyable. The child wants to interact with the activity not because he/she is told to but because of a desire to (Bundy, 1991).

- When children play, their focus is on the activity as they have chosen to structure it. Their only concerns are having fun and the challenge of the activity as they have organized it.

- A safe and supportive environment is essential to facilitate play and development. Vandenburg and Kielhofner (1982) state that "the value of play is that through its imaginary or quasi-reality property it can create contexts with rules and consequences that are not seriously consequential. Because the player is free to create situations and try them out and because he can do so without fear of repercussions, play is a most efficient means of organizing the ongoing development of the child."

- The child is an active participant in play (Bundy, 1991) and finds it rewarding (Pratt 1989). The more invested in a task one becomes, the more meaningful and organizing it is for the individual, adult or child. Berlyne's theory of arousal proposes that the conditions for play exist in a "just right" challenge between the person and environment (Berlyne, 1960; Vandenburg and Kielhofner, 1982). Most children seem adept at finding this balance and the "just right" challenge for themselves.

- Play occurs within its own time and space boundaries (Florey, 1981), intermixing fantasy and reality. Newman referred to this state as a suspension of reality. Children should be free to transform or pretend themselves and the activity into anything desired (Bundy, 1991; Florey, 1981). This is a truly wonderful and magical aspect of play; the children appear to be absorbed in their other world yet are very much aware of the here and now.

- Play has been identified as a primary occupational role in childhood (Schaaf, 1992; Neville 1985), and the positive effects of play on the development of physical, emotional, social, and cognitive skills have been researched and documented by many

(Rast, 1986). Play itself follows a sequential, developmental progression (Florey, 1981, Bundy, 1991). Numerous researchers have identified various developmental sequences related to play, some of which are discussed later in this chapter.

Characteristics of Play Activities

Play activities are specific activities, tasks, toys, or games chosen or suggested by the therapist, teacher, or parent as a method of intervention. Play activities tend to follow a therapeutic or educational plan. The child is told to play on the roll or use the pegs and very often even how to interact with the materials. Therapists try hard to design play activities that are enticing and with which the child will want to interact. This is challenging with some children, especially those who have experienced difficulty or failure when interacting with standard age-appropriate materials or carrying out activities from the therapist's standard bag of tricks. New and different media frequently may be needed to entice and motivate.

Throughout this book various treatment ideas are given to address specific motor and sensory skills of the hand. When used in therapy, they may or may not be considered playing by the child. Many children, especially bright or older children, view these contrived activities more like work than play.

When engaged in a play activity, children may focus on an activity they have chosen, but a structure or modification may have been made by the therapist. For example, a preschool child with poor shoulder stability may play with blocks, towering them in front of him/her while sitting back on the heels. This becomes a play activity when the therapist asks the child to make a tower while lying on the stomach. The child's focus may remain on the task chosen—towering the blocks—but the external structure has changed the activity, and it may or may not continue to be fun for the child.

By changing the child's focus, also, playing can become a play activity, and what was fun may become more like work. For example, when the child playing with blocks is told he/she should keep the thumb in the "up" position or that two hands should be used rather than one, the focus will change from playing with blocks to a specific skill or task (hand position and bilateral coordination). Although the activity appears the same, it is now very different.

In therapy it is typically less threatening and more motivating for the child to have an activity of play restructured by the therapist, rather than diverting focus to a specific skill. The child is more cooperative, for example, when allowed to continue towering blocks simply from another position than when asked to divert focus to hand skills and hand positions. He/she may even be more cooperative about changing play activities altogether, rather than refocusing on specific skills; for example, shooting marbles or thumb wrestling, which intrinsically require the thumbs-up position, might be suggested instead. Generally, the older or brighter child tolerates more changes of focus in play activities than the younger child.

The concept of a safe and supported environment is especially important in the therapeutic setting. Many children with motor problems experience failure or frustration throughout the day. The therapy room can offer a nonjudgmental safe haven in which these children can learn and develop. Bundy (1993) discusses engaging clients in activities for which the consequences have been somehow diminished or suspended. Children do not have to fear eating because the spoon may drop or refrain from playing catch because they might miss the ball. The definitions of safe and supported vary from child to child. For some it may be a place where they try out new tasks or practice old ones without the eyes of peers watching. For others it may be a place where they can play on the sensory-motor level they need, without being ridiculed or told to grow up. Each child is different.

As therapists designing play activities, encouraging the child's active participation and investment in the task is one of our greatest challenges. The "just right" activity must be challenging enough to interest the child, yet not so difficult that success is beyond capabilities. As previously mentioned, creating a safe environment helps reduce anxiety and reluctance to participate, and the "just right" activity sparks active participation and investment in the task.

Therapy sessions and play activities may at times attempt to imitate or even encourage suspension of reality; however, the time during which we engage children follows more practical lines. Although some flexibility should be part of any treatment plan, there are schedules to be followed and certain objectives to be accomplished. There are also some children who use their ability to fantasize as a means of avoiding other activities and work. These children would rather play than engage in more therapeutic play activities.

Play activities also follow a developmental sequence. As progress toward a goal area is made, the play activities designed and chosen reflect that progress and are changed accordingly. Most play activity plans reflect patterns of normal development.

As can be seen, both play and play activities are complicated processes. Each can have a significant impact on development. Each also has a definite place and purpose in the therapeutic setting. Clarifying the difference between play and play activities should help clarify what occupational therapy does and why.

THEORIES ON PLAY AND DEVELOPMENT

Just as cognition and hand skills follow a documented developmental sequence, the development of play skills has also been shown to follow a sequence documented by researchers such as Florey, Takata, and Parten. A few of the theories of play development more commonly recognized by occupational therapists follow:

Parten's Social Play Hierarchy

Parten (1932, 1933) identified six levels of social participation in play.

- *Unoccupied.* Plays with own body/random activity.
- *Solitary.* Plays with different toys than the other children; interested only in own play; individual play.
- *Onlooker.* Watches others but does not participate.
- *Parallel.* Plays independently beside, but not with, other children but is aware of others' play. Frequently wants the other child's toy. Learning to share and take turns.
- *Associative—group.* Play with clear recognition of a common activity. Take turns; share materials willingly.
- *Cooperative—group.* Organized activity with division of labor for a common goal; controlled by one or more children.

Parten also identified degrees of leadership.

- *Following.* The child follows the lead of others ("Can I play too?").
- *Independent pursuit.* The child chooses an activity, then attempts to invite others to play ("Want to help me make a fort?").
- *Following some but directing others.* The child may join a play group following the lead of another, but then may take a directing role to a third child ("Okay, I'll be the mommy, Eddie you be the baby.").

- *Sharing leadership with another.* The child accepts another as also a leader and director of the play ("Yeah that's a good idea, but let's pretend to make lunch first.").
- *Directing alone.* The child prefers to direct the play situation. This may lead to frequent arguments with others who also may want to direct or lead the group.

It's important to remember that children can and do move back and forth between these levels, depending on the task presented and the social situation. Kenny, for example, is a very bright 8-year-old boy seen in occupational therapy for fine motor difficulties, poor tactile discrimination, and dyspraxia. He easily plays on the associative-cooperative level with the therapist in occupational therapy and also at home with friends and siblings. The family recently went on a vacation to a beach resort. There were several boys Kenny's age teaching themselves to body-surf in the waves. Although Kenny was obviously interested and motivated to try, his mother reports that he would not join them, only watched and occasionally talked to them as they came out of the surf (onlooker). Later that day Kenny went into the water and tried to body-surf but far from all the others (solitary). After practicing all afternoon, he swam over to where all the others were and joined them in their games (associative).

Parten's social play hierarchy may be used in occupational therapy both as a goal of treatment and as a treatment modality (or tool). Kenny is already able to play with peers on an associative-cooperative level. So the goal of treatment should focus more on the motor skills he needs to function within his peer group on that level. Kenny, for example, was very interested in soccer. He knew all the rules, enjoyed playing the game, and desperately wanted to be on a recreational team with his friends. But he also knew his soccer skills were not up to par with those of his friends, and he did not want to be ridiculed. So instead he assumed an onlooker position. In occupational therapy his desire to be on a soccer team became a functional goal of treatment. The soccer skills he needed to develop were broken down into the following motor components for treatment: equilibrium reactions, response speed, sequencing of movements, visual tracking and scanning, overall endurance, and body awareness. Initially, Kenny worked on these areas alone in treatment, but as his skills and confidence developed, a second child was introduced into the sessions. Treatment continued but now on a parallel level. Each client, for example,

had his own therapy ball to work with while practicing wall-ball patterns for sequencing, response speed, and grading of movements. Over time, the clients chose to work together on activities (associative). In this case the social play hierarchy was used as a treatment tool. (Yes, Kenny did make the team.)

For another child the goal of treatment may be to facilitate actual social-play growth. Becky is a 4 ½-year-old preschooler. She has age-appropriate verbal and cognitive skills but refuses to talk more than a whisper in school. She prefers to spend much of her day as an onlooker, watching others but not participating. Playtime is the only time during the day that Becky will actively participate. She prefers to play in the kitchen area and will do so even if others are there, but she plays on a solitary level. She plays with only her materials by herself. Frequently another child, Jackie, who is at a socially higher developmental level, attempts to interact and play with Becky, sharing materials or suggesting that they make lunch together. During these times Becky stops playing and watches Jackie or moves to another area of the kitchen to play alone. Therapist or teacher interaction assists Becky in her play skills. Asking questions and giving her some control in the situation frequently help Becky play with Jackie and others. These questions might include: "Becky, how about making me lunch?" "Can Jackie help?" "Jackie, what would you like to make for lunch? Becky will you help her make that?" Both children are encouraged to repeat the same interactions again during the next play time, reinforcing positive interactions and growth.

Takata's Play Taxonomy

Nancy Takata (1974) also developed a taxonomy or hierarchy to examine the contents of play and to help identify areas in need of intervention. She proposed that play develops through a series of age-related epochs, following a specific sequence.

- *Sensorimotor epoch (0 to 24 months).* Play involves exploration and manipulation of self, others, and common objects in the environment. Play is for its sensory experiences and knowledge of basic actions and properties of people and objects. It begins as the infant explores himself/herself and enjoys sensations (such as watching his/her hand move, making noises, moving hands and feet to mouth to suck and feel). The infant then learns how to produce effects on objects in the environment, with each repeated effect being the same (shaking a rattle makes a noise each time). As the infant gets older and develops a better repertoire of skills, this cause-and-effect learning continues through active trial-and-error processes, and problem-solving skills begin to develop. The infant now enjoys activities such as rolling an object, watching objects fall, making splashes in water with objects, filling and emptying objects, and placing objects under, over, beside, in, or out.

- *Symbolic and simple constructive epoch (2 to 4 years).* As language skills develop, the child develops symbols for the objects (car), properties (hard), and actions (pull) explored during the sensorimotor period. Play during this stage is influenced by several key developments: greater growth and mobility, developing language skills, and improved manual dexterity. As a result symbolic play and parallel play with others begin. Play may now include running, climbing, digging, building, and tearing apart things. Make-believe and pretend play also are developing. What happens in the child's life may now be repeated in play. Blocks may be used to make houses and buildings; cars become the school bus. The child's play is no longer centered or focused upon the body but rather on a group of manageable toys.
- *Dramatic, complex constructive, and pregame epoch (4 to 7 years).* Increased socialization is the key development of this period. The child seeks playmates and will share materials and toys with them. Increased motor control and hand dexterity skills allow for participation in small muscle activities. The child now enjoys activities such as hammering, sorting, putting things together (such as small Leggos), and simple arts and crafts projects that can be completed in a short time. This is when the child is proud of accomplishments, and productions need to be saved and displayed. During this period the child also learns to role play. The child is able to imagine himself/herself being in different social roles, environments, and situations (e.g., Mommy feeding the baby at bedtime). Dramatic play emerges and takes

the place of fantasy or imaginative play used during the symbolic epoch.

- *Game epoch (7 to 12 years).* The school-aged child is involved in many new things and areas. He/she is curious about nature and science; attempts to attribute a value to everything; develops speed, coordination, and precision in sports activities; develops new social relationships; and is very focused on games, rules, and mastery. Friends become very important to the child. He/she enjoys being part of a group and becomes concerned about how others view him/her. The child now enjoys playing with others in an organized manner (team sports) and also against others in competition. The rules of games become important to follow and to master; then the child makes up new ones with peers.
- *Recreation epoch (12 to 16 years).* This period focuses on mastery of previously learned skills through the use of games that challenge and assist the child in developing skills and strengths both physically and mentally. Most activities are group based. Many are competitive (such as team sports), some are cooperative groups (such as choir), and others are reflections of developing social roles (such as SADD [Students Against Drunk Driving]).

For example, Jamie is a 4-year-old preschooler referred for occupational therapy for autistic behaviors. The teacher reports that he is unable to focus on, attend, or participate in any classroom activities. It is determined that he is functioning primarily in the sensorimotor epoch and that attention and participation could be sustained for several minutes if the activity were on his level. Some examples of his play behaviors are feeling the sand fall through his fingers at the sandbox, shaking the can of pegs, pulling things and being pulled, and climbing up bookshelves and hanging by his arms.

Intervention began at this level but also focused on developing more interactions with objects and people, especially those related to cause-and-effect learning (a later skill developed during the sensorimotor epoch). Activities include pouring sand into his hands from a container, then filling the container using his hands; dropping pegs into a metal can to make a noise, then removing the pegs from a board to drop them into a container; pushing and pulling to ride a scooter or Sit' N' Spin; and climbing the schoolroom slide and sliding down. Education of classroom staff also was a focus. Jamie could not participate in some classroom activities, such as doing the weather chart or calendar. He could, however, sit with the group during this time, if he was involved with a sensorimotor-level activity such as being hugged and rocked in an assistant's lap or sitting in thick blankets in a child-size rocking chair.

John, at an older age level, is a 13-year-old student with a medical diagnosis of muscular dystrophy. He is being seen by occupational therapy once a week for maintenance of skills and medical management. The school's child study team requested a full team meeting to discuss some incidents in the cafeteria and hallways between John and another student. The other student had been teasing John, stealing his money, and also pushing his head. John in return had been name calling and spitting and recently had cornered the student against the wall with his powered wheelchair. The other student was reprimanded and given detention. The meeting was to discuss how to help John fit in more. Staff all expressed concern that John has only one or two friends, both of whom have lunch at a different time. The occupational therapist, being aware of the age-related epochs, was able to present several suggestions based on the knowledge of play development at John's age. Peers were developing new social relationships out of their participation in sports, but John's physical limitations limited his opportunities for developing new social relationships. It was suggested that a coach meet with John and discuss whether there was a specific sport he enjoyed watching and followed professionally. He would then be invited to join the team as a statistician. If interested, John would also be invited to write a sports article about the team for the school newspaper. Other play suggestions were to encourage John to join the chess or computer club, which emphasized strategy and planning skills rather than physical abilities. It was also recommended that John receive detention for his actions just as the other student had.

Florey's Classification of Play Characteristics

Florey (1971) discussed play based on the earlier works of White and delineated four main principles.

- *Play is learning*. It's a spare-time behavior that is part of the learning process. Play is considered to be the child's principal method of discovering what effects he/she can have on the environment, and what effects the environment may have on him/her. Florey also believes that therapists must remember to consider play a kind of learning that takes place every day and is not just limited to treatment sessions or home programs.
- *Play should be nurtured*. Certain environmental conditions (including biologic) can facilitate play, and others may inhibit it. Being hungry, fearful, or anxious may contribute to the inhibition of play and play activities. An environment with novelty and opportunities for exploration, risk taking, and imitation may facilitate play and play skills.
- *Personal constitution influences play in terms of the degree of satisfaction the child may feel as a result of his/her efforts.* In therapy this may be influenced by the child's dysfunction or areas of deficit.
- *Play is action on human and nonhuman objects*. This includes feelings, perceptions, thoughts, and active physical actions. These actions change with the age of the child. Human objects include parents, peers, siblings, and the child's own body. Nonhuman objects are divided into three subcategories.

  Type 1: Creative or unstructured media that seem to change shape and form when manipulated (such as paint, clay, sand, water).
  Type 2: Objects that seem to change shape or form when combined with another object (such as beads + string = necklace; blocks + cars = highway).
  Type 3: Objects that do not seem to change shape or form (such as dolls, bicycles, balls).

Children's actions in play can be related to their active actions with these human and nonhuman objects, and these actions change over time with development. For example, a 2½-year-old's play actions may be as follows:

- *Parent action*. The child insists on hearing the same bedtime story over and over again.
- *Peer action*. Parallel playing; defending play objects, fighting for toys.
- *Self action*. Practicing motor skills such as balancing and hopping.

The 2½-year-old's nonhuman play objects may include the following.

- *Type 1 objects*. Exploring with finger paints; making marks with crayons and pencils.

- *Type 2 objects*. Stringing beads, building vertically with blocks.
- *Type 3 objects*. Kicking balls, learning to climb; imaginary play with objects, such as "feed the baby."

Relevance to Occupational Therapy

As can be seen by this wealth of research and information, play is serious business and can be used as a serious therapeutic tool. Most researchers agree that play can facilitate development (Bundy 1991; Florey 1981; Neville 1985; Takata 1974). They also agree that objective observations of play and play skills reflect a developmental level of the child (Florey 1971; Takata 1974; Bundy 1992).

In occupational therapy the child's play level should be determined and considered in the intervention plan, regardless of which theory of play is chosen as a reference. Many children with developmental delays also exhibit social-emotional delays as a result of poor play skills. Furthermore, these limited play skills may also interfere with the child's relationships with peers and siblings and also with performance in the classroom since teachers frequently require children to share materials and play and work cooperatively on projects. As much as possible toys and play activities should be selected to meet the individual child's varying developmental levels in the areas of social-emotional, cognitive, and motor abilities.

Play Assessments

The use and selection of a play activity as a therapeutic tool *must* take into consideration the child's developmental play skill level. You would never give a client a 50-pound barbell to lift without first knowing his/her range of motion, muscle tone, endurance, and strength levels; nor should you choose an activity, toy, or game without first knowing the child's play skill level! Although this seems minor, the frustration, ego damage, exhaustion, and possible physical injury experienced by children working at an activity above skill level are very real.

Several play scales can help establish a child's developmental play and play skill level. These include, but are not limited to, the following.

Takata's Play History

This is an interview or questionnaire that looks at previous as well as current play skills (Takata 1974). The play history is divided into three sections.

- *General information*. Name, date of birth, and presenting problems.
- *Previous play experiences in specific areas*. Solitary play, play with others, play with toys and materials, gross physical play, pretend and make-believe play, sports and games, creative interests, hobbies, collections and other leisure time activities, and recreational social activities.
- *Actual play examination*. What does the child play with and how? What type of play is avoided or disliked? With whom does the child play and how? What body postures does the child use during play? What is the length of play? With what and where does the child play?

Also considered are which activities and areas are encouraged or discouraged by caregivers. A play prescription is developed through analysis of all information presented, considering the child, the environment, and the caregiver.

Knox Play Scale

This scale was based on the earlier works of Erikson. It analyzes play in four dimensions over yearly increments: space management, material management, imitation, and participation skills. It involves observing the child within a range of activities and comparing behaviors and skills to a developmental scale. Point values are assigned to each level, and a play age can be obtained for use in conjunction with other developmental testing procedures.

- *Space management*. How children learn to manage their bodies and the space around them through experimentation and exploration.
- *Material management*. How and why children handle materials.
- *Imitation*. How children learn to understand the social world and express and control feelings. It includes mimicking actions and speech of others.
- *Participation*. The amount and type of interaction with others, including independence and cooperation.

The scale can also be used as a profile of play behavior. It can show trends of behavior, areas of abilities and limitations, gaps, and unusual behaviors (Knox, 1974).

Preschool Play Scale

This is a revised version of the Knox Play Scale. Revisions include adding a mathematical component to the scale for comparisons and development of reliability and validity studies (Bledsoe, 1982).

Play Skills Inventory

The Play Skills Inventory was developed by J.M. Hurff at Children's Hospital in Los Angeles for use with children approximately 10 years old (middle childhood). It is administered using readily available materials. Four areas are analyzed:

- *Sensation.* Including the ability to detect changes in touch and visual and auditory stimuli.
- *Motor Skills.* Basic strength and flexibility, motor control, motor planning and accuracy, balance, and fine motor coordination.
- *Perception.* Figure-ground, design copying, spatial sequencing, auditory sequencing.
- *Intellect.* Visual sequencing, ordering, egocentricity, decision making, problem-solving skills, and group goal achievement.

Scoring guidelines and performance expectations are given for each area for scoring and interpretation (Hurff, 1974, 1980).

TOYS, TECHNOLOGY, AND HAND SKILLS

Just as modern technology has changed the way we cook, watch movies, communicate, and listen to music, it has also had an impact on how we and, more importantly, how our children play. Today's technology changes rapidly. A new development today may be common in 6 months and obsolete in a year or two. Children, unlike their often rigid parents, are much more flexible and fearless in the face of change and the use of new technologies. Perhaps this is because this generation of children has always known advanced technology. Most have grown up with remote control televisions, VCRs, camcorders, compact disc players, microwave ovens, and computers, all of which are operated with the mere push of a button. The same is true of many modern games. From Nintendo, to computer games, to switch-activated battery-run toys, the hand skills needed to play have changed. This has been a wonderful change for children with limited motor skills. Now, by pushing a button, pressing a key, or wiggling a finger, cars move, firemen climb ladders, music plays, and whole worlds unfold.

With controlled movements of any one body part a child can now play. Computers and battery-operated toys can be fitted with a variety of different types of switches. Switches are available that respond to a squeeze, push, pull, poke, sip, puff, eye blink, or slight movement of a body part. These electronic toys and computer-based games put all players on equal ground, allowing disabled children to interact and compete in the play environment with nondisabled peers and siblings. This assists in the development of social competencies, self-esteem, and self-worth, which in turn foster personality development and maturation. As previously discussed, children practice skills in all areas of development as they play. With the assistance of technology, play and subsequently the practice of skills are fun and willingly repeated. Control and mastery soon result, reinforcing the pattern of interest, effort, practice, and success. This is an important pattern to be learned, a foundation for all other learning and future success. New technologies allow all children—including the physically disabled and the less coordinated—the opportunity to experience, through play, the self-motivating pattern of effort, perseverance, and mastery.

There are other benefits of these ever-increasing toys of technology. Although they require only minimal hand skills, they can be used to develop and refine specific hand skills. This can be accomplished through the careful selection and positioning of the different switches and specific games. Switches can be chosen and positioned to develop or facilitate wrist extension, isolated finger movements, basic pinch patterns, gross grasp, and elbow movements as well as build strength and bilateral hand use. Although these are important skills, far more refined and functional skills can be developed through play with more traditional toys and games.

Nintendo, Sega, and other video-computer games have become very popular and are readily available at local toy stores. Most standard control pads require the use of both hands and isolated thumb movements. These movements, however, are not ideal since they facilitate thenar flexion rather than thenar opposition, but they are isolated movements. For some this may be the next developmental step for their skills. For others, however, it reinforces poor motor patterns that then may be used at inappropriate times, such as when writing, grasping, or manipulating small objects. These "Nintendo thumbs," as coined by Benbow, are hard patterns to alter because of their continued reinforcement through endless hours of play. This illustrates the possibly negative impact technology-based games can have on the development of hand skills in children. In addition to reinforcing patterns of hand use, which do not readily translate to other functional skills, the endless hours some children spend in front of the television or computer screen, moving only one or two fingers, leaves less time available for playing with other toys and games, toys that require movement and coordination and encourage more refined and mature hand skill development.

TIPS FOR PLAYING IN THERAPY

Children (and adults) automatically view toys and games as play and therefore as fun, motivating, and nonthreatening. "Without playfulness all activities become work" (Bundy, 1993). As adults it has been a long time since our main occupation has been play. The principles outlined below may assist in bringing playfulness into therapy sessions.

- Play *with* the child, don't just observe! Consider yourself the child's playmate and friend, while also being the therapist.
- Give the child a sense of control. Ask the child to choose which game he/she would like to play. Limited choices may be given. ("Should we play with the pegs or blocks now?")
- Remember to ask the child at times for direction and permission. This helps to maintain the child's sense of control. ("What should *I* do? Should I hold this for you?")
- Try to keep up with the terms of the times. ("Cowabunga" or "radical" vs. "cool" or "neat"). Use these and other playful noises ("zoom," "wee") appropriately (Parham, 1992).
- Choose your words carefully. Most children know if they've done well with a task or not. Telling them that they've done well or "did a good job" when they've done "just okay" doesn't necessarily fool them or encourage them. Using phrases such as "you tried hard," "good job trying," and "not quite, but much better" are still positive but more honest, encouraging, and believable.
- For some children accepting your attempts to grade an activity they are involved in can be difficult. This is especially so if the child is reluctant to change or if he/she perceives that you are making the task too difficult. For some, changes can be made

with no comments made at all; others need more information. A question can at times be used almost as a challenge. "Do you think you can pick up 10 pegs in one hand?" (Using this technique can be tricky—it does give the child the chance to say no, and you should accept this if it happens.) Another approach is to discuss what other children like to do. "Sometimes, the other children I see like to try to hold 10 or 11 pegs in one hand" (Parham, 1992). Still another approach is to be a model for the child, encouraging them to meet your skills. ("Look, I have 10 pegs in my hand; you do it now.") For very fearful children, those with poor self-confidence, and those resistant to change, the most successful approach may be the "Let's try" statements. "Let's try to hold 10 pegs in one hand." This conveys that an attempt will be accepted, even if they are unable to complete the task successfully. It also may convey that you are going to try, too, as a partner in play and also might not be successful.

- Cooperation vs. competition. Most therapy situations are meant to be cooperative: partners working toward a single goal. But there also is a definite place for competition. In everyday situations children must face competition, so this skill needs to be practiced and refined in therapy—both winning and losing. Most children, of course, enjoy winning, but for many children seen in therapy this is an infrequent occurrence. Therapy can offer them a chance to experience the satisfaction, self-esteem, and confidence that comes with winning. Most children, however, are very perceptive and do not want you to just let them win. They must feel that they won the game fairly, with a challenge.
- Be creative and imaginative. Again, try to stay current. For some children just introducing a name for a game can begin the playing process and bring out the imagination of the child. ("Let's play Ninja Turtles or Supermarket.")
- Remember that few situations must be approached as a matter of life or death! "The person who approaches problems in a flexible, playful fashion is much more likely to find the solution than is the person who thinks there is only one right approach" (Bundy, 1993).

STRUCTURING PLAY IN SCHOOL AND AT HOME

As discussed throughout this chapter, play is an important part of development. Why, then, do so many parents and teachers underestimate the importance and significant potential of play?

In schools, teachers frequently use playtime as the main focus of a behavior management program. Good behavior, completing assignments, and doing homework are rewarded with permission to participate in playtime. Playtime and lunchtime recess are usually the first to be reduced or eliminated for disciplinary reasons or because of time constraints. When playtime is permitted, it is frequently structured arbitrarily, only allowing children to interact with specific materials and toys and possibly even choosing play partners. As playtime is cut short or inappropriately structured, children lose important time that might otherwise have been used to learn to structure, to independently challenge themselves, and to practice developing skills.

In view of the research (Rast, 1986; Schaff, 1992; Neville, 1985), it would appear that children, especially the younger child, are better served if play and play activities are incorporated into daily programs and lessons. For example, fine motor coordination games could be incorporated into handwriting lessons and curricula; gross motor activities could assist in teaching spatial and directionality concepts; and building sets could be used for math concepts.

The same barriers to free play that exist in the school setting are also seen at home. Homework requirements, chores, poor behavior, time constraints, and a lack of interest on the part of some parents make play an expendable activity in the course of daily routine. Play is too important to be pushed aside, especially for children who might be experiencing delays in development. As part of our assessment of a child, occupational therapists should consider and make recommendations concerning the amount of play and the play environment at home. Are there siblings and peers available as playmates, or is the child playing only with adults (parents, grandparents, or other caregivers)? The therapist must help caregivers learn to truly play with the child. Many adults feel the need to choose the game or toy that would be "good" for the child as opposed to what would be "fun." Parents should allow their child to lead in choosing play activities. This gives the child the freedom to select games and toys that are motivating and likely to be at the appropriate skill level.

TOY ANALYSIS
Matching Toys to the Child's Needs

As previously stated, toys and games are an important part of childhood and therefore of development. Many of us can trace our own development through the toys and games with which we played: rattles, teething rings, and mobiles as infants; blocks, push and pull toys, rocking horses, and stuffed animals as toddlers; building sets, paints, crayons, dolls, and puzzles as young children; bicycles, roller skates, simple board games, and beginning card games as older children. As social and motor skills continued to develop, games became more complex. We used smaller balls or markers in combination with complex motor patterns for the "A my name is . . ." game, jacks, and hopscotch. We played larger group games like tag, hide and seek, follow the leader, and statues. What a thrill when your skills were considered good enough to join the older children in their "big kid" games. Eventually adult games like bridge, solitaire, Scrabble, and chess replaced war, go fish, Bingo, and checkers.

A similar progression can also be identified when looking specifically at hand skill development and play. In infants uncontrolled arm and hand movements become more purposeful and directed as they play with busy boxes, rattles, and squeeze toys. As toddlers, large popbeads, toy pianos, and hammer and workbench toys help develop bilateral hand skills, finger isolation, and arm and hand strength. For school-age children peg sets, building sets, tops, and Barbie toys (with clothes of course) help grasp patterns mature and manipulative skills improve. In adolescence and adulthood, hand skills are refined, fine tuned, and maintained by play and recreational activities such as model building, sports, sewing crafts, calligraphy, woodcarving, stained glass work, and learning magic tricks.

Toys are so much a part of childhood that simply remembering them usually evokes fond and happy memories. Try asking friends or parents about what their favorite toys and games were growing up. While their answers will be somewhat affected by regional, cultural, and economic factors, you may be surprised by the answers. Frequently it is not the costliest or largest toys that are remembered; these may have been forgotten and abandoned shortly after being purchased. Every year millions of dollars worth of toys and games are purchased but forgotten in the back of closets and the bottom of toy chests. The most common reason for this is that the toy or game does not match the developmental skill level of the child for whom it was intended. Most often parents or relatives purchase toys that are too advanced. This can lead to frustration, a lack of interest, and broken toys.

Toys and games are best received and most used when they fit the children for whom they are bought. Children tend to be motivated to try or do something they perceive as being attainable, neither too hard nor too easy. They want a challenge, but one that is in their realm. If too easy, interest is quickly lost and the toy becomes classified as mastered. The challenge for toygivers and therapists is to find a toy challenging enough to hold interest without leading to excess frustration and failure.

This challenge is heightened when the toys are for children with deficits or delays in development. To meet this challenge, toys and games should be looked at from different angles and analyzed before being purchased. Looking at the manufacturer's intended age recommendations is not enough. The child's physical capabilities, motor coordination, sensory processing, perceptual skills, cognitive abilities, and social-emotional levels need to be matched with the demands of the toy or game.

We do not, however, want to challenge the child in all these areas at one time since this may make the toy seem impossible to master. Instead, try challenging one or two areas while reinforcing already learned or mastered skills in another area. For example, if you want to work on improving fine motor skills, including pinch, transitional movements, and developing the arches of the hand, and perceptual skills are basically good, the game "Battleship" by Milton Bradley may be a good choice. But if perceptual skills are also weak, the game may prove too challenging, and motivation and effort will soon be lost. Many times the toy that appropriately challenges or even under-challenges one area may be more challenging in another area. This can work to your advantage by distracting the child while he/she continues to work on the weaker area. A game like Battleship may be so perceptually and socially rewarding that the child does not realize how hard his/her hands and fingers are working.

When buying a toy or game, read the directions, look at and feel the playing pieces, and study the design of the board. Are the pieces too big or too small? Are the required movements too complex? Is it sturdy, durable, and made well? What cognitive skills are needed? Beyond the instructions given for using the toy or game, also consider how you can alter or modify the toy and broaden the use of the materials. Can it be made easier or more difficult by changing positions, adding or subtracting pieces, making your own designs? Battleship can be made easier by reducing the size of the playing board and the number of ships used or by giving the child one of the coordinates of the opponent's ship. The game can be made more difficult by altering positioning, requiring the players to hold all or a number of their position-marking pegs in one hand and use the same hand for placement, and by using all ships given with no cues added.

Formal Toy Analysis

By thinking through the various components of a toy or game before purchasing or before choosing it as a play activity during therapy, you can avoid some frustration for the child and adult involved. The three toy analysis forms in the boxes on pp. 234 to 239 are designed to assist therapists, parents, and teachers choose more appropriate and beneficial toys and games; it is hoped that the result will be finding the "just right" toy or game for the child.

The first toy analysis is designed for parent and teacher use. Professional jargon and terms have been purposely avoided. Occupational therapists may use this form to assist parents and teachers in selecting appropriate toys and games. The whole form or only selected parts of it may be used. Note that there are two columns to be completed ("Child needs" and "Game requires"). The "child needs" column is meant to reflect those areas in which the child demonstrates delays. A check mark or plus sign is placed next to all those areas needing to be developed. A minus sign may be used if this area is not of concern at this time, or it may be left blank. Leaving blanks may be most useful if the form is to be updated at a later time. It may be most helpful to parents and teachers if the therapist completes the "child needs" column, highlighting the areas of priority.

The "game requires" column is completed while analyzing a specific toy or game. A check or plus sign again may be used. Adaptations should also be considered in this column and may be denoted with a star.

The second and third toy analysis forms are designed for use by occupational therapists and may be helpful in treatment planning. The second form is an overall toy analysis, and the third form is specific for hand development.

Parent-Teacher Toy Analysis

Sensory Systems	Child Needs	Game Requires
Movement/gravity		
Touch		
Hearing		
Vision		
Smell		
Taste		
Perceptual Aspects		
Color recognition		
Size recognition		
Shape recognition		
Counting		
Reading		
Spatial relations		
Body scheme		
Social Skills		
Independent play		
Turn taking		
Cooperative play		
Play with one other person		
Play with small group		
Play with large group		
Direction following		
Competition		
Communication, verbal		
Physical contact		
Motor Requirements		
Movements of entire body		
Large movement of arm(s)		
Large movement of leg(s)		
Smaller controlled movement of arm(s)		
Smaller controlled movement of leg(s)		
Controlled movement of hand(s)		
Gross grasp and manipulation		
Refined grasp and manipulation		
Right		
Left		
Dominant		
Nondominant		
Bilateral coordination		

Parent-Teacher Toy Analysis—Continued

Positioning Options	Child Needs	Game Requires
Standing		
Sitting on floor		
Sitting in chair		
Lying on stomach		
Lying on back		
Side sitting to right		
Side sitting to left		
Alternating side sitting		
Games: Physical Characteristics		
Playing board		
Playing markers		
Many other small pieces needing manipulation		
Dice		
Timer: sand or windup		
Spinner		
Popper		
Ages specified		
Space required		
Sex identification		
Safety precautions or possible damage/mess		
Anatomy Involved		
Head		
Legs/feet		
Right		
Left		
Arms		
Both		
Right		
Left		
Hands		
Both		
Right		
Left		
Dominant		
Nondominant		
Fingers		
Right		
Left		
Specific fingers		

Occupational Therapy Toy Analysis

Anatomy Involved	Child Needs	Game Requires
Head		
Legs/feet		
Both		
Right		
Left		
Arms		
Both		
Right		
Left		
Hands		
Both		
Right		
Left		
Dominant		
Nondominant		
Fingers		
Right		
Left		
Specific fingers		
Positioning Options		
Standing		
Sitting in chair		
Sitting in chair with work surface		
Sitting on floor		
Sitting on floor with work surface		
Kneeling		
Half kneeling		
Lying prone		
Lying supine		
Side sitting		
Right		
Left		
Alternating		
Tailor sitting		
Social Skills		
Independent play		
Turn taking		
Cooperative play		
Play with one other person		
Play with small group		
Play with large group		
Direction following		
Competition		
Communication, verbal		
Physical contact		
Sensory Input		
Vestibular		
Rotary		
Linear		
Axillary		
Combined		
Tactile		
Stimulation		
Discrimination		

Occupational Therapy Toy Analysis—Continued

Sensory Input (Cont'd)	Child Needs	Game Requires
Kinesthesia		
Proprioception		
Auditory		
Stimulation		
Discrimination		
Olfactory		
Stimulation		
Discrimination		
Ocular		
Stimulation		
Discrimination		

Motor Planning

	Child Needs	Game Requires
Ideation		
Construction		
Two-dimensional		
Three-dimensional		

Bilateral Integration

	Child Needs	Game Requires
Symmetric		
Asymmetric		
Doer/stabilizer		

Perceptual Aspect

	Child Needs	Game Requires
Visual		
Figure-ground		
Position in space		
Form constancy		
Color perception		
Size/shape perception		
Body scheme		
Stereognosis		
Reading		
Counting		
Spatial relations		

Motor Requirements

	Child Needs	Game Requires
Shoulder flexion		
Shoulder abduction		
Shoulder adduction		
Elbow flexion/extension		
Forearm supination		
Forearm neutral		
Forearm pronation		
Wrist extension		
Wrist flexion		
Ulnar deviation		
Radial deviation		
Gross grasp		
Mass grasp		
Three-point grasp		
Radial digital grasp		
Pencil grasp		
In-hand manipulation skills		
Tool use		
Repetition		
Strength		

Occupational Therapy Toy Analysis: Hand Skill Development

Range of Motion	Child Needs	Game Requires
Shoulder		
Flexion		
Extension		
Abduction		
Adduction		
Elbow		
Flexion		
Extension		
Forearm		
Supination		
Pronation		
Neutral		
Wrist		
Flexion		
Extension		
Deviation		
Finger		
Flexion		
Extension		
Abduction		
Adduction		
Opposition		
Strength		
Arms		
Hands		
Fingers		
Midrange Control/Joint Stability		
Shoulder		
Elbow		
Wrist		
Fingers		
Reach		
Gravity assisted		
Gravity eliminated		
Against gravity		
Release		
Voluntary		
Placement/accuracy		
Grasp		
Gross		
Mass		
Hook		
Power		
Spheric		
Cylindric		
Disk		

Occupational Therapy Toy Analysis: Hand Skill Development—Continued

Pinch	Child Needs	Game Requires
Lateral		
Radial digital/3-point		
Standard palmar/2-point		
Tip/superior		
In-Hand Manipulation		
Separation of the hand		
Development of arches		
Proximal transverse/carpal		
Transverse/metacarpal		
Proximal phalangeal transverse		
Longitudinal		
Translation		
Fingers to palm without stabilization		
Fingers to palm with stabilization		
Palm to fingers without stabilization		
Palm to fingers with stabilization		
Shift		
Horizontal		
Vertical		
Rotation		
Bilateral Hand Use		
Symmetric		
Stabilizer		
Doer/helper		
Tool use		
Pencil		
Scissor		
Other		
Pencil Grasp		
Mass		
Quad-tripod		
Static tripod		
Dynamic tripod		
Adapted		

Table 13-1 reviews the therapeutic properties of many commercially available toys and games as they relate to hand and finger development. It is meant only as a guide or a starting point for selecting more appropriate toys and games. It is in no way a definitive toy list or endorsement of any specific product. The final column of Table 13-1 identifies four interest levels as identified by Frantzen (1957). The interest levels are: *1*, toys that are very basic and mostly simple in design and that tend to engage on a sensory level with minimal motor output (e.g., rattles); *2*, toys requiring some basic motor skills but with success depending mostly on chance (e.g., Hungry Hippos); *3*, toys requiring some planning to perform well but that can still be played without planning (e.g., Kerplunk); *4*, toys requiring strategy and planning to play well (e.g., Battleship). Interest

Table 13-1. Therapeutic properties of some commercially available toys

TOY/GAME	TACTILE EXPLORATION/STIMULATION	ARM CONTROL/REACH/EYE-HAND	GRASP	THUMB-FINGER GRASP	WRIST MOVEMENTS	THUMB ISOLATION	FINGER ISOLATION	BIMANUAL SKILLS	IN-HAND MANIPULATION	TOOL USE	WRITING	TACTILE DISCRIMINATION	INTEREST LEVEL*
1. Vibrating busy boxes/switch plates, vibrators	X	X	X		X		A	A				A	1
2. Rice, macaroni, split peas, puffed rice, sand, beans in buckets	X	X	X	A				X	A			X	1
3. Shaving cream; foam in a can	X	X			A	A	X	X			A		1
4. GUK	X	X	X					X					1
5. Koosh balls, Krinks, Softee	X	X	X					A				A	1
6. Sticky creatures/materials/objects	X	A	X					A				A	1
7. Snowball	X	A	X	X				X	A			A	1
8. Framed mobiles/hanging mobiles	X	X	X					A					1
9. Water mat games	X	X						A					1
10. Busy boxes; rattles	X	X	X	X	X		X						1
11. Tabletop mazes/roller coasters		X	X	X	X		A						2
12. Pecking chickens/climbing gingerbread man (counterweight toys)		X	X										2
13. Magnet/felt/Velcro boards		X	A	X	A				A				2
14. Snatchers; reachers; grabbers		X	X		X			A		X			3
15. Stacrobats; Don't Monkey Around		X	X	X									3
16. Top Choice		X	X	X	X			X					4
17. Block building sets; block towering games (Jenga)		X	X	X				A	A				3-4
18. Fishing games (battery operated)		X	X	X						X			2-3
19. Pegboards		A	X	X	A				A				1-4
20. Popbeads			X	X				X					2-3

Toy/Game								Age*
21. Water squirt toys		X	X					2-3
22. Air squirt toys		X	X					2-3
23. Pig Pong		X	X	X				2-3
24. Stamp sets/stamp blocks	A	X	X	A				2
25. Colorforms sets	A	X		A				2-4
26. Pearler Beads/Hama Beads	A	X						4
27. Squiggle worms	A	X	X		X			2-3
28. Mini clothespins; mini hair clips; mini squeeze clips	A	X		A				2
29. Lite Brite	A	X		A	A			2-3
30. Battleship; HiQ; Chinese checkers; Mastermind	A	X		A	A			4
31. Don't Spill the Beans	A	X			A			2-3
32. Kerplunk	X	X		X	A			3
33. Thin Ice	X	X	A	X			X	2-3
34. Bed Bugs/Crocodile Dentist/Operation	A	X					X	3
35. Work benches/hammer games (Tap-A-Chap)	X	X	X	A	A		X	1-2
36. Electronic drumsticks	A	X	X	X	X			1-3
37. Hands Down	A		X	X				2-3
38. Don't Break the Ice	A	X		X			X	3
39. Yo-Yos/Yo-Yo Ball/Koosh Yo-Yo	X	X	X					2-3
40. Water-filled toys	X	X	X	X	X			2-3
41. Sliding puzzles		X	X	X		X		3-4
42. Etch-A-Sketch		X	X	X	X			2-4
43. Wind-up toys	X	X	X	X	X			2

*See text, p. 239
X, skill interest in toy or game.
A, skill obtained by adapting toy or game.

Table 13-1. Therapeutic properties of some commercially available toys—Continued

TOY/GAME	TACTILE EXPLORATION/STIMULATION	ARM CONTROL/REACH/EYE-HAND	GRASP	THUMB-FINGER GRASP	WRIST MOVEMENTS	THUMB ISOLATION	FINGER ISOLATION	BIMANUAL SKILLS	IN-HAND MANIPULATION	TOOL USE	WRITING	TACTILE DISCRIMINATION	INTEREST LEVEL*
44. Electronic keyboard/gloves		A				X	X	X					1-4
45. Tricky Fingers/Super Fingers			X				X	X					4
46. Musical accordion toys/toys using accordion or bellows-type action		X	X	X	X			X					1-2
47. Building sets		X	X	X				X	A				3-4
48. Mr. Potato Head		A	X	X				X				A	2-3
49. Clay; putty; dough	X	A	X	X	A	A	A	X	A	A		A	1-4
50. Mini finger going				A									4
51. Juggling scarves		X	X		X			X					4
52. Tops: doodlers, musical, square, egg, hologram, lighted				X	X				X				3-4
53. Eye-hole lacing projects, Pegs for Lacing		X	X	X					X				2-3
54. Splat	X		A	X				X	A				2-3
55. Stencil rubbing pictures	X		X	X	A					X	X		1-2
56. Magna Doodle; Ghost Writer, Glo-Doodler		X	X	X						X	X		1-3
57. Motorized pens	X		X	X	X					X	X		1-4
58. Shape sorters		A	X	X					A			X	2-4
59. Tactilo		A	X	X					X			X	3-4
60. Tactile form boards		A	X	X					X			X	2-3
61. Tactile dominoes		A	X	X					X			X	3

*See text, p. 239.
X, skill inherent in toy or game.
A, skill obtained by adapting toy or game.

level is an additional guide in toy selection and, combined with skills required, is a much more functional method of selecting toys than by manufacturer's recommendation. Toy adaptation can also be used to obtain other interest levels.

More specific information or each toy, including the manufacturer, a brief description, and how it may be adapted for additional skill development may be found in Appendix A. Some lesser-known toy distributors for some of these products may be found in Appendix B.

REFERENCES

Berlyne, D.E. (1960). *Conflict, arousal, and curiosity.* New York: McGraw-Hill.

Bledsoe, N., & Shepherd, J. (1982). A study of reliability and validity of a preschool play scale. *American Journal of Occupational Therapy, 36*(12), 783-788.

Fisher, A., Murray, E., & Bundy, A. (1991). *Sensory integration: Theory and practice.* Philadelphia: F.A. Davis.

Bundy, A. (1993). Assessment of play and leisure; delineation of the problem. *American Journal of Occupational Therapy, 47*(3), 217-222.

Frantzen, J. (1957). *Toys . . . the tools of children.* Chicago: National Society for Crippled Children and Adults, Inc.

Florey, L. (1971). An approach to play and development. *American Journal of Occupational Therapy, 25*(6), 275-280.

Florey, L. (1981). Studies of play: Implications for growth, development and for clinical practice. *American Journal of Occupational Therapy, 35*(8), 519-524.

Hurff, J. (1980). A play skills inventory. *American Journal of Occupational Therapy, 34,* 651-656.

Hurff, J. (1974). A play skills inventory. In M. Reilly (Ed.). *Play as exploratory learning.* Beverly Hills, CA: Sage Publications.

Knox, S. (1974). A play scale. In M. Reilly (Ed.). *Play as exploratory learning.* Beverly Hills, CA: Sage Publications.

Neville, P., Kielhofner, G., & Royeen, C. (1985). Childhood. In G. Kielhofner (Ed.). *Model of human occupation theory and application.* Baltimore, MD: Williams & Wilkins.

Parham, L.D. (1992). Strategies for maintaining a playful atmosphere during therapy. *Sensory Integration SIS Newsletter, 15*(1).

Parten, M.B. (1932). Social participation among preschool children. *Journal of Abnormal and Social Psychology, 27,* 243-269.

Parten, M.B. (1933). Leadership among preschool children. *Journal of Abnormal and Social Psychology, 28,* 430-440.

Parten, M.B. (1933). Social play among preschool children. *Journal of Abnormal and Social Psychology, 28,* 136-147.

Pratt, P.N. (1989). Play and recreational activities. In P.N. Pratt & A.S. Allen (Eds.). *Occupational therapy for children* (2nd ed.). St. Louis: Mosby.

Rast, M. (1986). Play and therapy, play or therapy? In C. Pehoski (Ed.). *Play—A skill for life.* Rockville, MD: American Occupational Therapy Association.

Schaff, R., & Burke, J. (1992). Clinical reflections on play and sensory integration. *Sensory Integration SIS Newsletter, 15*(1).

Takata, N. (1974). Play as a prescription. In M. Reilly (Ed.). *Play as exploratory learning.* Beverly Hills, CA: Sage Publications.

Vandenberg, B., & Kielhofner, G. (1982). Play in evolution, culture, and individuals' adaptation; implications for therapy. *American Journal of Occupational Therapy, 36*(1), 20-28.

A

Descriptions of Commercially Available Toys and Games and Their Sources

---

MAJOR FUNCTIONS ELICITED BY TOYS (SEE TABLE 13-1)
Tactile Exploration/Stimulation, #1-7
Reach/Arm Control/Eye-Hand, #8-18
Grasp, #19-23
Thumb-Finger Grasp, #24-32
Tool Use, #33-35
Wrist Movements, #36-40
Thumb Isolation, #41-44
Finger Isolation, #45-46
Bimanual Skills, #47-52
In-Hand Manipulation Skills, #53-55
Writing, #56-58
Tactile Discrimination, #59-61

Tactile Exploration/Stimulation

Product name: Vibrating busy boxes/switch plates; vibrators (1)
Description: Several electronic busy boxes now offer a plate that vibrates when pushed, which many children find rewarding. Various types and strengths of personal vibrators are also commercially available. These also vary in size from hand-held pocket models to models designed to wrap around specific body parts (e.g., neck).
Adaptations: Many of these toys may be placed vertically to promote shoulder movements.

Product name: Rice; macaroni; split peas; puffed rice; sand; beans (2)
Description: Buckets filled with these materials offer a stimulating environment in which to practice hand skills through tactile exploration. Small objects (beads, cars, coins) can be hidden and searched for within the materials. Buckets can contain only one substance or materials can be combined. Covers should be airtight.

Adaptations: Materials can be chosen and presented in a graded sequence of choice (soft to hard; smooth to rough; one texture to several). Materials can also be used for development of various hand skills depending on therapist structuring of the activity (pouring material through cupped hands; raking with fingers; picking up one kernel/piece and storing it in the palm).

Product name: Shaving cream; foam in a can (3)
Description: Foam products in a can that are spread onto a playing surface: mirrors, walls, tables, etc. Fun to spread, then draw in with an isolated finger or practice finger movements in. Can also be spread on arms, hands, and fingers. After some time, the cream begins to dry. Rubbing hard helps to make the cream dry and disappear.
Adaptations: Various hand and finger patterns can be incorporated into play (e.g., cupping hands to hold foam).

Product name: GUK (4)
Registered trademark of: Chieftain, Inc.
Description: Colored powder in a resealable bag. Add water as directed on package to make GUK. GUK is an unusual nonsticky slimelike material. It feels somewhat rubbery and somewhat wet. If kept moving, it can be shaped into a ball, but it "melts" when movement stops. Facilitates finger and hand movements. Dries back to a powder that can be saved and used again.

Product name: Koosh balls; Krinks; Softee (5)
Registered trademark of: Oddz On, Inc.
Description: These balls offer a variety of textures: soft, fuzzy, stringy, light, and heavy; they are also colorful. Sizes range from 1½ to 8 inches.
Adaptations: Can be used in a matching texture game without vision for developing tactile dis-

crimination. Also can be used for throw and catch activities and ball/racket games. Kooshes do not roll when they hit the floor.

Product name: Sticky creatures/materials/objects (6)
Description: Available in many shapes and sizes from many companies. Balls, dinos, slugs; rope; also seasonal novelties such as eyeballs for Halloween. These very sticky, colorful materials can be flattened, pulled, and stretched to great lengths and will resume their original shape.
Adaptations: Can be used in a matching texture game, without vision, to develop tactile discrimination.

Product name: Snowball (7)
Registered trademark of: Cap Toys, Inc.
Description: Interesting nonsticky material. Pleasantly fragrant. Ideal for rolling, squeezing, pulling, and shaping. Leaves little residue but needs occasional refreshening with water or lotion. Much like clay or putty in its uses, but finished products cannot be dried. Reusable if stored in an airtight container and refreshened occasionally. Assorted colors available.
Adaptations: Can be used for development of various hand skills depending on therapist structuring of the activity. Can also be used in a matching texture game without vision for developing tactile discrimination.

Reach/Arm Control/Eye-Hand

Product name: Framed mobiles/hanging mobiles (8)
Description: Various forms of play mobiles are available. Some allow the objects to be changed by the caregiver for a variety of stimulation. Others are designed to be used while lying or sitting on the floor, for use in a playpen, crib, bed, or wheelchair.

Product name: Water mat games (9)
Description: Plastic or vinyl water-filled play mats. Most have sponged or glitter objects floating within, encouraging reaching and touching to make the objects move.
Adaptations: A white or other solid-colored background may be less visually distracting than a clear background; vary water temperature.

Product name: Busy boxes; rattles (10)
Description: Various types and sizes of busy boxes and rattles are now available. Many may be attached to playpens or cribs. Some rattles and busy toys are secured to tabletops with suction cups.

With these types of toys reach is usually rewarded with sound and/or movement. Electronic switch busy boxes are also available. Other arm/hand patterns are also facilitated through the use of busy boxes. These may include poking, patting, pushing, pulling, and sliding. Each busy box should be carefully analyzed for the specific hand patterns encouraged.
Adaptations: May be used in various planes and positions.

Product name: Tabletop mazes/roller coasters (11)
Description: Various versions of these three-dimensional games are available. Each is somewhat different but is still designed to address reach and shoulder development. There are usually one to five bent wires that intertwine with each other. Each is fastened into the playing base at both ends. One or more cars, trucks, animals, or beads are at the ends of each of the wires. The child must grasp an object and try to slide it along its path to get to the opposite side.
Adaptations: Young children especially like these games. Adaptations include races between players and races between two hands/objects. The position of play also greatly affects the area of shoulder and arm development being addressed (e.g., sitting vs. lying).

Product name: Pecking chickens/climbing gingerbread man (counterweight toys) (12)
Description: These old-time toys are usually constructed from wood. Child holds handle and gently moves arm in small circles, starting movement of counterweight, which causes chickens to peck or gingerbread man to climb.
Adaptations: When elbows are stabilized on a surface, isolated wrist movement is facilitated to start the counterweight moving.

Product name: Magnet/felt/Velcro boards (13)
Description: Although the materials used are very different, the basic concept of all of these activities is the same. Pieces are attached to a playing surface that is usually vertical or angled to some degree. Arms and hands are repetitively brought up to attach or reposition objects on the boards. Whole stories can be displayed and words and letters can be constructed with most sets.
Adaptations: The use of these sets is unlimited.

Product name: Snatchers; reachers; grabbers (14)
Description: These come in a variety of styles and shapes, such as alligators, parrots, dinos, sharks, and hands. A few look like robot claws. Basic

grasp and release movements are used to activate the snatchers. Shoulder stability is needed for placement and maintenance of the snatcher's position to grab objects.

Adaptations: Additional arm stability is needed to lift heavier objects with the snatchers. These may include objects such as Koosh balls (by Oddz On, Inc.) and small cars. Two hands can be used on the snatcher to increase stability.

Product name: Stacrobats; Don't Monkey Around (15)

Registered trademark of: Stacrobats by Ravensburg; Don't Monkey Around by Milton Bradley Co. *Description:* The object of these games is to be the first player to stack all his/her playing pieces onto the vertical stand, without having any fall off. Plastic monkey- or acrobat-shaped pieces have a number of holes from which they can be balanced and stacked.

Adaptations: Positioning of child during these games (e.g., sitting vs. lying) greatly influences the level of difficulty. The number of pieces can also be graded.

Product name: Top Choice (16)

Registered trademark of: Koeller Products

Description: Game consists of a flat playing board and a specially designed top. Object of the game is to keep the top spinning while also directing it to various places marked on the board. Top is kept spinning by moving the board smoothly in a wave-like pattern.

Adaptations: Once basic movement is mastered, try flipping top in the air and catching it back on the board while still spinning. Also try walking or turning the board around. When four people are playing, each holds and controls a different side of the board. Can also be done on larger surfaces, such as a card table.

Product name: Block building sets; block towering games (e.g., Jenga from Milton Bradley Co.) (17)

Description: Block towering games are always popular and come in various forms. One version has a tall tower of rectangular blocks. Players must remove one block at a time and carefully place it on the top of the tower without making any of the blocks fall. Another version of this game uses asymmetric pieces for towering.

Adaptations: Symmetric game pieces are easier then asymmetric ones. To make the game more challenging, blocks can be numbered with a pen or marker, then players must remove or place a specifically numbered block on their turn.

Product name: Fishing games (battery operated) (18)

Description: These battery-operated fishing games are available from a variety of sources and vary slightly in their design. Most have a round pond in which hungry fish bob up and down trying to catch something to eat. The player is the fisherman trying to catch the hungry fish with a fishing pole. Arm and shoulder stability is needed to center the fishing pole and lift the fish out of the pond.

Adaptations: The child's positioning for the game can be graded (sitting, lying, elbow on the table). Fish can also be grabbed with fingers if using the fishing pole is too difficult.

Grasp

Product name: Pegboards (19)

Description: Pegs and pegboards can be found in a variety of shapes, sizes, weights, and materials. The grasp pattern needed for holding and placement is most affected by the size of the peg being used (gross/mass grasp to mature pincer).

Adaptations: Hand positioning and grasp patterns used can be affected by the position of the child (prone, sitting, standing) as well as the board (horizontal, angled, vertical). Difficulty can be increased by using pieces that have more than one peg to be lined up with a hole for placement. (L-shaped pieces in Tile Pictures by AMAV). Using rubberized boards or pegs also increases difficulty by adding resistance when pegs are placed and removed.

Product name: Popbeads (20)

Description: Many available designs make popbeads fun and motivating to most children. There are ducks, unicorns, balls, geometric shapes, bears, stars, hearts, numbers, and popular theme characters (Mickey or Turtles). The size and shape of the popbead delegate the grasp/pinch pattern to be used. Sizes range from 4 inches to ½ inch.

Adaptations: Popbeads are naturally adapted by the size offered. Other components may be added for interest, such as sequencing by color, style, or number.

Product name: Water squirt toys (21)

Description: These water toys are generally made of colorful plastic or vinyl and vary in size and shape. Small, round shapes can be used to facilitate finer pinch patterns and palmar arches. Larger sizes may need the use of all fingers in a gross grasp.

Adaptations: Small crumpled pieces of tissue or a small eraser may be placed under the ring and little finger to facilitate separation of the hand. These squirt toys often can be used without water to play air hockey games with a cotton ball or small ball of tissue paper. Other games may include blowing pieces of confetti to a specific place or to clear a specific spot to see a hidden message or picture.

Product name: Air squirt toys (22)
Description: These toys are activated by repetitively squeezing a plastic bulb attached to the toy. There are jumping frogs, rabbits, horses, and monkeys who bang on drums.
Adaptations: The bulb mechanism of these toys makes them especially adaptable for use in hand skill development. The bulb is sensitive enough to be activated through individual finger opposition, abduction-adduction of individual fingers, or isolated wrist flexion-extension.

Product name: Pig Pong (23)
Registered trademark of: Milton Bradley Co.
Description: This air puff game has two hand-sized rubber pigs. When they are squeezed, a puff of air is emitted and is used to keep a light ball up and passing over the net to the other player.
Adaptations: Keeping ball up in the air can be difficult. But air puff pigs or other squeezable air puff toys are great for blowing Ping-Pong balls, bits of paper, or cotton balls across a table surface. Great for grasp and release and for finger strengthening.

Thumb-Finger Grasp

Product name: Stamp sets/stamp blocks (24)
Description: There are many stamp sets available that mount the stamp design on a small block of wood or rubber. This requires the use of only two or three fingers to pick up the block and press it into the ink pad. (Use of only fingertips would be ideal, so fingers stay out of the ink.) Set designs include alphabet, faces, animals, numbers.
Adaptations: Wooden toothpick pieces or large push pins can be put into the backs of rubber stamp pieces to make holding pegs.

Product name: Colorforms sets (25)
Registered trademark of: Colorforms, Inc.
Description: This classic game is still around and available in various forms, including theme character sets. The original set includes large sheets of

Colorforms pieces in four colors that contain many shapes and sizes, and five individual playing boards. "Making Silly Faces" is a preschool board game. Players take turns using spinner to determine playing pieces. First to complete their funny-face person wins. Theme sets include different types of clothes and accessories for popular characters and are frequently updated. The thin, flimsy nature of Colorforms requires the use of a fine pincer grasp.
Adaptations: The original set can be used to tell stories or copy designs, or as a classroom manipulative. Playing boards easily lend themselves to vertical positioning.

Product name: Pearler Beads/Hama Beads (26)
Registered trademark of: Pearler Beads by Novacon Corp., Hama Beads by Cilis, Inc..
Description: These small cylindric plastic beads are placed over small plastic points that hold them securely in a frame. Frames come in many different shapes and beads in many different sizes and colors. Beads range in size from approximately ⅛ to ½ inch. Choose bead size to facilitate pinch refinement needed. Once all points have been filled with beads, the tops of the beads are melted together with an iron, after which the bead design can be removed intact from the frame. Frame can then be reused.
Adaptations: A similar product is available that includes a small pencil-like tool to assist in placement of the beads. Beads are approximately ⅛ inch in diameter. A tool to assist in the placement of the larger beads can be fabricated from splinting material.

Product name: Squiggle Worms (27)
Registered trademark of: Milton Bradley Co.
Description: A large apple is full of smiling worms that bob up and down as the apple turns. Players must grasp bobbing worm and turn it over. The tail of each worm has a color painted on it. Players must match the tail colors to colors on their playing cards or return them to the apple. The first to fill his/her card wins.
Adaptations: The small size of the worms and their bobbing movements make this an ideal activity for developing purposeful reach and grasp patterns. The game may also be structured so the child is weight bearing on an arm or holding the playing card so that only the dominant hand is available to both grasp and manipulate the worm. The movements used when turning the worm over can be structured to facilitate in-hand manipulation.

Product name: Mini clothespins, mini hair clips, mini squeeze clips (28)

Description: The small size of these mini clips requires the use of a fine pincer grasp. Items can be clipped together, or put on clothes, around a box top, or on a suspended clothes/yarn line. Some types of clips are slightly more resistive than others (mini clips vs. mini clothespins). Each type of clip is also available in several different sizes. These sizes can be chosen for specific grasps or mixed to require spontaneous use of an assortment of grasp patterns.

Adaptations: The surface that the clips are to be placed on will vary the amount of force needed. A thinner surface such as a paper requires less effort and strength than to place them on a cardboard cigar box or plastic container. A crumpled small piece of tissue or small eraser can be placed under the ring and little fingers to assist in facilitating separation of the two sides of the hand as the child works.

Product name: Lite Brite (29)

Registered trademark of: Milton Bradley Co.

Description: This favorite game is still loved by children of all ages. A black pattern sheet is placed under the Lite Brite screen and the toy is then plugged in. Small colored, translucent pegs are then pushed through the screen and pattern sheet, illuminating and creating a design. Extra design packs are available in a variety of current popular themes and characters.

Adaptations: The small pegs lend themselves to developing separation of the two sides of the hand and use of a three- or two-point pincer grasp. Further structuring can be done to require that pegs be stored in the palm of the hand and moved to the fingertips using translation and shift movements. By design the Lite Brite screen is vertical, which facilities wrist extension. For perceptual work, rows of pegs can be placed in a sequence; then the child is asked to repeat or continue the pattern.

Product name: Battleship; HiQ; Chinese Checkers; Mastermind (30)

Registered trademark of: Battleship and HiQ by Milton Bradley Co.; Mastermind by Chieftain.

Description: All of these games involve the use of small pegs or marbles, but focus is based upon a strategic plan. Cognitive skills and planning are used to develop a course of action to win the game. These games are more appropriately used with the older child.

Adaptations: The small pegs lend themselves to developing separation of the two sides of the hand and use of a three- or two-point pincer grasp. Further structuring can be done to require that pegs be stored in the palm of the hand and moved to the fingertips using translation and shift movements. For perceptual work, rows of pegs can be placed in a sequence; then the child is asked to repeat or continue the pattern.

Product name: Don't Spill the Beans (31)

Registered trademark of: Milton Bradley Co.

Description: This classic game is still ideal for developing hand and finger skills. The total number of small playing beans is divided among all players. The bean pot is balanced on the special playing tray as players take turns carefully placing their beans one at a time onto the pot. The first to use all their beans without spilling the pot is the winner.

Adaptations: Small cans are included with the game to hold players' beans. If these are not used, players can be required to hold beans in the palms of their hands and use palm-to-finger translation movements before placing one bean in the pot.

Product name: Kerplunk (32)

Registered trademark of: Tyco, Inc.

Description: Kerplunk is a wonderful toy for developing hand skills. Before starting, players need to set up the game. This involves poking the pick-up type sticks horizontally through little holes in the middle section of a Plexiglas cylinder. After all sticks are in place (approximately 20), marbles are dropped through a hole in the top of the cylinder and are suspended by the sticks. Now the game begins. Players take turns removing a stick one at a time, trying to dislodge as few marbles as possible. The player with the least marbles at the end wins.

Adaptations: Larger marbles may be substituted.

Tool Use

Product name: Thin Ice (33)

Registered trademark of: Pressman

Description: Children of all ages enjoy this prescissor game. A standard tissue is secured into a suspended hoop. This is the ice. Players then use cardboard tweezers to place a marble on top of the ice until the ice breaks (tissue rips).

Adaptations: Other tools could be used to manipulate the marble, instead of the provided tweezers.

Additional tissues may make the ice stronger and more difficult to break.

Product name: Bed Bugs/Crocodile Dentist/ Operation (34)
Registered trademark of: Milton Bradley Co.
Description: Each of these games uses a tweezer-type tool. Bed Bugs and Crocodile Dentist are for younger children. In Bed Bugs players attempt to pick up as many bed bugs as possible from the vibrating bed. In Crocodile Dentist players take turns removing teeth from a large mechanical crocodile without getting snapped; some resistance is offered. Operation is for older children due to the increased control needed to be successful. Players use a small tweezer to remove designated "body parts" without setting off the buzzer.
Adaptations: Each of these games can be played without the electric or windup connections made. This prevents the bugs from jumping, the crocodile from snapping, and the buzzer from buzzing. This also reduces auditory input, resulting in less fear and excitement.

Product name: Work benches/hammer games (Tap-A-Chap)
Registered trademark of: Ambi, Inc. (35)
Description: There are many of these types of games available. Construction is usually of wood or plastic and most contain child-size tools, including pliers, screwdrivers, and hammers. The child is encouraged to screw and unscrew, pound, pull and push, providing plenty of opportunity for arm, hand, and finger use. Smaller versions usually contain only a hammer and pegs to pound through. Tap-A-Chap may be more visually appealing and motivating. As the large button is hit with the hammer or a hand, a plastic "chap" pops out of his hole. Hit the button hard enough and the chap comes all the way out.
Adaptations: The child's position (sitting, standing, lying prone, or kneeling) changes the arm and body responses used. There are also some versions that use thin nails pounded into styrofoam or corkboard. These require finer grasp and manipulation skills.

Wrist Movements

Product name: Electronic drumsticks (36)
Description: These drumsticks have plastic-coated tips and are attached to a small speaker. Tapping on a surface produces a drumming sound.
Adaptation: Care in positioning can result in isolated movements of the wrist, especially if tapping against a vertical or slanted surface. Sticks can be used either unilaterally or bilaterally.

Product name: Hands Down (37)
Registered trademark of: Milton Bradley Co.
Description: The real action of this game centers around a special playing board with four movable hands. Players take turns playing a basic card game, then try to be the first to hit their colored hand down.
Adaptations: Player positioning can be altered to require various isolated movements. Sitting with elbow on table requires isolated elbow extension. If the forearm is supported on the table, wrist movements can be isolated (small arm weights or beanbags could assist in stabilizing forearm). The playing board may also be used in other situations, perhaps to determine who gets to answer a teacher's math question.

Product name: Don't Break The Ice (38)
Registered trademark of: Milton Bradley Co.
Description: Players take turns using a small hammer to tap out individual blocks of ice from an elevated tray, trying not to be the one to drop the most ice.
Adaptations: Placing elbows on the tabletop or other surface assists in isolating wrist movements when using the hammer. A small bolster, half bolster, or block may be used as a surface to support the elbows. Small blocks or beanbags may be taped to the hammer's handle to increase its weight.

Product name: Yo-Yos/Yo-Yo Ball/Koosh Yo-Yo (39)
Registered trademark of: Yo-Yo Ball by Marchon; Koosh Yo-Yo by Oddz On, Inc.
Description: Yo-yos are a motoric challenge to children with motor planning, sequencing, and/ or isolated wrist movement difficulties. Modern yo-yos come in many designs and styles. There are soft-sided ones, some that light up, and some with popular theme characters printed on them. The Yo-Yo Ball has a special mechanism designed to automatically retract the ball on the string. As a result, it takes purposeful movement and force to drop the yo-yo down. It will not just drop when released. The Koosh Yo-Yo is a mini Koosh ball attached to an elastic cord with a finger loop. There is no winding of the string. The Yo-Yo Ball is useful for learning the wrist movement needed to push the yo-yo down. The Koosh Yo-Yo is useful for learning the turning and wrist movement needed to jerk the yo-yo back up.

Product name: Water-filled toys (40)
Description: There is a wide assortment of these toys available today. They come in both standard and travel size, unilateral and bilateral, and range from simple basketball games to more difficult ring toss games. The specific hand pattern required for the game greatly depends on the specific size of the activation button and its particular location. Some travel versions, for example, are thin and promote distal finger extension with MCP flexion and the use of thenar flexion to press the buttons. Some are spherical, which promotes arching of the hand with active thumb movements. Careful attention must be paid to the specific location of the activation button. Some are set off to one side. This usually dictates which hand is to be used.

Thumb Isolation

Product name: Sliding puzzles (41)
Description: These travel-size puzzles are still available in their simple form and also in more elaborate designs. The original puzzle designs are approximately 2 × 2 inches and have eight small squares that slide but cannot be removed. Pieces generally are numbered or make a simple design when placed in the correct order. Isolated thumb movements are generally used to slide pieces around. More elaborate designs include mind teasers with many pieces and may come in cylindrical shapes.

Product name: Etch-a-Sketch (42)
Registered trademark of: Ohio Art
Description: Toy consists of a drawing screen with two knobs. The right knob controls vertical movement of line, and the left knob controls horizontal movement. Controlled alternating movement of the knobs creates simple to complex designs on the screen. Simultaneous movement of both knobs makes angled lines, but this is difficult. Knobs are turned using either wrist or finger movements. There are travel and pocket sizes available. The Doodle Dome (by Tyco, Inc.) works in a similar manner, but the drawing surface is a globe shape.
Adaptation: Placing Etch-A-Sketch in the vertical position alters the arm, wrist, and finger movements used.

Product name: Wind-up toys (43)
Description: There are hundreds of varieties of wind-up toys available. Most, however, fall into one of five categories.

- Walkers/movers: These tend to move at a standard speed in a straight line.
- Move and twirl: These wind-ups usually move along a straight line, stop, spin in place, then continue in a straight line.
- Key wind-ups: These most closely resemble the original old-fashioned wind-up. They often are metal and larger in size. The key may be attached or removable.
- Ledge huggers: These wind-ups have a small leader in front that senses or feels the table edge and redirects the toy.
- Speciality wind-ups: These toys perform a variety of tricks: some jump, flip over, bang a drum or cymbal, or open a secret compartment. Movements frequently are erratic.

Most wind-ups use a standard spring device to activate them. The knob is quite small and requires a fine pinch. Winding is a bilateral task because the toy will spin if not stabilized while winding. The movement pattern used to wind the toy can be one of two: isolated thumb–index finger movements are usually the preferred pattern, but bilateral wrist ulnar and radial deviations may also be used.

Product name: Electronic keyboards/gloves (44)
Description: New technology has resulted in more portable, lightweight musical keyboards. The size, number of keys, and specific features vary between manufacturers. Most have at least 10 keys to allow each finger to operate in isolation. Musical gloves are also available and work in a similar manner.
Adaptations: A keyboard is also an excellent activity for developing sequencing and repetitive movements.

Finger Isolation

Product name: Tricky Fingers/Super Fingers (45)
Registered trademark of: Regey Industries
Description: This perceptual-motor game is also useful for developing finger isolation and kinesthetic awareness of the fingers. Tricky Fingers comes with two sealed plastic game boards, each containing 16 colored balls (four each of four colors). The balls are manipulated through individual holes under the board to reproduce patterns. Pattern cards are provided. Super Fingers is a single game board, just like Tricky Fingers, except there is only one empty space in the board. As a result, more motor planning and finger control are needed.

Adaptations: If the pattern cards provided are too difficult, the child can be asked to make rows of each color or design his/her own pattern cards. Assistance can also be provided to help keep the board level and keep the balls from rolling for children with bilateral difficulties.

Product name: Musical accordion toys/toys using accordion or bellows-type action (46)
Description: These toys require the accordion to be held at both ends. By pushing hands together, the bellows become smaller; they then get larger when hands are pulled apart. Depending on the toy, music, a squeak, a clicking noise, or bubbles are produced.
Adaptations: Grasp patterns used depend on the shape of the toy. Wrist stability facilitates success in pushing together the bellows.

Bimanual Skills

Product name: Building sets (47)
Description: There are many varieties and sizes of building blocks, which interlock when pushed together. The smaller the pieces, the more refined the hand grasp needed.
Adaptations: Building a number of smaller projects in the lap, rather than a large piece on a table, will encourage greater use of two hands together. Increased use of two hands may be further seen when constructions are taken apart, so encourage children to do this. The degree of resistance also changes from building set to building set, and between the sizes used. Larger pieces may not always be easier or less resistant than smaller ones.

Product name: Mr. Potato Head (48)
Registered trademark of: Playskool
Description: Classic game requiring one hand to hold potato body while other hand pushes body parts into body. Can also be done with a real potato or clay.
Adaptations: It now is available with Velcro pieces and a soft body. This newer version may be easier for children to grasp and stabilize while working.

Product name: Clay; putty; dough (49)
Description: Many varieties of clay and putty are available. There are also many recipes for making your own. These materials are so versatile, any hand or finger movement can be facilitated.
Adaptations: Try scented doughs. Use tools for cutting, rolling, and making designs. Each tool

encourages different hand patterns, as well grading of pressure and movements.

Product name: Mini finger going (50)
Description: This mini plastic football shape on a string is slipped over fingertips (usually thumb and index or middle fingers) of each hand. By the coordinated extension of the fingers on one hand and the simultaneous opposition of the other hand, the football is propelled to the other side of the string. As these hand patterns are repeated, the football moves back and forth. A high degree of motor planning is also needed.
Adaptations: This can also be used by two players, each holding two strings on one side. One player then separates strings quickly on his/her side and the football flies to the other player, who then separates his/her strings to send it back. The length of the string may be altered as needed. There are also larger versions of this game with strings 15 and 21 feet long with rigid handles attached to the strings.

Product name: Juggling scarves (51)
Description: A wonderful way to develop the use of both hands and arms at the same time. Can easily be adapted to all skill levels by using only one or two scarves. A grabbing action with hands pronated is used to catch and throw scarves.
Adaptations: Try throwing with one hand and catching with the other. Throw one scarf up with each hand at the same time and catch the same way. Hold two scarves, one in each hand; throw scarf with nondominant hand first and then other one. Next catch the first thrown with the dominant hand, then the other one. Repeat. Next step would be three-scarf juggling. When trying this, it is important to start the throwing with the hand that has two scarves (nondominant hand). The holding and release of just one scarf at a time are easier by holding one scarf in a three-point pinch and the other under flexed ring and little fingers. Separation of the two sides of the hand is facilitated.

Product name: Tops: doodlers, musical, square, egg, hologram, lighted (52)
Description: Tops offer a challenge to children with hand skill limitations. One of the varieties of tricks they are now able to perform is sure to motivate clients of every age. Tops that are musical or light up tend to be especially motivating to older children. These tops have a minimum speed with which they need to be spinning in order to activate the music or lights. Doodlers, egg tops, and

hologram spinners tend to be easier and more successful for beginning spinners.

Adaptations: Using a concave surface with a raised lip around it also assists those having difficulty. The concave surface facilitates a longer spin, and the raised lip keeps tops contained.

In-Hand Manipulation Skills

Product name: Eye-hole lacing projects, Pegs for Lacing (53)

Registered trademark of: Pegs for Lacing by Ideal, Inc.

Description: These unique lacing boards have vertical eye holes to lace with string or yarn. Their vertical orientation tends to facilitate shift movements of the fingers. This same activity is also done with cylindrical pegs with holes that are inserted into a rubber mat.

Adaptations: A stiffer string makes this task easier. Lanyard lacing (plastic) may be good for this.

Product name: Splat (54)

Registered trademark of: Milton Bradley Co.

Description: This is a special board game for children 6 and up. Before playing, players choose a color dough and *make* their playing piece using the special bug maker tool included with the game. (Bilateral hand use and some strength required to use tool). These game pieces are then used as players. The object is to try to be the first to get home without being "splat" by the big foot.

Adaptations: Players can make their own creations out of the clay for their playing piece. Being splat is a good reason to make several game pieces. For specific hand movements, shapes (e.g., balls, snakes) can be required to be the game pieces.

Product name: Stencil rubbing pictures (55)

Description: Children can make creative pictures simply and with almost guaranteed success with these coloring kits. A plastic case has a frame that lifts up, templates with raised designs are set in, and a sheet of paper placed on top, then the frame closed. The child then colors across the top of the paper with a crayon or pencil, making the picture emerge. Various theme characters are available. Most pictures are made using three templates, which can be mixed and matched to create humorous pictures.

Adaptations: This is a wonderful activity for learning grading of pressure, and for developing grasp and arches of the hand if crayons are held horizontally. The playing surface can also be held vertical to facilitate wrist extension.

Writing

Product name: Magna Doodle, Ghost Writer, Glo-Doodler (56)

Registered trademark of: Magna Doodle by Tyco Co.; Ghost Writer by Ohio Art; Glo-Doodler by Colorforms, Inc.

Description: Each of these toys is a modernized magic slate. A metal-tip pen or magnetic stylus is moved across the screen to write and create drawings. Most maintain the image until you remove it, by lifting a shield, sliding an eraser bar, or turning the slate upside down.

Adaptations: These toys are especially appealing to the writing-phobic child and the child developing prewriting skills. Most can be used vertically to promote wrist extension and shoulder stability (except Ghost Writer, which slowly "melts" when held vertical).

Product name: Motorized pens (57)

Descriptions: Most of these pens run on an AA battery or two and come with interchangeable colored ink cartridges. The size, shape, and weight of the pen barrel vary between brands. The vibrating sensation created by the pen is enticing and stimulating to most children. It increases awareness of the hand and fingers and may increase muscle tone.

Adaptations: Using tighter or looser grips on the pen changes the writing pattern. This may assist in grading of grip strength.

Product name: Shape sorters (58)

Description: Basic preschool activity of varying complexity, produced by many companies. Traditionally the child simply places shapes into corresponding holes. By occluding vision this becomes a game of tactile discrimination. The child may only feel the shape, before pointing to the hole into which it will fit. For older children the game Perfection (by Milton Bradley Co.) can be used in this way.

Adaptations: This activity can be graded by limiting the number of pieces used and/or the possible answers.

Tactile Discrimination

Product name: Tactilo (59)

Registered trademark of: Fernando Nathan, Inc.

Description: The object of this game is for players to identify small wooden shapes by feel and match them to their corresponding picture. Toy comes with a fabric feely bag, 36 small objects, and six picture-matching cards.

Adaptations: Can be graded by limiting the number of shapes and pictures from which to choose. It may also be used like a bingo game.

Product name: Tactile form boards (60)
Description: Pieces must be matched to corresponding place on form board by texture, not by shape. Activity can be done with or without vision depending upon the skill of the players.
Adaptations: Grade number of pieces and/or choices.

Product name: Tactile dominoes (61)
Description: Played like any domino game, but textures are matched instead of dots or pictures. Can be played with or without vision depending upon the skill of the players.
Adaptations: Grade number of pieces and/or choices.

B

Sources of Toys

Pocket Full of Therapy, Inc.
P.O. Box 174
Morganville, NJ 07751

OT Ideas, Inc.
111 Shady Lane
Randolph, NJ 07869

Therapro, Inc.
225 Arlington St.
Framingham, MA 01701

Toys to Grow On
P.O. Box 17
Long Beach, CA 90801

PDP Products
12015 North July Ave.
Hugo, MN 55038

Sensory Integration International
1402 Cravens Ave.
Torrance, CA 90501

World Wide Games
P.O. Box 517
Colchester, CT 06415

Kapable Kids
P.O. Box 250
Bohemia, NY 11716

Toys for Special Children, Inc.
385 Warburton Ave.
Hastings-on-Hudson, NY 10706

Local toy stores
Scientific specialty stores
Educational toy stores

14

Principles and Practices of Teaching Handwriting

Mary Benbow

In human history the use of tools was a major breakthrough, extending our ability to control our environment. The first tools were natural objects—sticks, stones, and bones—requiring gross motor skills such as pushing, striking, and throwing. It took thousands of years for humans to develop a tool as precise as a pen or pencil, requiring intricate fine motor skills. Because we take the simplicity of a pencil for granted, it is easy to overlook the complexity of its operation. From a motor skills perspective, a pencil is more difficult to use than the most powerful computer.

It is no wonder that children, their parents, and their teachers are often frustrated with the results of early experimentation with this advanced tool before the fine motor muscles are ready to function. Boys, whose fine motor development is typically behind that of girls, have greater difficulty managing writing tools and tend to prefer simpler motor tools, such as computer keyboards, Nintendo games, and TV remote controls. Girls face a different problem. Many of them begin to "write" as early as age 2½, often without proper adult attention or supervision. Lacking sufficient hand development or guidance, they may adopt pencil grips that are inefficient or even harmful as they pursue their fascination with the letter shapes Big Bird shows them daily.

The overall management of handwriting training can be conceived as a kind of triage, in which some children (group A) learn to write well regardless of the method(s) of teaching. At the other extreme a few (group C) are unable to learn the skill no matter what interventions are employed to alleviate their difficulties. Most children (group B) fall between the two extremes and readily benefit from good teaching strategies. Therefore group B should receive the greatest concentration of effort from teachers, occupational therapists, and other professionals. It is simple to distinguish between groups A and B, but much more difficult to separate group B from C. For this reason it seemed appropriate to develop teaching and treatment strategies around the combined needs of groups B and C. Appropriate compensatory or intervention strategies should enable most of these children to gain functional writing skill.

In the current educational environment, which requires the inclusion of children with widely differing developmental levels being taught together in the classroom, handwriting instruction demands attention and investigation. Professionals must focus on the subskills necessary to ensure more consistent success with this high-level skill. They must strive to teach all schoolchildren more efficiently, thoroughly, and permanently.

All students, especially the great variety of children who are subtly delayed, can be helped by developmentally ordered physical, visual, kinesthetic, and fine motor learning. A better understanding of the constellation of skills that enable one to write efficiently must guide professionals in developing more systematic ways to prepare children for handwriting and to teach handwriting. Occupational therapists are frequently called on for motor evaluations, consultation, and remediation for public school children, and nonfunctional handwriting is a common reason for referral. For an evaluation to be useful for effective curriculum implementation or intervention, professionals must understand the multiple subskills that enable a student to write comfortably, automatically, and with accuracy.

The purpose of this chapter is to describe hand skills that are most adept in operating a pencil. The chapter presents not only the optimal skills—the way the hand should work to produce efficient handwriting—but also problems that arise when motor components for the skill are absent or less dexterous motor patterns are used. Techniques to promote the development of the foundation skills are presented, along with ways of remediating or compensating for related problems that arise. A discussion of pencil grip includes the description of a promising new method of research in handwriting. The final section on the teaching and remediation of handwriting presents the rationale and method for the kinesthetically based instruction of cursive writing. It should be noted that this chapter does not address language components such as word finding, sentence formulation, punctuation, and spelling but is limited to the mechanical aspects of writing and cognitive-associative mental processes.

Handwriting instruction in schools typically begins with manuscript writing (printing) and shifts to cursive writing in the third grade. My experience has shown that the development of functional handwriting can be fostered by an earlier introduction to cursive script. Therefore the discussions of prewriting and writing skills emphasize cursive writing. The cursive vs. manuscript writing issue is discussed more fully in a later section of this chapter.

MOTOR AND PERCEPTUAL COMPONENTS OF WRITING SKILL

To be effective in promoting efficient graphic skills, developmental therapists must often address ergonomic factors (postural, tonal, and stabilizing) as well as fine motor intervention. Graphomotor learning difficulties usually cluster under one or more of the following classifications: (1) incomplete utilization of the proximal joints of the upper extremity, (2) immature wrist and hand development with clumsy distal manipulation skills, (3) insufficient visual control, (4) incomplete bilateral integration, (5) inadequate spatial analysis and/or synthesis skills, and (6) insufficient somatosensory input with failure to develop kinesthesia. Each of these areas is discussed as it relates to optimal handwriting skills.

Upper Extremity Support

The development of dexterous hand skills depends on the interaction of all joints of the upper extremity: scapulothoracic, glenohumeral, elbow, and wrist. Each component must be developed and move freely into its mature patterns. In children experiencing fine motor delays it is not uncommon to find the shoulder joint slightly biased toward internal rotation, adduction, and/or flexion; the elbow joint toward flexion and/or pronation; and the wrist toward flexion and ulnar deviation.

In addition to fluid range of motion, each upper extremity joint must provide a stable base of support for the control of the joint(s) distal to it. When a therapist finds functional limitations in proximal joints, he/she should include weight bearing, traction, and compression activities for scapula, shoulder, and elbow joint control. Specific proximal joint needs are most naturally incorporated into therapeutic or adapted physical education goals.

For example, jumping rope backward requires the simultaneous involvement of all upper extremity joints moving into their mature patterns. Since this activity fully incorporates all upper extremity joints, it should be included in developmental hand therapy programs for children who show dysfunction or inefficiency in proximal joints. A younger or less coordinated child should first learn to turn one end of a long rope with a partner using the dominant hand while a third child jumps. The initial goal is to develop external rotation in the shoulder on the dominant side and secondly full range of the nondominant shoulder. The third step is for the child to swing a jump rope backward over his/her head and step behind it when he/she hears the rope strike the floor. Finally, the upper and lower body should be coordinated in reverse rope jumping.

The case of Zachary demonstrates the value of an integrated upper extremity program for hand skill development. This 6-year-old boy was referred to occupational therapy for difficulties with printing and sloppy paperwork. Initially a program of hand activities was prescribed that specifically addressed the referral request. Zachary faithfully practiced his prescribed program. He made little progress because the hand activities felt so unnatural and were so difficult. Client resistance became a new and serious deterrent. After assessing his upper extremities more thoroughly, the therapist found some limitation of motion in external rotation of the shoulders and incomplete supination at the elbows. After a progressive program for upper extremity range and stability, his hand skills followed naturally and resistance to fine motor activities lessened. Zachary's case is fairly typical. The often overlooked component of proximal development proved to be the key in unlocking distal skills.

Wrist and Hand Development

In addition to a developmentally based gross motor program, early education curricula should stress developing the entire upper extremity with particular emphasis on the hands. The goals are (1) to stabilize the wrist with fine manipulation of small tools, objects, and writing implements, (2) to open and stabilize the thumb-index web space, (3) to increase and stabilize the arches of the hands, (4) to separate the motor functions of the two sides of the hand, and (5) to develop two aspects of precision handling—precision translation and precision rotation. These hand functions are fundamental for all higher-level tool skills.

Stabilize the Wrist

Bunnell (1970) states that the wrist is the key joint of the hand, and wrist limitations cannot be compensated for by any other upper extremity joint. Wrist movements are inseparable from the hand as a single physiologic unit, so therapists should combine wrist and hand activities. Capener (1956) noted that the position of the wrist influences the tension of the extrinsic muscles. The origins of the extrinsic muscles of the hand are in the forearm and generally move the digits in gross flexion or extension patterns. Extrinsic tendon length does not allow simultaneous maximal flexion or extension of the wrist and fingers, so an interplay is seen with wrist and finger movements.

Long (1970), using electromyographic studies, found that intrinsic muscles (whose origins are in the hand) guide and grade the multiple intermediate finger and thumb patterns and control all rotary movements of the thumb and metacarpophalangeal (MP) finger joints used in precision handling. Tubiana (1981) pointed out that no single articulation in the hand is an isolated mechanical entity. Instead, each articulation functions as part of a group arranged in kinetic chains. Each articulation depends on the equilibrium of forces acting at its level, and this equilibrium is subject to the position of the immediate proximal articulation. Mobile balance is realized through the interdependence between the elements in the same osteoarticular chain. That interdependence includes both passive and active components. The active component is the dynamic balance between antagonistic muscles. The passive components include the restraining action of ligaments and muscular viscoelasticity that facilitates coordination of motion (Smith, 1974). Therefore the wrist influences the position of the MP joint, and the MP joint influences the position of the proximal interphalangeal (PIP) joint, which in turn influences the distal interphalangeal (DIP) joint. These anatomic principles provide a foundation to analyze, design, and sequence hand activities that is more effective in developing the constellations of motor patterns for fine motor skills. Any tool is an extension of the hand that uses it. Developmental logic dictates that a hand must be skilled before it can skillfully manipulate a tool as an extension of the hand.

Activities that facilitate wrist stabilization in extension with precision finger skills can best be done on vertical surfaces above eye level. Such positioning automatically positions the wrist into its optimal posture and facilitates abduction of the thumb to work distally with the fingertips. Working above eye level requires holding the arms at a level where their weight strengthens the muscles and stabilizes the joints of the scapula and shoulder. Enjoyable proximal joint activities include painting on chalkboards with brushes dipped in water or more colorful tempera painting on paper at an easel. Many commercially available toys can be vertically positioned to develop wrist stabilization with distal finger skill. Magna Doodle, Etch-A-Sketch, pegboards, and eye-hook boards can all be fastened onto a wall, set in a chalk rail or on an easel ledge, and secured with an elastic cord if necessary.

Open and Stabilize the Thumb-Index Web Space

Muscle tightness on the ulnar side of the wrist (flexor carpi ulnaris) limits range of motion and reduces stabilization of the wrist in extension for distal digital manipulation. The carpometacarpal (CMC) joint located at the base of the thumb column should fully rotate so the thumb pulp can be pronated and positioned diametrically opposite each of the four finger pulps. Incomplete abduction and rotation at this mobile thumb joint result in a posture that cannot be well stabilized for distal manipulation (Kapandji, 1982). A well-expanded web space between the thumb and index finger allows dexterous digital manipulation. According to Elliot and Connolly (1984) this leads to economy, variety, and convenience of movement since it requires minimum involvement of the upper extremity when moving a prehended object. Input from the intrinsics regulates grip pressure on the shaft of the tool and provides ongoing kinesthetic feedback to the nervous system for rapid automatic correction of motor programs. When the hand is in a power grip with the fingers flexed, the lumbricals do not contract, so the hand loses much of its joint-balancing potential and proprioceptive guidance (Long, 1970).

Increase and Stabilize the Arches of the Hand

The hand's great adaptability depends on its fixed and mobile units. Fixed elements include the distal row of carpal bones and the central attached metacarpals to digits II, III, and IV. The small degree of movement at the fixed junctures allows stability without rigidity (Tubiana, 1984). The mobile elements include the five digits and the peripheral metacarpals of the thumb and little finger (Littler, 1960). The mobile units of the thenar and hypothenar eminences cup or arch the hand, providing balanced isolated intrinsic activity within the hand.

Activity papers with circles to fill or shapes to circle or outline before coloring can be designed for this purpose. The papers can be graded by decreasing the size of shapes as refinement of skill progresses distally. When papers or coloring book pages are secured in a vertical orientation (fitted onto a vertically mounted clipboard or taped up on a wall or easel), the oblique arch of opposition can more easily manipulate the pencil or marker. The most refined use of finger control with crayons or markers is in outlining the shapes before coloring them in. The diamond coloring sheet shown in Figure 14-1 requires both dynamic finger skill to outline and static finger skill to color in the shapes.

Primary school children are self-motivated to draw and practice numbers and letters on the blackboard when their efforts on this surface yield satisfying results. For one nursery school child, working on a vertical surface magically transformed his clumsy attempts to color at the table into performances that delighted him and his teacher. It may be worth noting that the first products of human use of an advanced tool, in the cave paintings at Lascaux, are on a vertical surface at or above eye level, as are the petroglyphs made by Native Americans on the canyon walls of the Southwest. Without knowing why, these primitive tool users maximized shoulder stability, wrist posture, and visual and hand dexterity for their expressive needs. Today skilled artists rarely draw or paint on a horizontal surface.

Separate the Motor Functions of the Two Sides of the Hand

Capener (1956) noted the coupling action of the two ulnar digits (IV and V), which function together in power grips and precision handling. In precision handling, when the ulnar digits are flexed against the palm, they provide stability at the MP arch while isolating control of the radial digits for manipulation with the thumb. Separation of the ulnar from the radial side of the hand and the counterbalance of the MP arch for higher-level skills or holding weighted items, such as a teacup, is achieved by abduction and extension of digits IV and V. The radial digits (II and III) are isolated and stabilized from the arched posture to perform their function more precisely with the opposed thumb.

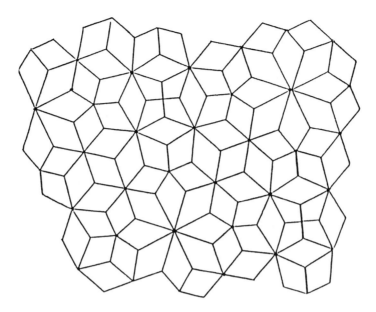

Figure 14-1. Diamond coloring sheet.

(Copyright: Mary Benbow.)

The proper handling of scissors requires the separation of the motor functions of the two sides of the hand, with flexion and extension of the tripod digits acting simultaneously. The ulnar digits should be flexed and stabilized against the palm. With the wrist stabilized in extension, the child should place the distal joints of the thumb and middle finger into the loops (oval loops stabilize easier). The loops should be small enough to enable the child to stabilize the handles at the DIP joints of the long finger and the IP joint of the thumb. The index finger should be placed against the shaft of the handle to support the scissors in a vertical position and help to close the blades. The ulnar digits (IV and V) should be flexed and pressed against the palm to add stability to the MP arch. If it is frustrating or difficult to remember to flex and stabilize digits IV and V, have the child press a small flat sponge against the palm with the two ulnar digits as shown in Figure 14-2. This motor separation of the functions of the two sides of the hand isolates control in the two radial digits to work in combination with the thumb. Initially a child should practice simply opening and closing the blades. After intended blade movements become rhythmic, introduce tiny straws (which take almost no control from the recessive hand) to be cut into tiny segments. Advance to oaktag or old playing cards and finally to paper, which requires the most skill. The nondominant hand must hold the paper taut enough for cutting without tearing.

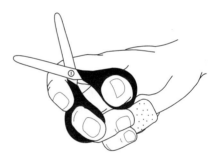

Figure 14-2. Small hand scissors designed by author shown with small sponge gripped by the ulnar digits.

(Available from OT Ideas, Inc.; copyright: Mary Benbow.)

Develop Two Aspects of Precision Handling: Precision Rotation and Precision Translation

Precision handling requires full range of motion at the CMC joint of the thumb so its pulp can be flexed and placed diametrically opposite each of the finger pulps. From this stable position the multiple variations of the two precision handling skills—precision translation and precision rotation—should be developed and refined (Landsmeer, 1962). Translation movements require that the thumb and index or the thumb, index, and middle fingers move in synchrony in a toward-the-palm or an away-from-the-palm pattern (Long et al., 1970). Needle threading uses a translation-away pattern from the fully flexed translation

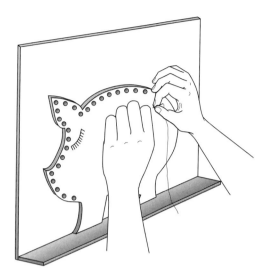

Figure 14-3. Threading shape designed by author.
(Available from OT Ideas, Inc.; copyright: Mary Benbow.)

toward the palm. Pulling a thread through a needle is an example of translation toward the palm-finger pattern.* Writing in a cursive hand requires rapid alternation of toward and away translation patterns to produce letter strokes.

Bead stringing is the classic preschool activity for developing speed and dexterity in the alternate use of translation patterns. However, children who most need to develop this skill often adopt an efficient substitute system. They place the bead over the lacing tip rather than inserting (translation away pattern) the tip through the bead. For development of this skill, eye-hook lacing boards were designed to prevent this movement substitution and provide a more motivating activity for young children (Figure 14-3). Because children tend to be self-driven to stay with this lacing board activity, it is effective and efficient in developing the alternate moving finger prewriting skill.

Precision rotation skill is used when strength demand is low, in activities such as opening and closing loosened tube or jar lids, turning knobs, and turning over small objects for inspection. When a person substitutes less efficient forearm rotation for digital rotation, an evaluation for range of motion and stabilization of the thumb is indicated.

*The term *precision translation* is used by Long and his associates (1970) to describe the movement of an object toward and away from the palm while the grip on the object is maintained. The term has also been used to describe the shifting of a small object such as a piece of lint from the fingertips into the palm (Exner, 1992; see also Chapter 8).

The child must have functional range of motion at the CMC joint to position the thumb diametrically opposite the third digit. Snapping the fingers provides the therapist with a simple nonthreatening skill test for evaluation of range of motion at the CMC joint. When there is limited separation between the thumb and index metacarpals, physically expanding the web space by joint mobilization and progressive stretching may be indicated. Expansion of the joint-supporting structures can often bring the thumb CMC joint into a position where it can be stabilized for distal manipulation with the index or index and middle fingers.

A simple activity to promote precision rotation is rolling tiny balls (⅛-inch diameter) of clay or therapy putty between the pulps of the thumb and index finger. Another is in playing tug-of-war with a small-diameter object such as a coffee stirrer or plastic lace. Digital rotation at the MP joint is necessary to shape the grip snugly enough so the extrinsics can effectively provide strength for distal power pinch. Holding a coffee stirrer or plastic lace between the index and thumb pulps enhances position contact of finger pulps for strength.

An engrossing group activity is turning over a row of 25 pennies from heads to tails in a race against classmates or a stopwatch. A more sophisticated activity is holding and shuffling a deck of cards at their distal ends. A tiny moving picture flip book or small deck of cards requires full CMC expansion in the hand of a primary school child. Adequate range and stability at the CMC joints are required for both card shuffling and distal dynamic pencil control. With middle school or high school students shuffling a standard size deck of cards is a challenging activity that promotes better range of motion and stability at the thumb CMC joint. Tactile sensitivity of the thumb pulps needs to be refined to manage the intermixing of the cards from the two hands.

Visual Control

Manuscript and cursive writing use vision differently in the guidance of movement. In manuscript writing the hand's output depends almost entirely upon the input and ongoing guidance of the visual system. In cursive the visual system should play a less significant role. For this reason many children with visual motor problems should be advanced to cursive instruction as soon as written work is required. The reduced demand for visual motor integration yields more satisfactory results. When using kinesthetic teaching strategies for cursive training, visual control becomes secondary to proprioceptive guidance during the first lesson. An accomplished handwriter limits visual control to staying on the writing line, to guiding retrace lines, to properly spacing between words, and to serving as a neatness checker of written work.

Most American schoolchildren learn to print their names before entering kindergarten. A few children master the whole alphabet. Imitating family members, early education teachers, or educational television shows, they rely heavily on visual control in drawing their block letters. Close visual monitoring of the pencil point is required for them to control stroke length and angle, to find the intersecting or joining points, and to inhibit pencil movement at the intended stopping place.

In any mainstreamed primary classroom one can observe many accommodations to insufficient eye-hand skills. Children who have difficulty focusing when ocular alignment or extraocular control are affected adapt by turning the head far to one side to isolate use of one eye while diverting the other eye from the paper. Warren (1993) explains that this head position eliminates the second image. Neger (1989) cautions therapists that tilting or turning the head in a certain position may not indicate poor head control in the strabismic patient so much as an adaptive maneuver initiated to reduce visual confusion. A child who has difficulty moving the eyes downward or converging the eyes will continue to draw circles, write numbers and letters from bottom to top, and fail to adopt the cultural pattern of top to bottom stroking of letters and numbers.

In the early grades figure copying tests such as the Developmental Test of Visual-Motor Integration (Beery, 1989) are used to determine a child's visual-motor integration age level. Beery cites Piaget (1952) and others (Compton, 1958; Lamme, 1979) who have explored the underlying visual-motor skills that determine a child's potential for mastering manuscript formations. Beery states that it is prudent to postpone formal pencil and paper writing until at least such time as a child can easily copy the VMI Oblique Cross (form 8). The oblique cross requires the child to have the ability to cross the midline using diagonal visual guidance. This high-level perceptual-motor skill is necessary to produce several manuscript letters.

A recently developed assessment tool, the Observation of Visual Motor Orientation and Efficiency (Benbow, 1992), can be a practical supplement to observe visual control of the hand as the eyes guide the pencil in various orientations. To

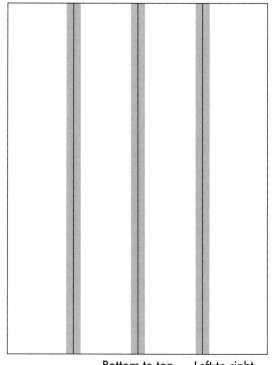

Top to bottom

Bottom to top **Left to right**

Figure 14-4. Form used to observe visual control of hand movements.

(Copyright: Mary Benbow.)

observe visual-motor efficiency in various orientations, the instructor should prepare an unlined sheet of paper ($8\frac{1}{2} \times 11$ inches) with three lines $\frac{1}{8}$ inch wide and 11 inches long. Ruled lines should be drawn with a highlight marker and spaced 2 inches apart. The child is directed to draw a continuous controlled line with his/her pencil along the middle of each brightly colored line. With the paper positioned vertically (it may be slanted for better viewing), the child is instructed to draw the first line from top to bottom and the second line from bottom to top (Figure 14-4). The accuracy of control is noted as the child visually guides the hand into upward and downward space and is asked which direction is easier to do. The paper should then be turned horizontally to observe eye-hand coordination across the visual midline as the child draws along the third line, moving from left to right.

If the child appears stressed while doing the preceding task on a desk top, a second sheet can be taped on the wall or chalkboard in the vertical plane with the middle of the sheet of paper positioned at eye level as the child stands to work.

This placement requires the child to elevate and lower the eyes along the first two lines. If he/she does poorly on trial 1 (desk top) and better on trial 2 (wall or chalkboard), it will be advantageous for him/her to stand while practicing numbers and letters on the blackboard or at an easel. The child's ability to control a pencil in the various orientations is a clear demonstration of the visual system's control of the hand for graphic skill training. Tracking comfort and skill often clarifies the reason some children are unable to conform to writing numbers and letters from top to bottom.

When poor efficiency in visual-motor orientation is noted in the classroom, a child should be further evaluated by physical educators since ball and game skills are often impaired as well. Remediation for visual scanning problems is not to be found in paper and pencil activities but in vestibular based, visually demanding gross motor activities. If the child has difficulty tracking upward, include activities that require upward gaze such as tossing a ball straight up and catching it at chest level, gently tapping a ball suspended above eye level, racket games, volleyball, and flying kites or airplanes. Alternatively, if the child has difficulty tracking downward, bouncing a ball and catching it at waist level is advised. A line or pattern drawn on the floor or sidewalk can make bouncing on a hippity-hop ball or riding a scooter board or bicycle more interesting and organizing. A rapidly moving activity demanding visual guidance helps integrate visual tracking with body skills.

In cursive writing, problems in tracking downward result in the poorer control of the loops that continue below the writing line (*f, g, j, p, q, y,* and *z*). Alternatively, when children are stressed by elevating the eye, they may have trouble with the ascenders of tall letters (*h, k, b, f, l,* and *t*). Temporarily averting the gaze while producing the stroke is usually a satisfactory compensation once the child has developed the kinesthetic feel for the length of the stroke.

When a child can complete a single stroke line but has trouble retracing segments, the problem may be a near-point focusing insufficiency. A therapist can most easily detect a focusing problem on the retraced segments of *a, d, m,* and *t*. When these errors are consistently seen, a referral for a visual examination is indicated.

Bilateral Integration

Bilateral integration and sequencing (BIS) dysfunction is a common cause of motor deficits (Ayres, 1991). In addition to well-documented gross motor deficits (such as postural, equilibrium, and body side coordination), a child with BIS dysfunction is slow to establish a good division of labor between the two hands. By the time most peers are performing well in the graphomotor area, the child is still using the hands interchangeably to do far less sophisticated activities. On paper and pencil tasks the child usually experiences an interruption in crossing the visual midline and produces reversals long after other classmates have resolved this issue. The child is unable to change stroke direction in a continuous flow pattern. This is evidenced as an inability to shift the right under-curving lead-in stroke to the left when approaching the line top while writing letters *h, k, b, f* and *l*. Functional graphomotor work remains far beyond the child's reach. Unfortunately additional paper and pencil practice will not solve these developmental issues.

A child who is not bilaterally integrated neglects to stabilize the paper with the nondominant hand when writing or coloring. Until the dominant hand assumes a definite leadership role, the nondominant hand does not sense and perform its assisting role. Instead of cooperation between the two body sides, there is residual competition. Synkinesis (motor overflow) is usually observable, which supports the finding of inadequate central nervous system inhibition of the nondominant hand as the dominant hand is being programmed by the brain (Bradshaw and Nettleton, 1983). When older children must produce written assignments, it is prudent to provide a visual (e.g., a colored hand design on the left side of the page) or verbal reminder to cue the child to steady the paper with the nondominant hand. Having the nondominant hand placed on the edge of the paper visually defines the working area while promoting more consistent sitting posture.

Directionality confusion is suspected when a child continues to write wraparound letters after instructions are given to stop at a specific point and retrace a letter segment. When this wraparound pattern, as seen in the letters *a, d, g, q,* and *o,* is the only immature pattern noted, one can logically assume that the motor behavior was generalized from self-taught incorrect formation of manuscript letters at an earlier stage. A typical example is seen in Figure 14-5.

When a child with incomplete bilateral integration draws horizontal or diagonal lines, a hesitation or jerk is often seen along the pencil line where the eyes crossed their midline while guiding the pencil. This interruption is more visible and disorganizing when the child draws diagonal lines.

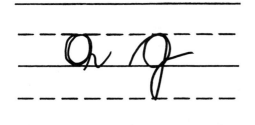

Figure 14-5. Example of the incorrect formation of the wraparound letters *a* and *g*.

(From *Loops and other groups* by Mary Benbow, copyright 1990 by Therapy Skill Builders, a division of Communication Skill Builders, Inc., P.O. Box 42050, Tucson, AZ.)

Typically the child substitutes near-vertical lines for diagonals without being aware of it. The child's cursive writing appears near vertical. Vertical letters are more slowly produced because the wrist is not in a position to efficiently make the long diagonal down strokes.

A later sign of a problem with bilateral integration is the writing of mirror-image letters or numerals. These output errors are more commonly seen when a symbol is produced in isolation. An evaluation of 900 middle school writing samples revealed that the most typical residual reversals of letters in cursive writing were limited to three left-moving capital letters: *3* for *E, f* for capital *J,* and horizontally expanded reversed lowercase *b* for capital *I* (Figure 14-6) (Benbow, 1990).

Averting the gaze is an effective accommodation to writing letters that reverse directions abruptly across the visual midline. In writing capitals *D, G,* and *S,* the child should be taught the place to stop the pencil progression and shift visual focus. The focal place is usually where the stroke ends, as seen with directions for capital *D* in Figure 14-7. The child must avoid visually monitoring the pencil point where it recrosses the visual midline to write these letters successfully.

A very enigmatic problem associated with BIS dysfunction is seen in a child's inability to change

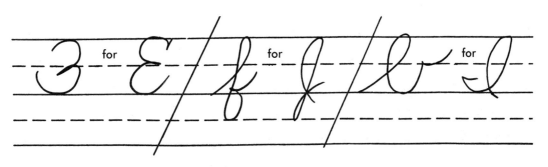

Figure 14-6. Typical reversal of capital cursive letters.

(Copyright: Mary Benbow.)

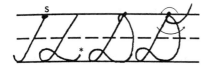

D

1. Start at top line. Make a straight left-slanted downstroke to the writing line.
2. Make a small underhand loop on the writing line and round a stroke right to place a "fat belly" on the writing line.
3. Stop at star.
4. Look at the starting point(s) on the top line and move pencil quickly to them without watching the pencil.
5. Make an overhand left loop at top line and curve up slightly for release.

Figure 14-7. Special instructions given to children learning to write a capital *D*.

(From *Loops and other groups* by Mary Benbow, copyright 1990 by Therapy Skill Builders, a division of Communication Skill Builders, Inc., P.O. Box 42050, Tucson, AZ.)

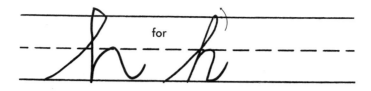

Figure 14-8. Illustration of the problem in changing direction with a continuous flow pattern.
(From *Loops and other groups* by Mary Benbow, copyright 1990 by Therapy Skill Builders, a division of Communication Skill Builders, Inc., P.O. Box 42050, Tucson, AZ.)

stroke direction in a continuous flow pattern. The child feels the need to touch the top of the line and pause before being able to shift line direction. When writing the long ascenders of the loop letters (*h, k, b, f,* and *l*), it is nearly impossible for these children to shift the flow of the right ascending lead-in stroke to the left while approaching the top of the line (Figure 14-8). In these tall loop letters the change of direction is required to prepare for the immediate down stroke once the line top is touched. Changing directions in a continuous flow pattern proves to be a most intractable writing problem. To change direction the child needs to see a demonstration, to hear verbal descriptions of the stroke, to talk about how to move as he/she uses shoulder movements while writing in the air, particularly for the inhibition of the right ascending stroke. Consistent practice to the point of overlearning is necessary for reliable success. The child's inability to change stroke direction in a continuous flow pattern causes a related problem in producing the alternating swoop line used to top capital *F* and capital *T*.

Spatial Analysis

Children with nonlanguage learning disabilities (NLDs), including difficulties with math, nonphonetic spelling, and visualizing (Rourke, (1989), usually lack strategies to analyze geometric shapes, numbers, and letters. These children require detailed letter analysis to learn to write. Small incremental steps (including starting place, pencil progression, distance to move, and place to stop) must be examined and explained and reexamined and reexplained. Retraces, the point of intersection with lead-in strokes, and instructions for the release stroke or connector unit require a great deal of emphasis and repetition. The instructor should emphasize the similarities of letter forms within the letter groups or they will be missed. Visual and verbal images that give letters their identity are required to aid memory and cue the lead-in stroke.

All motor learning requires that speed be matched to task difficulty and the learner's level of skill. Children acquire functional writing more easily when they are speed coached. A therapist can reduce learning time and trial-and-error frustration by explaining where the child should move the pencil slowly and quickly (Benbow, 1990). To hasten developing this sensitivity for all students in the room, initial letter instructions should include speed tips: the lead-in strokes flow more naturally when done quickly; retraces require some visual guidance, so slowing down is advised; speed should be resumed for any single line segment or release stroke that follows. These instructions seem most logical and are usually understood and followed by most second graders. Speed coaching is helpful for children who are struggling with any type of gross or fine motor skill learning.

NLD children can learn cursive writing with their peers when the entire class is given very detailed verbal directions for writing each new letter. The relatively good language skills of NLD students should be called on to support this motor learning.

Writing instructors should be precise in their use of the word *line*. It is confusing to the student to use the same word to describe top and bottom lines and the space between lines. Instructing the student to make a letter "half a line high" only adds to the confusion. If instructors consistently refer to the *top line*, the *writing line*, and the dotted *middle marker*, they will not confuse their students. The area between the lines should always be called a *space* (or *half space* for letters ascending only to the middle marker). It is also helpful to the child if the writing line is darker than the top line for initial learning and practice sessions. Using the designations *writing line*, *top line*, and *middle marker*, the instructor can easily describe what space the letter should fill. For example, all lowercase cursive letters lead in from the writing line and ascend to the middle marker or to the top line.

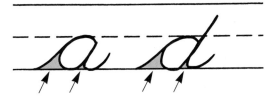

Figure 14-9. Showing negative shapes created between writing lines and letter strokes.

(From *Loops and other groups* by Mary Benbow, copyright 1990 by Therapy Skill Builders, a division of Communication Skill Builders, Inc., P.O. Box 42050, Tucson, AZ.)

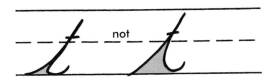

Figure 14-10. Knowing that the triangle should be small prevents a premature release of the down stroke.

(From *Loops and other groups* by Mary Benbow, copyright 1990 by Therapy Skill Builders, a division of Communication Skill Builders, Inc., P.O. Box 42050, Tucson, AZ.)

Seven letters descend to the middle marker below the writing line. Only four letters occupy more than a whole space: lowercase *f*, and capitals *J, Y,* and *Z*.

Negative shapes are created between lines and letter strokes. If students are made aware of them, these negative shapes can aid in determining whether the letters are written correctly. For example, a triangle is created on the writing line by the lead-in stroke and the lower rounded segment of the letters *a* and *d* (Figure 14-9). Contrasting it with the smaller triangle made on the right side of these letters before the release stroke proves to be an intriguing challenge to the novice for quality control. Readily identifiable negative shapes can help the child recognize letter accuracy and serve as a guide for self-correction. These visual cues control for line contact as well. Producing the small triangle at the bases of *i, u, w,* and *t* (Figure 14-10) prevents releasing the down stroke too soon for a good connection or release unit.

Kinesthesia

Writing is a motor skill and, as with other motor skills, efficient writing depends on kinesthetic input. Motor skills developed kinesthetically, such as riding a bike, touch typing, or handwriting, are the most permanent. In writing, an internal sensitivity that a letter movement feels

correct reduces a child's need to visually monitor the fingers or pencil point while moving across the line. This security enhances speed in learning and confidence in cursive writing. Kinesthetic writing naturally accelerates over time to functional speed without the reduction of performance quality seen with visually guided writing. The visual system is far too slow and mechanical to monitor the serial chain of finger movements required for note-taking much beyond fourth grade. Slowing a child down to visually monitor writing temporarily results in more legible paperwork. However this remedy is not practical beyond middle school, when greater speed is required in lecture settings. Therefore kinesthetic training is important whether or not a child has a visual-motor or kinesthetic problem. This is an area of training that should be explored and further developed by early educators.

Kinesthetic skill development is most beneficial for children experiencing visual-motor deficit and for children with diminished kinesthesis. In the former, kinesthesia is the effective compensation for eye-hand coordination difficulties and can be a powerful builder of motor confidence. Kinesthetic training enables these children to bypass their problem area and become efficient writers by concentrating on kinesthetic feedback. If diminished kinesthesis is not enhanced, a child continues an over-reliance on visual monitoring, with a subsequent slowness in the production of writing. Kinesthetic activities are an essential aspect of both prewriting and writing programs.

Kinesthetic skills usually intrigue young children. Elementary kinesthetic activities can be done on desk tops, at the blackboard, or in the gymnasium. A sample for each location follows.

- *Desk top:* Place an object (such as a coin or cube) anywhere on the desk surface within the arc of the child's reach. Withdraw the child's hand to a resting position and ask him/her to close eyes and reach directly to the object. Grade the activity by having the child place the object with one hand and retrieve it with the other.
- *Blackboard:* Sports that have a spatial component (baseball diamond, golf green) can be sketched on the blackboard. After the child visually and motorically senses the size and shape of the display, have him/her close the eyes, visualize the display, and draw with chalk a run from home plate for a single, double, or home run (Figure 14-11).

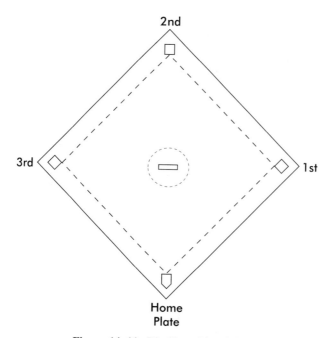

Figure 14-11. Blackboard baseball.
(Copyright: Mary Benbow.)

- *Gym:* After gaining the feel of movement of pitching like objects into a container, have the child close the eyes and use kinesthetic sense to continue the activity. It is important that the child not alter orientation or distance and that the objects be identical in weight and size. The most challenging position for this activity is seated on a one-legged stool.

As noted earlier, kinesthetic writing should use limited visual motor control. Shape copying tests such as VMI (Beery, 1989) are useful in predicting the child's potential ease or difficulty in learning manuscript. They are less helpful in predicting the ease a student will experience in learning cursive writing.

A Production Consistency Sheet (Benbow, 1992) can be used to informally observe a child's kinesthetic aptitude in writing and spacing cursive letters in words using the kinesthetic sense. Model shapes are displayed in the upper left-hand corner of a half sheet of unlined paper (5½ × 8½ inches). Each model is ½ inch high. The models include a square, a circle, a triangle, and a cursive capital *A*. Instruct the students to duplicate the printed model using a fluid moving stroke(s) rather than a rigidly controlled stroke(s). The four shapes should be drawn in three evenly spaced rows of five figures. On completion of the fifteenth figure, the child is told to close the eyes or avert gaze and complete a fourth row that looks like and is spaced like the rows above. The quality of the first three rows reveals the child's visual-motor control of horizontal, vertical, diagonal, or circular lines. The consistency of the fourth row is a graphic demonstration of the child's kinesthetic learning potential for both configuring and spacing. The two examples selected in Figure 14-12 were drawn by 10-year-old boys who were classmates in a third grade classroom. Consistency in shape, size, and spacing is a high indicator of potential for learning cursive writing. In comparing these two samples one can predict that the child who drew Figure 14-12, *A*, will learn to write with less difficulty than the child who drew Figure 14-12, *B*.

Summary

Children who benefit from ongoing diagnostic handwriting training usually have identifiable problems in one or more of several early childhood prewriting foundation skills. First is gross and fine motor readiness for cursive instruction. Output or production problems can include difficulties with visual control, bilateral integration, and spatial analysis and synthesis. Feedback difficulties include inadequacies in visual and kinesthetic reafferent systems.

Developmentally sequenced hand activities should be the major fine motor focus in preschools

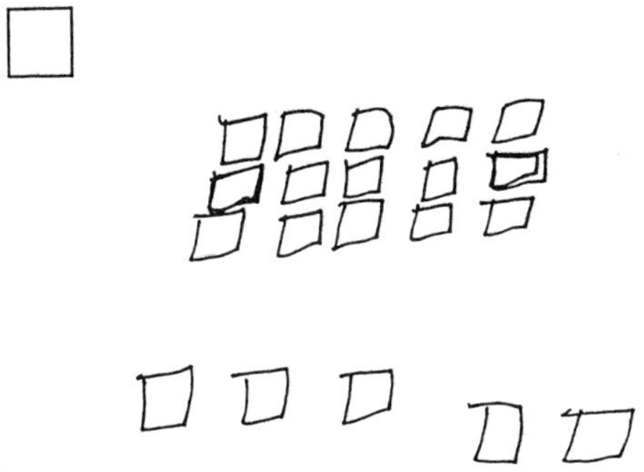

Figure 14-12. Production consistency of an average writer (**A**) and a poor writer (**B**).

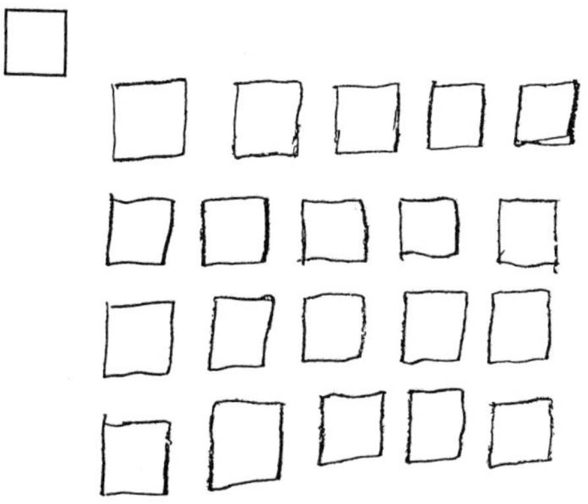

(Copyright: Mary Benbow.)

and early elementary education. Early educators should develop the full potential of children's hands for all skills since the remediation of prewriting hand skills greatly facilitates the learning of graphic skills. The following sections of the chapter now turn to two specific aspects of handwriting training, pencil grip and kinesthetic writing.

HANDWRITING TRAINING: PENCIL GRIP

Letter production in children can be influenced by the way they grip a writing tool. This section includes a description of pencil grips, a report on a research study of the influence of pencil grip on writing speed and pressure, and a discussion of the limitation imposed by maladaptive grips, with some remedial strategies.

Tripod Grip and Alternative Grips

Handwriting is the most complex and utilized motor skill required in education, yet little attention is paid to how, when, or where pencil practice best enhances the development of this skill. Adults

seem to assume that children will somehow know the best way to hold a pencil or that they will acquire the ability through incidental experience (Connolly, 1973). Rosenbloom and Horton (1971) found 89 of 92 British children and Saida and Miyashita (1979) found 151 of 154 Japanese children to have developed a dynamic tripod pencil skill by 72 months.

Benbow (1987) found only 33 of 68 American children of the same age who used this grip. The other 35 children were managing in school with a grip that was less efficient to maladroit. Any grip, efficient or inefficient, that has been used over time becomes kinesthetically locked in. An immature tool grip that is kinesthetically locked in inhibits a student's ability to advance to a higher level even after hand development has progressed.

Among 7-year-old normal children in a Boston suburb, more quadrupod grips—four digits (three fingers and the thumb) on the pencil shaft—were found than tripod grips, where three digits are on the pencil shaft (Benbow, 1987). This open thumb web alternative to the normal tripod grip most likely develops with premature use of pencils and/or low joint stability in the hand. The additional finger on the shaft adds power for stroking as well as a wider bridge to stabilize the pencil shaft. Many quadrupod grips do progress to become dynamic and fully functional (Kaplin, 1990). The two slight disadvantages of this grip are reduction in pencil point excursion and reduced stability of the MP arch when the little finger is used alone rather than being functionally coupled with the ring finger.

A few children assume an adapted tripod grip (Figure 14-13) in which they stabilize their pencil within the narrower web space between the middle and index fingers. This is an effective anatomic adaptation when joint stability is insufficient for controlled mobility. All of the skilled muscles of the classic dynamic tripod manipulate the pencil, and the MP joint of the thumb receives little if any stress. This posture is the most readily accepted alternate grip when a child or an adult is having motor or orthopedic writing problems.

Connolly (1973) states that joint stability in the hand is not necessarily related to force but depends on ligaments and fixed structures. Working with schoolchildren, one sees evidence that the functional use of the hand depends more on joint stability than joint mobility. Children adopt many ways to make their hands work for them when they lack joint stability. If the MP joint of the thumb is unstable, the web space collapses when

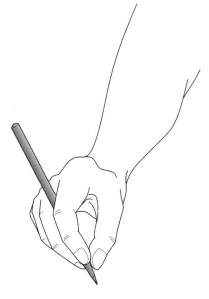

Figure 14-13. Adapted tripod grip.
(Copyright: Mary Benbow.)

the pulp of the thumb is used to stabilize a tool in the distal fingertips or against another digit. A child will unknowingly substitute the adductor pollicis for the three more highly skilled muscles of the thenar eminence: abductor pollicis brevis, flexor pollicis brevis, and opponens (Cooper, 1960). This substitution causes the thumb to supinate due to the angle of pull from its insertion on the internal sesamoid bone (Tubiana, 1981, citing Cruveilher). When using a pen or pencil, this individual wraps the thumb over or tucks the thumb under the index finger to control the stroke. Either grip provides a distal point of stability with the challenge to devise a system to mobilize the pencil proximally. When the web space is closed snugly over the pencil shaft, the MP joint support structures are stressed in an outward direction, and the proprioceptive feedback used to guide and grade fine motor muscles is reduced.

Study of Pencil Grip

A promising area of new research involves the use of a WACOM digitizer, which records a user's pen position 200 times each second during handwriting. The data are transmitted to a computer for processing and printing as a Graphogram.* Graphograms illustrate the continuous variations of the writer's axial pen force against the writing surface;

*The Graphogram representation was developed by Meeks Associates, Inc., Lincoln, MA, which has a patent pending on the commercial use of this method for displaying handwriting.

alternatively they illustrate the instantaneous stroke speed and pauses while the person is writing. These variables are represented by the varying width of an envelope surrounding the writing trace.

Sixty-seven grade school children ages 6 years 6 months to 10 years 8 months participated in a study designed to develop norms for the axial pen force exerted during name writing. The range of axial pen pressures was divided into 100-g intervals from 50 to 650 g, for the three age groups. In this study the children exerted a mean axial force of 301 g, with a standard deviation of 101.7 g (Benbow, 1991). Figure 14-14 illustrates the axial force distribution of this population.

The correlation of pencil grip with pencil axial force was not found to be significant within the average range of axial force. However, an adducted grip (closed web) was recorded in 10 of the 11 subjects whose axial force was above average (>350 g). Only one of the high axial force group used an open web or tripod grip. In the 12 subjects whose axial force was below average (<250 g), eight had tripod grips and eight had variations of nonopposition or partial web openings. However, the low force group was limited to the younger age ranges. In examining the graph in Figure 14-14 note that no subject between 6½ and 7¾ years was recorded above 450 g.

The Graphograms in Figures 14-15 to 14-18 display dynamic axial pen force, speed, and pauses while writing a connected series of letters—*lelele*—within ½-inch divided-line paper. The upper displays show that axial pen force changed as each student wrote the letter series. The wider the envelope around the line, the heavier the force against the writing surface. The bottom displays indicate ongoing speed of the pencil strokes. The wider the envelope, the faster the stroke. The circles show location and length of pauses during the writing sequence. The larger the circle, the longer the pause. These Graphograms were produced by four mainstreamed students at the completion of their second grade. All subjects had received kinesthetic cursive instruction for 9 months as part of their second grade curriculum and had been using cursive handwriting for all of their written work. Interestingly enough, the written series of all four students looks essentially the same.

Figure 14-15 was written by a girl using a dynamic tripod pencil grip. The axial force of 301 g was the mean pressure in the study noted previously. Total writing time for the six letters was 8.7 seconds. The only pause, indicated by the circle, is noted on initiation of the lead-in stroke.

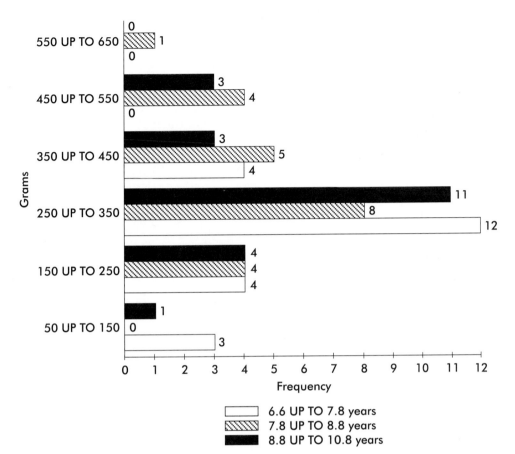

Figure 14-14. Distribution of average axial force.

(Courtesy Meeks Associates, Inc., Lincoln, MA.)

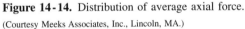

FILE: 208   PRESSURE   Scale (grams): ■301

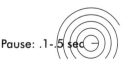

PEN SPEED   Scale (cm/sec): ■5.1 ■2.6   Pause: .1-.5 sec

Time (total): 8.7 sec   Time (pause): 0.2 sec

Figure 14-15. Graphogram: dynamic tripod pencil grip.

(Courtesy Meeks Associates, Inc., Lincoln, MA.)

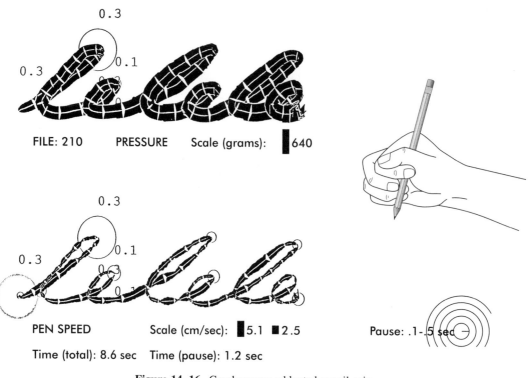

Figure 14-16. Graphogram: adducted pencil grip.

(Courtesy Meeks Associates, Inc., Lincoln, MA.)

Figure 14-16 was written by a girl using an adducted grip with the thumb pulp stabilized over the index finger. Her average axial force was 640 g. Total writing time was 8.6 seconds. Note the multiple pauses (circles) and irregular modulation of speed with this less adaptive grip.

Figure 14-17 was written by a boy who assumed the unique tripod grip pictured on the right of his Graphogram. The thumb is flexed at the IP joint to hold the pencil against the radial aspect of a curved middle finger. The straight index finger extends beyond the other two digits along the pencil point. The videotaped analysis of this child revealed that his middle and index fingers were motionless throughout the series. Movement at the thumb IP joint was minimal. Essentially all movement was produced by the wrist flexors and extensors and elbow rotators. His reliance on less adaptable larger joints is probably what slowed his writing time to 15.3 seconds for this simple exercise.

Figure 14-18 was written by a boy with a rigid static tripod grip. The video record shows no movement at any joint of the three radial digits. This rigid posture is frequently observed in children who write fairly accurately but lack the adaptability to develop functional speed. The lack of distal joint mobility in his writing hand probably caused the multiple pauses and the slow writing time of 16.6 seconds.

Note that the pen speed varies smoothly in Figures 14-15 and 14-16, where finger movements were used in stroking. However, in Figures 14-17 and 14-18, where minimal or no finger movement was observed, the Graphograms indicate a series of rapid bursts of movement.

Remediation of Pencil Grip

A number of prosthetic devices pictured in Figure 14-19 have been developed to help position the digits for efficient distal manipulation of writing tools. These devices are sculpted to position the distal aspects of the radial digits into an open thumb/index web posture. Fitting writing tools with positioning grips when preschool children are first exploring pencil use is the most sensible and effective use of these devices. Early implementation of these devices should eliminate the struggle to correct the inefficient grip after it has been reinforced and kinesthetically locked in.

When a child's hands are developing well and the pencil grip is variable or poorly postured, a finger placement device will often promote an open web posture in 4 to 6 weeks in primary age children. Flat triangular grips and triangular pencils are helpful but less exact when the goal is to open the web space for distal manipulation of the pencil.

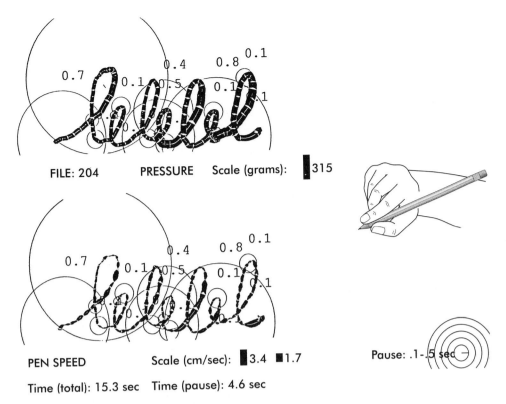

FILE: 204   PRESSURE   Scale (grams): ▮315

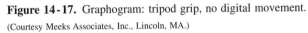

PEN SPEED   Scale (cm/sec): ▮3.4 ■1.7   Pause: .1-.5 sec ⊖

Time (total): 15.3 sec   Time (pause): 4.6 sec

Figure 14-17. Graphogram: tripod grip, no digital movement.

(Courtesy Meeks Associates, Inc., Lincoln, MA.)

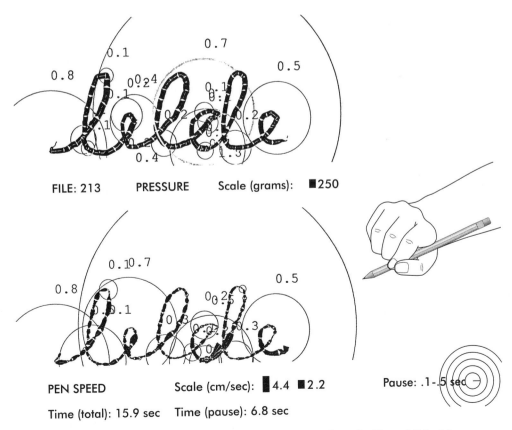

FILE: 213   PRESSURE   Scale (grams): ■250

PEN SPEED   Scale (cm/sec): ▮4.4 ■2.2   Pause: .1-.5 sec ⊖

Time (total): 15.9 sec   Time (pause): 6.8 sec

Figure 14-18. Graphogram: static tripod pencil grip. (Note: the "bow tie" in this graphogram is an artifact of the computer readout.)

(Courtesy Meeks Associates, Inc., Lincoln, MA.)

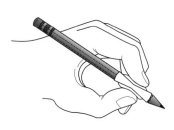
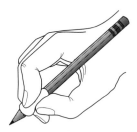
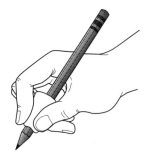

Figure 14-19. Prosthetic writing devices.

(Copyright: Mary Benbow.)

Success in advancing a child from a proximal power grip to a distal precision grip by means of a positioning device depends on the underlying cause(s). When limited rotation or abduction at the MP joints of the radial digits forces the fingertips distally beyond the device, specific therapeutic techniques should be implemented to increase intrinsic control of these two digits. In these cases the therapeutic goal should be to develop radial rotation at the index MP, abduction between the long and index MP joints, and more complete arching of the transverse metacarpal arch. A positioning device can be an effective reminder to maintain the advanced posture.

Joint hyperextension (white knuckle) at the DIP joint of the index finger is typically seen in combination with hyperflexion at the PIP joint (Figure 14-20). This hyperflexion reduces the equalizing control of length and tension between the finger's flexor and extensor system. With PIP hyperflexion the flexor digitorum profundus slackens by the pull from its lumbrical and is unable to exert flexor influence at the DIP joint. This finger posture allows the DIP joint to be easily pressed into hyperextension (Stack, 1962).

Limiting hyperflexion at the PIP joint or hyperextension at the DIP joint can be accomplished by taping or blocking PIP hyperflexion with a tape support, a neoprene joint jig, or a ring splint. With smaller, weaker, and less experienced hands tape support is often an adequate supplement to the extensor system. Microfoam surgical tape by the 3M Company increases joint awareness while adding stability to the extensor system. A ⅛-inch wide strip of Microfoam tape is affixed to the middle dorsal aspect of the index finger while the digit is positioned in full extension. The distal end of the tape should be attached to the nail and continue proximally over the DIP, PIP, and the MP joints to the midmetacarpal level (Figure 14-21). The tape should be adjusted to give the joint(s) stability without rigidity. Some children choose to use the tape when a large amount of written work

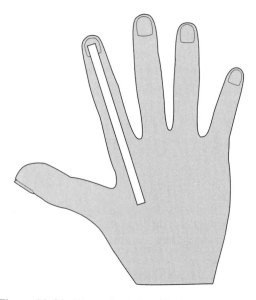

Figure 14-20. Pencil grip, showing hyperextension of the distal interphalangeal joint and hyperflexion of the proximal interphalangeal joint.

(Copyright: Mary Benbow.)

Figure 14-21. Illustration of positioning of Microfoam surgical tape on the back of the index finger to improve joint awareness and add joint stability.

(Copyright: Mary Benbow.)

is required, whereas others will insist on wearing the tape most of the day.

The ability to stabilize the CMC and MP joints of the thumb is critical for tripod manipulation of objects and tools. The IP joint will not be a functional mobilizer if the MP joint cannot provide it with a stable base of support. This stability/mobility problem renders the hand most dysfunctional, especially in the manipulation of coloring or writing implements. External support provided by taping the posterior aspect of the thumb in younger children with less severe cases often adds sufficient support to make this digit functional. Taping techniques outlined for the index finger can be applied to the thumb. When the MP joint of the thumb is moderately unstable due to ligamentous laxity, a positioning device helps hold and protect the joint while writing.

A forearm, wrist, and pencil grip adaptation to extreme laxity at the thumb MP joint is illustrated in Figure 14-22. The forearm is maintained in midrotation between supination and pronation and is solidly stabilized on the writing surface. The pencil shaft is cradled into the flexed index IP joint and extends distally across the third, fourth, and occasionally the fifth fingertips. The lead end of the pencil is pointed toward the writer's midline. Writing strokes come from a combination of wrist flexion and MP finger extension with minimal thumb IP flexion. Because the writer does not progressively slide the solidly stabilized forearm while writing, there is a need for the interplay between thumb IP hyperextension and wrist flexion. Writing into right space requires increasing flexion at the thumb IP joint and hyperextension at the wrist. When the wrist is fully hyperextended, a major right shift of the forearm is required for the next position from which to write additional letters or words.

Because this grip remains so nonfunctional over time, it is prudent to intervene as early as possible. Generally, when the joint support structures and extrinsic tendons cannot provide stability with the added support of the tape, the therapist should explore the use of a soft neoprene thumb abduction splint. This short glove-type splint positions the thumb in abduction and provides stability at the hypermobile MP joint when the thumb tip is positioned on the pencil shaft (Figure 14-23). Neoprene provides stability without the rigidity of a thermoplastic device. Wrist-length neoprene gloves designed to provide thumb positioning and stabilizing are commercially available in appealing colors and multiple sizes. Supplementing the splint with a wrist extension support is also possible with these gloves (Benik, 1992).

School therapists, knowledgeable in developmental hand functions, must use mature professional judgment in determining if, how, and when adaptations, motor interventions, or outside stabilization will be beneficial to the child. The expectations of the child, teacher, and parents must be fully appreciated and honestly incorporated into every child's educational plan. The therapist should include recommendations for short-term trials and offer periodic reassessments for their acceptability and effectiveness.

Many persistent persons write satisfactorily with horrible grips. Many of these grips require

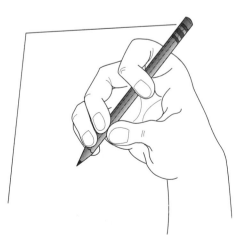

Figure 14-22. Pencil grip adaptation to extreme laxity of the metacarpal-phalangeal joint of the thumb.

(Copyright: Mary Benbow.)

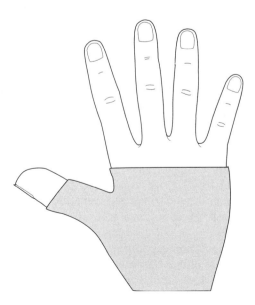

Figure 14-23. Neoprene thumb abduction splint.

(Copyright: Mary Benbow.)

the person to develop skilled use of proximal joints, which lack the precise control of the distal joints. A pencil held in a closed web grip by the adductor pollicis cannot move very far or use the rotary agility of the index MP joint in producing rounded strokes. Curving and rounding must be produced by more proximal joints requiring supination at the elbow and external or internal rotation at the shoulder. Wrist and forearm extensors must produce elongation of upstrokes, which is efficiently done using a digital translation away pattern and minimal wrist extension. A few writers use the entire skilled side (radial) of the hand to clutch and stabilize the pencil, and mobilize the pencil by extending and flexing the three joints of the power digits IV and V.

KINESTHETIC APPROACH TO TEACHING HANDWRITING
Cursive vs. Manuscript Writing

One of the difficulties facing anyone investigating handwriting teaching and remediation issues is the lack of longitudinal studies in the field. Studies of preparatory skills, curriculum techniques, and timetables for the consolidation of skill at an automatic level are scarce. Tradition rather than scientific investigation has guided the teaching of handwriting in America. For example, there are no studies to substantiate the practice of using manuscript throughout kindergarten and first and second grade. In fact there is considerable evidence showing that such teaching may impede the development of functional handwriting in some students. Cursive instruction is typically introduced at the beginning of grade three (Bergman and McLaughlin, 1988).

Several motor patterns adopted for printing and reinforced by 3 to 5 years of use are often resistant to change at age 8. In manuscript, children become accustomed to having the paper square to the edge of the desk in order to "write." Later, slanting the paper to the appropriate angle to accommodate the wrist for diagonal down stroking and up stroking in cursive is motorically disconcerting for many children. The D'Nealian manuscript program is unique in that letters are practiced with the paper positioned at an angle to take advantage of the wrist flexors in down stroking. Interestingly, this angling of the paper is beneficial only when the radial side of the hand is used to guide the pencil to write. However, this placement of the paper is usually demanded of all children regardless of grip. In addition, the eye-hand pattern of top to

bottom control of verticals needs to be shifted to bottom to top under curving diagonals.

The strategy for gaining an understanding of ball and stick manuscript letters requires whole-to-part analysis. The production of these letters requires the synthesis of the parts back into wholes. For many children it is perplexing to alter the process and analyze and integrate movement for the whole letter formation required for cursive writing. Again the D'Nealian manuscript program has been the most successful in reducing segmentation of lines for letter formations.

In my extensive experience in the teaching of handwriting I have found that second grade is an optimal time for most children to learn cursive handwriting. Student interest is high, and generally students have not yet developed faulty habits of inventive cursive before formal instruction begins. Training activities of combining letters into simple two- and three-letter words to practice letter formations and connector units are at a more appropriate cognitive level for second grade students. Initiating cursive writing instruction in the fall of second grade allows a full year for students to stabilize this motor learning before the higher volume of written work expected at the third grade level.

Curricula that use instructional techniques to accommodate for perceptual and motor delays and deficits should enable nearly all children to advance to cursive writing at an earlier age. In schools where cursive writing is introduced earlier and mastered kinesthetically, there is less confusion with and substitution of manuscript letters with cursive letters. Programming ample time to master cursive writing reduces the number of children who revert to manuscript in middle school when the output volume increases dramatically.

Motor Patterns in Cursive Writing

Motor output for cursive writing requires continuous stroke patterns. For this reason cursive letter analysis and instructions should be programed to maximize visualization of the whole. Mental formulation of the plan and verbalization of the entire motor sequence should be stressed. This elicits the child's proprioceptive and kinesthetic sense that supports the flow of the whole letter.

Most published handwriting programs currently in use employ a "copy the letter" scheme followed by visually guided reproduction of the letter within divided lines. Able or not, children are typically expected to convert to cursive writing during the fall of third grade. Many curricula introduce one or two alphabetically sequenced lowercase letters each week. Such slow progressions mean that the lowercase letters are unavailable for classroom work for 3 or 4 months, and the uppercase letters still remain to be learned. Other programs introduce the lowercase and uppercase of the same letter in tandem. Shifting unrelated motor patterns for lead-in strokes required when either alphabetical system is followed does not facilitate efficient motor learning.

Grouping letters according to common movement patterns overcomes many of these difficulties (Benbow, 1990). After the initial session of introducing the movement pattern, during which each child learns to verbalize the pattern and produce it kinesthetically, additional letters in the group can be learned expeditiously. The learning process is further hastened by reinforcement as all of the letters within the cluster are practiced together.

General instructions included in most handwriting manuals are inadequate for children experiencing visual-motor difficulties, incomplete bilateral integration, weak spatial analyzing ability, and attention or memory problems. Specific compensations for their special needs must be included with initial classroom instructions or their classroom practice periods will not be productive. In many schools the practice time is insufficient for all but the most skilled students to achieve functional output ability. Children are as frustrated by their handwriting failures as are their parents and teachers. Those with special needs, along with many who have simply not received enough help or time to master this complex motor task, resign themselves to poor handwriting or simply revert to manuscript, which received more teaching time and reinforcement in the lower grades.

Why Teach Writing Kinesthetically?

Writing is a motor skill that requires competent motor teaching and reinforced motor learning. Fitts (1964) believed the process of skill acquisition falls into three stages. The first, the cognitive stage, involves the initial encoding of the instructions for a skill into a form sufficient for the learner to generate the behavior to some crude approximation. He emphasized that rehearsal of information is necessary for the execution of skill. The second, the associative stage, involves smoothing out of the motor performance with gradual detection and elimination of errors and the dropping of verbal mediation. The third, the autonomous stage, is one of gradual improvement that may continue indefinitely.

It is important to distinguish these motor skill requirements for writing from other classroom learning. Learning to write is very different from learning to read. If it were not, more good readers would be able to write legibly. Learning to write is not a language skill, though language skills are required to supply the content of written production. Learning to write should not be coupled with learning the alphabet. Learning to write letters in alphabetical order is more likely to enhance alphabetizing skills than handwriting skills. As with all fine motor skills, a student must understand that the head learns to write faster than the hand. The hand requires hundreds of repetitions before writing is fast, easy, and automatic.

By its very nature a kinesthetic approach to handwriting provides children with a clear, enjoyable progression from (1) the placement of the letter within the three half-space vertical units, to (2) the precise motor analysis with verbal support of the motor plan, to (3) the appropriate variations in speed, to (4) the practice with eyes closed or averted and finally, to (5) the reinforcing or setting of motor and memory engrams at an automatic level.

The product of visually guided, or drawn, writing may be legible or even beautiful but will not be functional because its methodical execution is too slow and too consuming of cognitive power. The motor activity of writing must be fairly autonomous to free cognitive power for composing and spelling. The human nervous system can focus clearly on only one complex mental task at a time. Related skills, such as writing, must be sufficiently automatic to be carried out at an associative skill level. It is beyond the ability of most persons to compose a complex sentence and think about the way each letter in each word is executed. This failure in skill mastery is often the cause of a typical parent or teacher complaint: "My brilliant child's hand cannot keep pace with his mind."

Luria (1980) explains that

There must be a constant flow of afferent impulses, not only from external objects that are to be taken into account when the movement is constructed, but also, and primarily from the subject's own locomotor apparatus, whose every change in position alters the conditions of the movement. This is why the decisive factors in the construction of movement are not so much the effector impulses (which are of a rather purely executive character), as the complex system of afferent impulses that give precision to the composition of the motor act and that ensure that the movements are subjected to a wide variety of correction (p. 190).

Levine (1987) expands Luria's work in noting that

The complex motor action of writing is overwhelmingly dependent upon accurate, ongoing kinesthetic (reafferent) feedback. Before undertaking the written transcription of a word or sentence, the writer has a kinesthetic plan in mind. She or he compares ongoing kinesthetic feedback to the original plan in order to correct, persist in, or terminate the graphomotor pattern. A breakdown in the kinesthetic feedback to the original plan process is a common and insidious deterrent to writing. . . . Children with impaired kinesthetic feedback . . . often show no impairment whatsoever with other aspects of fine motor function. . . . This discrepancy can occur because nonwriting tasks consist of predominantly visual input and visual kinesthetic feedback . . . visual feedback during writing is far too slow and mechanical. It is not easy for them to monitor the serial chain of motor movements . . . writing becomes too slow and much too awkward; as a result, automatization of motor movement is delayed or absent (pp. 226–227).

Kinesthetic Teaching Method

Handwriting is a motor skill of the highest order. When kinesthetic teaching techniques are incorporated from the very beginning of handwriting instruction, the child will naturally develop a kinesthetic potential for writing and for other fine motor skills as well. The kinesthetic method of teaching cursive writing presented in *Loops and Other Groups* (Benbow, 1990) provides both general and compensatory instructions that are required for teaching in a mainstreamed classroom. It enables learning disabled students to progress with their normal peers. Compensatory instructions and tips are included for students with perceptual-motor delays or deficits including difficulty with visually producing diagonals, midline crossing interruptions, and fluctuating motor memory for configurations.

The group names for letters relate to familiar objects in a child's environment and promote visualization of the lead-in strokes. The first letter in each of the four groups must be mastered at the kinesthetic level before the child is allowed to advance to the next letter. As soon as any letter is mastered, instructions are given for connecting it to itself or other known letters. The student's awareness of and repetition of the common motor patterns within each group hasten mastery of the skill by reinforcing motor learning of the entire group.

I have conducted successful kinesthetic writing programs by dividing the learning of lowercase letters into six teaching blocks for classroom use.

The blocks are rapidly (6 weeks) but thoroughly taught in daily 30-minute sessions during September and October in the second grade. The lowercase letters are consistently reinforced with daily practice and used whenever possible (such as spelling tests when children have learned the required letters) to reinforce and stabilize this new skill. During the fall, manuscript capitals are used in combination with lowercase cursive letters for all written assignments. The cursive capitals are introduced after the winter holiday vacation. This interval allows time for lowercase to become stabilized before the capitals are introduced. This interim significantly reduces uppercase and lowercase confusion in children with weak memory for configuration.

Kinesthetic Remediation Techniques

Writing errors often tend to cluster and make a paper look sloppy. With older students, correcting one or two cluster errors is effective in producing an acceptable-looking paper. Overall appearance can often be significantly improved by gaining control of the seven loops that descend below the writing line to the middle marker. The three common cluster errors include these seven loop letters, whose loops are often huge, carelessly formed "sausages" that interfere with the lower line of writing. The second deciphering error is incomplete closure of the four round-over-the-top letters in the *a*, or clock climber, group (*a, d, g, q*). The third cluster error is failure to retrace letters to the writing line before the release stroke. This failure places the connector unit too high or too low to lead into the letter that follows it.

Cluster remediation is often more palatable for older students to undertake. Group letter analysis and speed coaching for segments to be produced quickly or slowly offers new hope that is motivating for these often discouraged students. With kinesthetic training, reinforcement, and moderate persistence most students will be self-motivated to improve their output quality and increase their writing quantity as well.

Line space should be compatible with the fineness or bluntness of the writing implement and distal digital excursion of the writing tool—not the grade, age, or height of the writer. Line space of ½ inch or more naturally elicits movement from more proximal, less skilled joints. Regardless of age, when fine motor muscles are to be trained for graphic skills, the letter, number, or symbol size to be learned must be within the excursion distance

Distal Finger Control

Rest side of hand on desk. Use one stroke to circle left from top around to top within the donut.

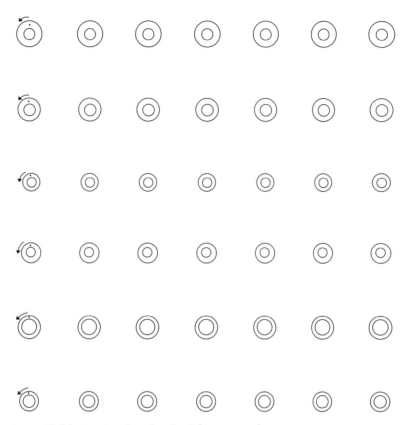

Figure 14-24. Practice sheet for distal finger control.

(From *Loops and other groups* by Mary Benbow, copyright 1990 by Therapy Skill Builders, a division of Communication Skill Builders, Inc., P.O. Box 42050, Tucson, AZ.)

of the digits that manipulate the pencil. A distal control sheet (Figure 14-24) can be used to determine the ideal line rule for older students. Accurate stroke excursion flows more naturally and shows better control when producing strokes within a compatibly ruled paper. Most learning disabled students and children with restricted grips produce their best writing on the ¼-inch ruled paper. In addition, this narrower ruled paper feels right for their motor system (Benbow, 1990).

An efficient way for the evaluator to detect well-formed letters that have not been learned to the automatic level is to look for connector breaks in the line at the point where the lead-in stroke is initiated. Figure 14-25 indicates breaks in writing the alphabet before the letters *f, j, r, s,* and *y*. These breaks generally slow the writer's overall speed. The interruptions, or think breaks, can also be detected within words, but a connected cursive

alphabet is the most thorough and efficient way to assess every letter of the alphabet. Specifically reinforcing the identified letters that follow "think breaks" to the automatic level can often convert nonfunctional output speed into functional skill.

Kinesthetic reinforcement of letters can increase writing speed while maintaining quality in a child who writes beautifully but has not developed functional speed. After carefully reexamining the line progression of any known letter and producing it with visual guidance, the child should close his/her eyes, visualize the letter, and write with fluidity on scrap paper 15 times before checking the results. Once the initial letter within a motor group is written reliably at an efficient speed, the remaining letters of the group should be brought up to speed one by one. A most popular time to suggest for children to increase their speed in writing is while watching television. The

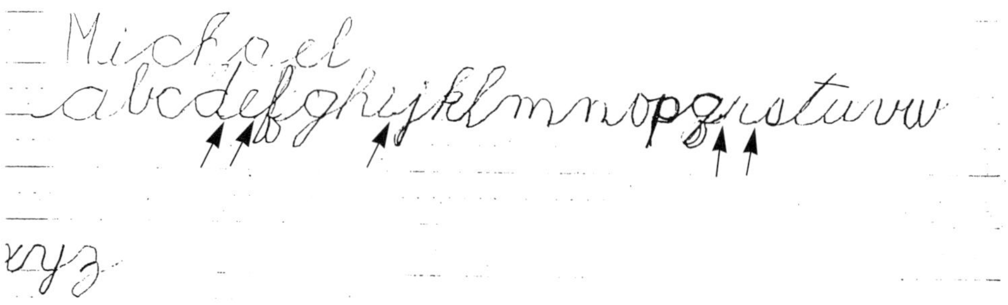

Figure 14-25. Think breaks in writing.
(Copyright: Mary Benbow.)

combination of these two activities diverts visual monitoring from the writing hand, and the student willingly extends practice periods.

Learning Sequence

The learning sequence for handwriting training in an mainstreamed classroom should be as follows.

Seating Posture and Classroom Arrangement

Properly fitted furniture is essential if children are to learn handwriting efficiently. If the chairs are too high and the child's heels do not touch the floor, he/she will be unable to counterbalance himself/herself for weight shift as the arm moves across the paper. If the desk surface is too high, the upper arm will be abducted too far to control the fingers effectively. Figure 14-26 illustrates a properly fitted student chair and desk for writing.

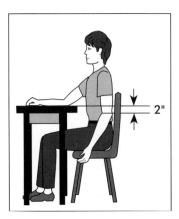

Figure 14-26. Correct sitting posture for handwriting. Knees and hips are flexed at 90 degrees and feet are flat on the floor. Writing surface is 2 inches above the student's bent elbow. Top of chair should be slightly below the student's shoulder blade.

(From *Loops and other groups* by Mary Benbow, copyright 1990 by Therapy Skill Builders, a division of Communication Skill Builders, Inc., P.O. Box 42050, Tucson, AZ.)

Every child's desk should face the blackboard where the teacher demonstrates the letters. There may be subjects that can best be learned in cluster or circular seating, but handwriting is not one of them.

Presentation of a Model

The instructor introduces every letter by producing a 15-inch model of it within the appropriate line space(s) on the blackboard. While demonstrating each new letter the instructor should speak aloud each step of the motor plan. Familiar objects in the student's environment are used to aid the students in visualizing the movement pattern as they motorically sense the stroke progression. For example, the lead-in stroke for the letter *a* should climb up and round over a clock face between the 11 and 1 o'clock positions and stop before retracing this lead-in to 9 o'clock (Figure 14-27). A popular visual image is to drop an egg on the writing line after the initial lead-in stroke for the letter *o* (Benbow, 1990).

Preparatory Exercises

Before using pencils, children perform two prepaper exercises. In each exercise they are to use the hand posture shown in Figure 14-28. Digits II and III are extended. Digits IV and V are flexed and held down with the thumb to reinforce separation of the two sides of the hand. For each exercise and each practice trial, verbal directions should be voiced by the teacher and the students.

The students should use shoulder movements and the hand postures described previously to trace the letter in the air. At the same time each student verbalizes the motor plan while following the shape of the blackboard model. Each student in the class must demonstrate the ability to verbalize the motor plan while following the line of the letter model.

When secure in an understanding of the motor sequence, each student closes the eyes to facilitate

Clock Climbers

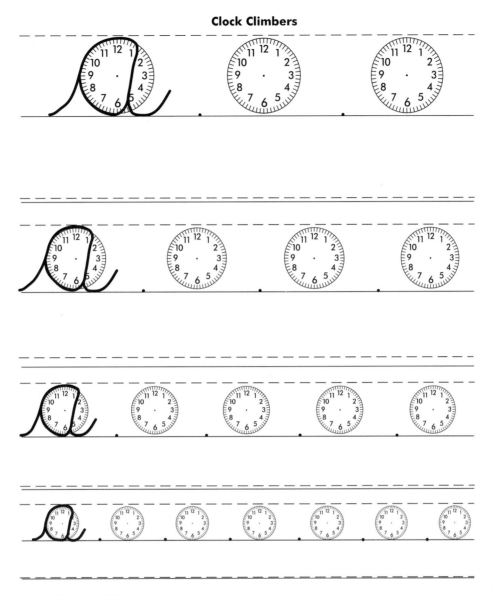

Figure 14-27. Practice sheet for clock climber group (*a, d, g, q, e*).

(From *Loops and other groups* by Mary Benbow, copyright 1990 by Therapy Skill Builders, a division of Communication Skill Builders, Inc., P.O. Box 42050, Tucson, AZ.)

visualization and the kinesthetic movement pattern. At this stage students place their elbows on the desk top to "write" using elbow and wrist movements. Again, they must recite the motor plan aloud as they move their hands to pattern the visualized letter.

These preparatory exercises are most essential to the initial learning of handwriting. In a mainstreamed classroom the instructor is able to see which children are unable to pattern the model letter, verbalize the motor plan, and visualize the letter with eyes closed or gaze averted. With a few additional minutes of coaching, nearly every student can be brought to a base level of skill before pencil and paper are introduced.

Paper and Pencil

Half-inch lined paper with a dotted middle marker is most satisfactory for early cursive practice with visual guidance. Using the newly learned motor plan, children complete ten trials of the letter. They are told to, "talk to your hand, and make it do what you tell it to do." It is important that children subvocalize the motor plan as they form the letter. The instructor should be sure that the letter is placed in the proper space(s) in relation to the writing line and the middle marker.

After 10 trials students should circle all of the letters that are correct. Among those, they should select the one that is the best and write 20 more from their own kinesthetic model.

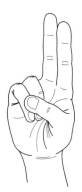

Figure 14-28. Hand posture used in preparatory exercises.

(From *Loops and other groups* by Mary Benbow, copyright 1990 by Therapy Skill Builders, a division of Communication Skill Builders, Inc., P.O. Box 42050, Tucson, AZ.)

When all children are confident in their ability to write the letter with eyes open, they should close the eyes to visualize and gain the feel of the smaller movement pattern. Children who have tracking, converging, or crossing the midline visual disorganization should spend a major portion of their practice time with their eyes closed or gaze averted to avoid visual interference.

CONCLUSION

Kinesthetic handwriting training takes the drudgery out of a task that is often difficult and time-consuming. For all children and for their teachers, this provides some benefit. For some children, kinesthetic training is the single most effective tool for learning handwriting.

Children who benefit the most from kinesthetic handwriting training usually have identifiable problems in one or more general areas. Developmental gross and fine motor foundation skills for cursive instruction may be less than optimal. Output or production problems may include difficulties with visual control. Feedback difficulties include inadequacies in visual reafferent systems.

Kinesthesia is the key to the lost science of handwriting. Properly understood, it is the basis for understanding handwriting problems and for preventing or remediating them. Kinesthesia can be either a curse or a blessing. When a complex motor activity is scientifically analyzed, appropriate foundation skills are set, teaching steps are properly sequenced, and the skill is practiced to the automatic level of performance, kinesthesia is a lifelong blessing in the performance of that skill. On the other hand, maladaptive kinesthesic patterns can be a curse. When a motor activity is

haphazardly acquired at an immature stage of development and reinforced to the automatic level of performance, the kinesthesic pattern can last a lifetime, blocking effective and efficient performance of the skill and frustrating any attempts to modify it.

One of the world's great artists, Henri Matisse, once confirmed the importance of what I have called kinesthetic learning (Bernier, 1991). A friend who visited him noticed a sketch in white chalk on the back of his living room door. Matisse explained, "I had been working all morning [drawing] from the model. *I wanted to know if I had it in my fingers.* So I had myself blindfolded, and I walked to the door and drew" (p. 30, italics added).

The process that worked for Matisse is precisely the kinesthetic learning that is most effective for training children in handwriting. In cursive handwriting, as in drawing from a model, if I don't have it "in my fingers" my work will be slow, crude, and unsightly. This approach allows children to discover what the great artist described.

REFERENCES

Ayres, A. J. (1991). Sensory integration and praxis tests. In A. G. Fisher, E. A. Murray, & A. C. Bundy (Eds.). *Sensory integration, theory and practice.* Philadelphia: F. A. Davis.

Beery, K. E. (1989). *Developmental test of visual-motor integration.* Cleveland: Modern Curriculum Press.

Benbow, M. (1987). *Sensory and motor measurements of dynamic tripod skill.* Unpublished masters thesis. Boston, MA: Boston University.

Benbow, M. (1990). *Loops and other groups. A kinesthetic writing system.* Tucson: Therapy Skill Builders.

Benbow, M. (1991). *An anatomist's view of pen grip and graphic production.* Paper presented at the International Graphonomic Society, Section on the Motor Control of Handwriting, October, 1991.

Benbow, M., Hanft, B., & Marsh, D. (1992). *Handwriting in the classroom: Improving written communication.* The American Occupational Therapy Association Self Study Series. Rockville, MD: The American Occupational Therapy Association Press.

Benik. (1992). *Catalogue of neoprene supports.* Silverdale, WA.

Bergman, K. E., & McLaughlin, T. F. (1988). Remediating handwriting difficulties with learning disabled students: A review. *Boston College Journal of Special Education, 12*(2), 101-120.

Bernier, R. (1991). *Matisse, Picasso, Miro: As I knew them.* New York: Alfred A. Knopf.

Bradshaw, J. L., & Nettleton, N. C. (1983). *Human cerebral asymmetry.* Englewood Cliffs, NJ: Prentice Hall.

Bunnell, S. (1970). *Surgery of the hand* (5th ed.). Philadelphia: J. B. Lippincott.

Capener, N. (1956). The hand in surgery. *The Journal of Bone and Joint Surgery, 38B*(1), 128-140.

Compton, C. (1985). *A guide to 75 tests for special education*. Belmont, CA: Pittman Learning.

Connolly, K. J. (1973). *Factors influencing the learning of manual skills in children*. London: Academic Press.

Cooper, S. (1960). Muscle spindles and other receptors. In G. H. Bourne (Ed.). *The structure and function of muscles* (vol. 1). New York: Academic Press.

Elliott, J. M., & Connolly, K. J. (1984). A classification of manipulative hand movements. *Developmental Medicine and Child Neurology, 26,* 283-296.

Exner, C. E. (1992). In-hand manipulation skills. In J. Case-Smith & C. Pehoski (Eds.). *Development of hand skills in children*. Rockville, MD: American Occupational Therapy Association.

Fitts, P. M. (1964). Perceptual motor skill learning. In A. W. Melton (Ed.). *Categories of human learning*. New York: Academic Press.

Kapandji, I. A. (1982). *The physiology of the joints*. New York: Churchill-Livingstone.

Kaplin, J. P. (1991). *Pencil grasp: Its relationship to handwriting*. Unpublished masters thesis. Boston, MA: Boston University.

Lamme, L. L. (1979). Handwriting in early childhood curricula. *Young Children, 35,* 20-27.

Landsmeer, J. M. F. (1962). Power grip and precision handling. *Annals of Rheumatic Disease, 21,* 164-169.

Levine, M. (1987). *Developmental variations and learning disorders*. Cambridge, MA: Educators Publishing Service.

Littler, J. W. (1960). The physiology and dynamic function of the hand. *Surgical Clinics in North America, 40,* 259-266.

Long, C., Conrad, M. S., Hall, E. A., & Furler, M. S. (1970). Intrinsic-extrinsic muscle control of the hand in power and precision handling. *Journal of Bone and Joint Surgery, 52A,* 853-867.

Luria, A. R. (1980). *Higher cortical functions in man* (2nd ed.). New York: Plenum Publishing.

Neger, R. E. (1989). The evaluation of diplopia in head trauma. *Journal of Head Trauma Rehabilitation, 4*(2), 27-34.

Piaget, J. (1952). *The origins of intelligence in children*. New York: International University Press.

Rosenbloom, L., & Horton, M. E. (1971). The maturation of fine prehension in young children. *Developmental Medicine and Child Neurology, 13,* 3-8.

Rourke, B. (1989). *Nonverbal learning disabilities*. New York: The Guilford Press.

Saida, Y., & Miyashita, M. (1979). Development of fine motor skill in children: Manipulation of a pencil in young children. *Journal of Human Movement Studies, 5,* 104-113.

Smith, R. J. (1974). Balance and kinetics of the fingers under normal and pathological conditions. *Clinical Orthopaedics and Related Research, 104,* 92-111.

Stack, H. G. (1962). Muscle function in the fingers. *Journal of Bone and Joint Surgery, 44B,* 899.

Thurber, D. (1983). *D'Nealian manuscript. An aid to reading development*. ERIC Document Reproduction Services No. ED 227 474.

Tubiana, R. (1981). *The hand* (vol.1). Philadelphia: W. B. Saunders.

Tubiana, R. (1984). *Examination of the hand and upper limb*. Philadelphia: W. B. Saunders.

Warren, M. (1983). A hierarchical model for evaluation and treatment of visual perceptual dysfunction in adult acquired brain injury. Part 2. *American Journal of Occupational Therapy, 47,* 55-66.

15

Treatment of Hand Dysfunction in the Child with Cerebral Palsy

Judith E. Freeman

The treatment of the infant and child with cerebral palsy is probably one of the most challenging tasks for an occupational therapist working in pediatrics. Although each child is unique in terms of sensory and motor abilities, there are some common problems most therapists face in planning and implementing programs. This chapter discusses those common factors in the development of a therapy program for fostering hand skills in the child with cerebral palsy. No chapter can hope to cover all of the possible problems a therapist might face in treating a child with significant motor handicaps. Therapists are cautioned about trying to fit their clients into the case studies presented. Rather, the therapist should view the approach presented here as a resource in devising treatment programs for children with hand dysfunction.

GENERAL PRINCIPLES

The initial stage of treatment is assessment, which is most fruitful if three areas are covered:

sensory processing, stability/mobility functions for support of the hand, and existing hand functions.

In the area of sensory processing, tactile functions can be evaluated by observation and by questioning the child's caregiver. When a variety of textured materials is presented (smooth cloth, terrycloth, fur, water, popcorn, sand, playdough), what is the child's response? It is most helpful if the textures are a part of an actual play activity. For example, quite often a swatch of material or a small sample of sand presented in isolation won't trigger a response one way or another in a child, but handling a stuffed animal or attempting to retrieve an object buried in a sandbox will elicit responses to the materials. In the very young infant, responses to being touched, particularly on the face and hands, are often the clearest ways of evaluating tactile functions. These include not only the response to human touch but also the response to the touch of clothing, bibs, washcloths, and bedclothes. The infant's response to the touch of the breast or bottle on the face is often the strongest clue to the organization of the tactile system.

An attempt should be made to evaluate vestibular functions. Reactions to head movement should be noted, particularly when the head is moved into and out of the upright position. Are responses to movement organized enough to allow freedom of arm motion in the seated posture, or are the upper extremities used to protect and position the neck and trunk? Ocular-motor control is an equally important function to observe. Eye control for both fixation and scanning should be evaluated in the horizontal, vertical, and circular directions. Since very young infants spend much of their time prone and supine, eye functions should be evaluated in these postures as well as while sitting.

When evaluating sensory processing in the multihandicapped child with cerebral palsy, other handicaps also need to be considered. This is particularly true of the child with visual impairment, who may startle at touch and movement while not being genuinely aversive to either tactile or vestibular input. This point becomes more important when planning treatment because the child with sensory hypersensitivity is treated differently from the child with sensory aversiveness.

Beginning with the neck, evaluate mobility/stability function in neck, trunk, shoulders, and hips. Depending on the child's age, this is done in at least one and usually several positions. Even the child who has mobility on all fours and can sit independently may continue to need the upper extremities for support from time to time when seated. For example, the young toddler with diplegia may demonstrate that he/she understands the concept of block stacking but cannot stack because he/she lacks stability in the trunk and must lean on the table for support. When this happens, the child's hands are not free to leave the support surface. It may even appear that the child is leaning on the blocks. He/she is continuing to use distal support for stability. Without assistance to make the shift to proximal stability, the hands are not free to develop skill and handle objects.

A final area of evaluation is the child's existing hand functions. In the infant this involves the assessment of the continuum from reflex to voluntary control of grasp and release, as described in earlier chapters. As the child grows, evaluation of grasp, pinch, and hand positioning is also required. Measurement should be taken of the ability to pronate and supinate the forearm, and substitution patterns should also be noted. For example, children who cannot pronate or supinate at the forearm often substitute humeral rotation. Although developmentally appropriate in a toddler, this substitution pattern represents immaturity and delay in a preschool child.

In evaluating the preceding functions in a child with cerebral palsy, abnormal patterns of tone and movement need to be observed as well. In the more involved child, infant reflexes, spasticity, and at times rigidity dominate motor patterns, interfering with normal development. Even in the less involved child reliance on components of primitive reflexes may persist if tonal support for stability is lacking. In some children there is chronic fixing of the shoulders in a retracted pattern and fixing of the spine in extension. These patterns are used to maintain an upright position, but they interfere with the ability to move the shoulder freely and strongly impede spinal rotation, both of which are required for bilateral and contralateral hand use.

Following this initial assessment the therapist will have some idea of the child's strengths and needs in the areas of function that support hand use. As the child's therapy program continues, additional information is gained during treatment. Evaluation of hand function is an ongoing process, which changes as the child's sensory and motor functions change.

CASE STUDIES

Case 1: Sam, 2 Years

Sam began therapy at 16 months of age. He initially presented with severe spastic quadriplegia, with poor neck and trunk tone, and increased tone in the extremities, most severe in the lower extremities. Sam had spent most of his life supine in a semireclined position and did not tolerate prone or supported sitting. His upper extremities were usually held tightly to his sides. His arms were adducted and internally rotated, elbows extended, and forearms pronated well past 90 degrees, with the wrists flexed and the hands fisted. Sam's head control was poor, and he did not appear to be able to see, although it was reported that he had vision. Sam had been a very irritable child until approximately 12 months, when he was diagnosed with a stress ulcer. When this was treated, he calmed down considerably. He remains sensitive to noise and is difficult to console when upset by fatigue, noises, or change in routine.

Sam enjoyed movement but appeared to be defensive to touch, particularly around the face and the hands. He was making no attempts to reach or bat at things and was unable to open his hands voluntarily. Grasp and release appeared to be reflexive although some grasp did appear to be voluntary; Sam was able to tighten his grasp on something placed in his hand.

Therapy goals began with a five-step approach. Sam's tactile defensiveness interfered with his ability to use his hands. He was uncomfortable touching objects or being touched. Sam's lack of postural control made it difficult for him to use both his eyes and hands. Postural control and mobility of the shoulders and upper extremities needed to be addressed as a preparation for the development of hand skills.

Step 1: Sensory Goals

The initial sensory goals were to decrease Sam's tactile defensiveness and to begin to build in tactile awareness. Heavy pressure brushing (Wilbarger, 1990) was applied in a modified technique. The usual technique combines brisk brushing, using a soapless surgical brush, with joint compression. In Sam's case the joint compression produced an unwanted increase in tone and extension. An alternative approach combined heavy brushing with joint rotation through the spine (Boehme, 1988). This technique produced both a normalization of tone and a reduction in tactile defensiveness.*

Following the reduction in tactile defensiveness, activities to increase tactile awareness were introduced. These activities included bringing Sam's open hands to his own body parts for grabbing and stroking. Reaching was first done without crossing the midline since Sam resisted contralateral contact. In normal infants the unilateral approach is also observed first. Eventually, he seemed to tolerate touching with his hand on the opposite side of his body but was initially upset by this approach. His caregivers were encouraged to help him to grab clothing, hair, and other objects infants commonly grasp during their early hand exploration activities. At the same time, objects were pulled slowly and gently through Sam's hands, from the ulnar to the medial side, to facilitate a voluntary grasp and to provide sensory input. Objects that were used included plastic necklaces of small beads, feathers, theratubing, serrated rhythm sticks, and pieces of textured cloth.

Step 2: Normalizing Muscle Tone

Simultaneously the therapist worked on the normalization of Sam's muscle tone. Positions that introduced trunk rotation or reduced the extensor posturing in the lower extremities appeared to be the most effective in reducing Sam's hypertonus. The first successful play position for Sam was to have him semireclining, straddling the therapist's lap, and leaning on her legs, which were flexed at the knees (Finney, 1975) (Figure 15-1). The therapist thus made a "chair" for Sam, which posi-

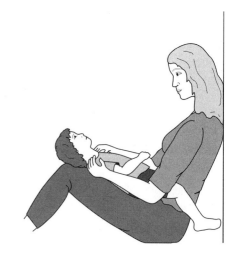

Figure 15-1. Child positioned straddling the therapist's lap.

tioned him almost in sitting, with hips abducted. This allowed the therapist to gradually bring Sam into 90 degrees of hip flexion for sitting upright and left the therapist's hands free to rotate the trunk or shoulders or to provide visual and tactile stimulation. Subsequently Sam began to tolerate side-lying on the ball, with trunk elongated and upper body weight on elbows (Figure 15-2) and sitting on the therapist's lap sideways with both feet on the floor (Figure 15-3). During all activities trunk rotation and weight shift onto and off of the upper extremities were stressed. Initially weight bearing was done mainly on the forearms to avoid locking at the elbows, with gradual progression

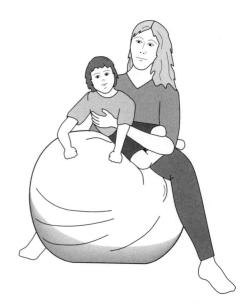

Figure 15-2. Child positioned side-lying on the therapy ball.

---

*Treatment techniques such as brushing and joint compression are highly specialized and require an understanding of the theoretical basis for their use.

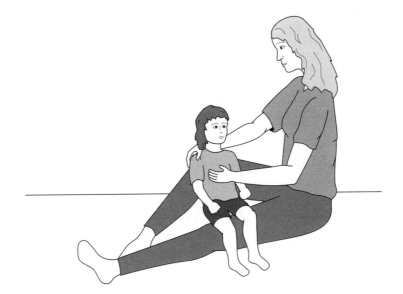

Figure 15-3. Child, with both feet on the floor, sitting on the therapist's lap.

onto the hands. As therapy progressed, Sam began to tolerate sitting on his buttocks and eventually could be seated on the floor, where he would prop his body up with his arms extended forward for support. He needed assistance to maintain this posture.

Step 3: Positioning Strategies

Because Sam had poor neck and trunk stability, it was difficult to feed him. He was not able to hold his head up consistently, which made hand use and interaction with the environment difficult. Various types of positioning equipment were tried to assist Sam and his caregivers. Sam had very poor tolerance for the positioning system that had been purchased for him as an infant and would cry when placed in it. It was found that feeding could best be accomplished with the "person as chair," as described previously. Eventually, as Sam became more tolerant of sitting upright, he was able to use a bolster chair (*TherAdapt Products, Inc. Catalogue;* see Appendix A). In addition to increased tolerance for sitting, Sam's reduced sensory defensiveness appeared to help his tolerance for positioning equipment. Initially Sam would extend if anything touched his face or head. As his sensory defensiveness was reduced, he began to tolerate equipment that touched his head, with the only exception being pressure to the occiput, which triggered the extensor response one usually sees with such a stimulus.

Step 4: Visual Skills

Work was also done on improving Sam's visual organization. With poor control of ocular scanning and fixation, Sam would not be able to use his eyes, even if his acuity turned out to be adequate. As his head control improved and his tolerance for being upright increased, attempts were made to stabilize gaze and eye tracking. It was found that Sam responded to black and white targets and also to other contrasting colors, such as a large worm made of 3-inch square yellow, green, and red sections. He was also provided with a black and white striped rotating drum (stripes ½ inch wide), which could be spun to initiate visual fixation. (This piece of equipment cannot be used with a child who has or may be having seizures; check with the child's neurologist before using it.) It is important to note that Sam's position had an effect on his eye tracking. When he was seated with his head in neutral or slightly flexed, he could fixate and follow a slowly moving stimulus. If his head was in extension, he could not fixate or follow with his eyes.

Step 5: Hand Spasticity

Sam had received neoprene hand splints to decrease thumb adduction and to improve range of motion in the hands (Joe Cool thumb splint, Pratt Medical, Inc.; see Appendix A). These were not initially successful, possibly due to the degree of spasticity in Sam's hands. A modified orthokinetic splint (Farber, 1974) was then made. This consisted of a firm surface, made from a hair roller combined with elastic webbing (a strip can be made from nylon stocking or very thin theraband) that went through the roller. The roller was placed in Sam's hand, with the elastic material secured by tying it over the dorsum of the hand, just proximal to the metacarpals. This provided a firm surface in the hand, to reduce flexor spasticity, combined with quick stretch to the extensors from the elastic surface. This splint worked well to reduce the spasticity in Sam's hands. When the splint was removed, Sam was able to bear weight with his hands flat and his fingers and MP joints extended. Weight bearing on the hands, with proper positioning of the arm, further facilitates hand opening.

During this time Sam was given bracelets with noisy, bright beads attached to them. His hands were guided gently into vats of beans, rice, and corn. Using a universal cuff with a Velcro attachment for toys, Sam was assisted in shaking, banging, and squeezing toys. Because of his interest in bells, he was assisted in pushing a large switch to activate a battery-operated chiming toy. A Mylar balloon was attached to his hand at times, with the sides alternating. Sam was encouraged to bring things to his mouth and was assisted in holding food to bring to his mouth (an unpredictable bite reflex precluded dipping his fingers in food to initiate hand-to-mouth activity). Activities to increase Sam's awareness of his hands and to facilitate active reach and independent grasp continue to be a vital part of Sam's therapy program. Sam is currently being fitted with a universal cuff so that he can hold objects such as finger foods, rattles, and simple toys.

Case 2: Dan, 2½ Years

Dan presented with mixed tone patterns, showing low axial tone, moderate tightness at the shoulders, and increased tone in the extremities. As an infant Dan was quite floppy, but increased tone was present by 12 months of age. The upper extremities showed bilateral fisting of the hands, with an indwelling thumb on the right side. By 18 months Dan showed quite a difference between the two sides of the body, with greater spasticity on the right side. Dan did not use his right hand in a prehension pattern until approximately 2 years of age. Dan was able to hold his head up but did this by holding his head in extension with the occiput resting on the upper cervical vertebrae. Dan had been diagnosed with visual problems, and surgery for strabismus was done at 16 months of age. Dan showed marked sensory defensiveness to touch in the upper extremities and oral/facial area and did not take solid foods in the mouth from a spoon until 2 years of age.

Dan shows a determined, curious personality, making strong efforts to explore his environment.

At 2½ years he now can sit and creep independently. He can pull to a stand and walks with the aid of a walker. He demonstrates awareness of cause-effect relationships, object permanence, and tool use. He can pretend and demonstrates representational play.

Therapy began with activities to reduce tactile defensiveness and promote tactile discrimination. Therapy then proceeded with activities designed to normalize muscle tone, promote stability, and develop the postural responses needed to support hand skills. The third step worked directly on the development of shoulder, arm, and hand skills.

Step 1: Warm-Up Activity

A warm-up time to normalize Dan's tone and reduce sensory defensiveness began each therapy session. Heavy pressure brushing with a surgical scrub brush (Wilbarger, 1990) was combined with shoulder, trunk, and hip rotation. Rotation was accomplished in several ways: holding Dan with his back to the therapist, with hands on Dan's ribcage and pelvis; seating Dan sideways on the therapist's lap and placing hands on chest and back to rotate the spine; placing Dan on the therapy ball, legs abducted around the therapist, with the therapist holding him at hips and rotating his spine as the ball counterrotated (Boehme, 1988, Finnie, 1975).

Step 2: Stability and Weight Bearing

Therapy proceeded with activities to promote trunk, neck, and limb girdle stability while facilitating rotation and elongation of the weight-bearing side. As often as possible, Dan was seated on equipment where he could hold on to vertical uprights, so that the tendency to pronate the forearms beyond 90 degrees was inhibited. This was particularly important since Dan showed limited active range of forearm supination. Examples of such equipment include the bolster swing and the platform swing, which can be used in combination with a bolster.

Weight bearing was also an important component of this second step. Weight bearing that is less than or equal to body weight reduces hypertonus of the shoulder, elbow, forearm, wrist, and fingers (Farber, 1974). Creeping over obstacles and down inclines provides the opportunity to normalize tone while simultaneously facilitating cocontraction in the shoulders. In addition, when surfaces are texture covered, tactile input is provided with pressure, which promotes tolerance for the input. Creeping downhill is particularly useful in facilitating cocontraction once the spasticity of the shoulders is reduced. In addition, both creeping and holding onto equipment by handles reduces spasticity of the forearm, wrist, and hand muscles while facilitating cocontraction at the wrist.

Dan previously used a modified orthokinetic splint (see preceding section for description; see also Farber, 1974), but currently he is not wearing any splinting.

Step 3: Working on Hand Skills

Positioning was of primary importance in working on hand skills with Dan. Several positions were used, including a bolster chair (TherAdapt Products, Inc., see Appendix A) supported kneel-standing, supported long sitting, and sideways sitting on the therapist's lap with feet on the floor. Side sitting was prohibited due to partial subluxation of the right hip. In addition, it was found that side sitting appeared to produce rounding of the trunk rather than elongation. It was found that Dan could not focus on the activity being presented unless he was in a very stable position with trunk support.

The next task was to work on shoulder and arm movements. Initially, this was done with Dan prone on the therapy ball, with the activity placed so that Dan could reach it when his hands were in line with his shoulders. At times a table was placed in front of the ball so that Dan could lean with one hand and reach with the other. Later this was done in the seated or kneeling posture. The therapist used her hands to support Dan through the upper trunk, to provide stability for the shoulders. The therapist's hands were placed on the upper trunk at the ribcage when he was prone and at the sides when seated. At times stability was given through the scapula, with the therapist assisting the forward movement of the scapula as Dan reached. Activities included stamping and painting on paper that was in the vertical plane to Dan, dropping golf balls down a chute maze, hitting a hanging balloon with a paper tube (the tube facilitates wrist cocontraction), throwing beanbags at a target, and pressing a lever toy to make a ball pop up.

To work on forearm movements, the therapist began by massaging the forearm, using a gentle vibrating motion between the radius and ulna to relax the forearm (Boehme, 1988). Beginning in prone, Dan was helped to stabilize his arm, leaning on his elbow. Gentle pressure on the forearms during lateral weight shift facilitated rotation. Thus rocking to one side to reach a toy while the therapist gave gentle pressure down on the weight-bearing surface began to facilitate rotation. Once Dan could stabilize his humerus in prone, he could

begin to play with toys that required the forearm to rotate in a non–weight-bearing situation. Turning a toy hourglass, putting rings on a stick, shaking a toy, and opening the doors of a toy box are all examples of activities that require forearm rotation if the distal end of the humerus is the point of weight bearing.

In the seated posture Dan was assisted in rotation by stabilizing the humerus against the ribcage. As more control was gained, the humerus was stabilized away from the ribcage, and eventually external stability was removed. At this time one of Dan's favorite activities became pouring, which was ideal for its rotational component. Tactile defensiveness was diminishing, and he was able to dig with his hands in bean, corn, and rice vats. He would pour into a bowl, using a 2- or 3-inch diameter cup. The firm surface of the cup helped to maintain normal tone in the hand by inhibiting flexor hypertonus. The cup needs to be large enough to inhibit spasticity in the ulnar border of the hand. If the hand shows ulnar deviation when holding the cup, gentle pressure and very slow traction to the ulnar border of the forearm bring the wrist into a more optimal posture. By stabilizing the wrist in this new position for the child, the muscles learn to cocontract in the new pattern. Dan attempted pouring with a ladle, which had the handle built up. Other toys that were used at this time included a glitter wand, a thunder-tube (when tipped from one end to the other, it makes a noise), a velcro board (strips of neon velcro he had to pull apart; rings on one end facilitated grasping), and a mystery box (which had two wide strips of sewing elastic secured to the top so that the opening was a slit where the two pieces of elastic met). To open the box, the elastic had to be pushed apart with both hands (American Printing House for the Blind, Inc.; see Appendix A).

Dan showed poor wrist extension, with the wrists usually held in flexion and ulnar deviation. Initially, the therapist worked with Dan in the prone position. A bolster was attempted, but Dan had difficulty with the pressure of the bolster on his chest and abdomen, so alternate methods were used. The therapist sat and held Dan "wheelbarrow" fashion, supporting him at the chest and abdomen. Because his legs were long enough, they were abducted around the therapist, maintaining good alignment of the spine and reducing the tendency for the hips to adduct in prone. With Dan in this position, his weight could be shifted laterally and forward and back on extended arms. This type of weight bearing on the hands provides for cocontraction at the wrist and elongation of the finger flexors. It also helps to stabilize the ulnar border of the hand as weight is shifted from side to side.

Dan is now creeping and has begun to pull to a stand. Pulling up and leaning on a wide variety of surfaces aid in developing the palmar arches. In addition, Dan is offered a variety of toys to assist in shaping the hand. Most of these toys are slightly weighted, to assist in grasp and release. It is found that, by stabilizing the forearm as Dan reaches, wrist extension can be facilitated and ulnar deviation limited. This allows for better and smoother release of objects. Initially Dan must contact the sides of the container or table surface before releasing the object, since his hand does not have the stability to open without support. Eventually it is hoped that wrist stability will develop to the point that Dan can release an object without external support.

Pincer grasp was initially worked on with large objects, such as golf balls and 1½-inch hardwood blocks, large washers, and very large jingle bells. Dan enjoys taking things in and out of containers, which is an age-appropriate play activity. He is beginning to enjoy sorting as well. Objects such as those mentioned previously can be used in sorting tasks, providing practice in cognitive and coordination areas.

To begin the development of isolated finger movements, the hand needs to be quite relaxed. After a weight-bearing activity, Dan and the therapist did water play in warm water (90° to 95°) to facilitate this relaxation. While in the water gentle pressure was applied to the wrist to maintain wrist extension. The therapist did gentle stroking in the palm to facilitate the palmar arches (Boehme, 1988). Following this, water play that invited poking activity was engaged in. For example, a large dry sponge placed in the water would give off bubbles when poked with a few fingers. This was very interesting for Dan (the container was clear acrylic, so bubbles could be seen). Following the water play, other finger activities were done: using fingers to draw in finger paint (since Dan was too defensive to touch the paint, the paint was placed inside a large Ziploc bag), playing with thick plastic stick-ons on a mirror, poking finger holes in thin cellophane stretched over an oatmeal box, and activating the keys of a musical toy.

Dan continues to make gains. His tactile defensiveness is diminishing, and he shows improved control of neck and trunk musculature. He is now being considered for computer training to assist with communication.

Case 3: Kristy, 2 Years

Kristy did not begin therapy until 18 months of age. She presented with fluctuating tone in the trunk, neck, and limbs. Low tone appeared to predominate much of the time, and choreoathetosis was seen distally in the limbs as Kristy attempted more skilled movements. She showed marked retraction at the shoulders when upright, with fixing of the spine in extension. Kristy could sit but did so with feet widely spread and knees locked in extension. Kristy could also pull to a stand and walk pushing a weighted cart. She could not creep, however, and attempts at supported creeping produced a homolateral creep with exaggerated lateral trunk flexion, rather than a cross pattern with trunk rotation. Kristy showed almost no active trunk rotation in any movement pattern.

Kristy's marked shoulder retraction prevented her from using her hands at the midline. In addition, when Kristy began therapy, she often showed a withdrawal pattern when presented with new objects, with arms horizontally abducted, elbows flexed, and hands held at shoulder height. Kristy also reacted negatively to noise when she first came to the therapy unit. She did not tolerate being in a group of children and would cry when anyone came near her. Given all of these factors, it was felt that Kristy might be experiencing sensory defensiveness in the tactile and auditory areas.

The initial evaluation also suggested that Kristy might have depressed vestibular functions. She showed poor balance responses and craved movement. Testing showed almost no postrotary nystagmus. Therapy began, then, with an attempt to reduce sensory defensiveness and stimulate the vestibular system.

Step 1: Normalizing the Sensory Systems

Heavy pressure brushing with the soapless surgical scrub brush was used on Kristy's arms, legs, hands, and feet (not the soles). This was combined with joint compression to the spine and extremities (Wilbarger, 1990). Brushing was done in a back-and-forth motion, with enough pressure to move the skin. Brushing began on one leg, and proceeded up the leg to the lateral trunk, the arm and hand, across the shoulders to the opposite arm and hand, down the side to the lower extremity. An attempt was always made to keep the brush on the body while brushing and to not jump around, but to do one side and then the other. This seems to be tolerated best by the children. Following this Kristy was seated in a standard plastic toddler swing and swung in a linear fashion (with padding to maintain her trunk and neck in alignment). The swing has vertical upright supports, which helps to diminish shoulder retraction as the children hold on while swinging. Kristy enjoyed swinging very fast. Initially there was an increase in extensor posturing of the legs, but this lasted for only a few minutes and could be modified by bringing the hips past 90 degrees of flexion while sitting in the swing. Within 2 weeks of beginning the program (mother brushing at home as well), Kristy was able to join the group activities without crying. She tolerated handling very well after a month in the program and showed a diminishing of the withdrawal response in the hands.

Step 2: Developing Proximal Support for Hand Skill

Initial work on the upper extremities began in the prone position. To prepare for reaching, we needed to work on trunk rotation to facilitate both lateral reach into space and bringing the hands forward in the midline. Kristy's shoulder retraction and limited spinal movement inhibited movement of her hands. Trunk rotation activities would assist the development of stability in the trunk, which would then decrease Kristy's need to fixate with shoulder retraction and spinal extension. Rotation of the trunk was carried out with three activities.

- With the therapist kneeling, Kristy was held with her back against the therapist. The therapist's hands provided stability at the ribcage and hips, while rotating Kristy at the spine, so that her hands came toward the ground (Figure 15-4). The movements were begun very slowly, depending on how much resistance was felt in the spine. Kristy enjoyed this activity; as she came toward the ground, she was encouraged to knock over blocks, hit a weighted inflatable toy, or pop bubbles with her hands. Movement in this position also facilitated protective extension as the speed with which Kristy came toward the ground was increased.
- Using a padded incline (very large wedge-shaped mat), Kristy rolled uphill and downhill, with the therapist facilitating rotation at the hips and shoulders. Kristy would carry beaded necklaces to a stuffed bear at the top of the hill and put them on the bear. The necklaces work well since they can be carried in one hand while rolling without getting in the way of the rolling pattern. It requires two hands, however, to put the necklaces on the bear, which helps facilitate bilaterality. To put

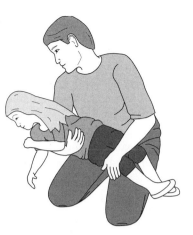

Figure 15-4. Therapist gently rotating the child so the child's hands reach toward the floor.

the necklace on the bear, Kristy would come up onto one elbow while the therapist assisted her in maintaining good elongation on the weight-bearing side.

- Kristy would sit on one of the therapist's extended legs, with the therapist providing stability at the chest and midback, to facilitate rotation. To encourage rotation and begin work on reaching, Kristy would put weighted objects into a container, with the container placed so Kristy had to rotate her spine to reach it. Other activities included hitting a hanging ball with a tube, sponge painting, putting necklaces on the bear, puzzles, which can be done on a small easel, and stamping. The stamps are adapted by attaching thick doweling or large knobs to the back of the stamp, so that the child is able to hold it easily. By using doweling for the stamps, flexor tightness can be inhibited. By using knobs, some molding of the palmar arches of the hand can be facilitated. In Kristy's case the knob-adapted stamps were used.

Weight shift over the shoulders was also used to support reaching. As a warm-up, Kristy was shifted side to side on the medium (36-inch) therapy ball. Following this Kristy was encouraged to reach with one hand while leaning on the other, bearing weight on the forearm. Support and gradual elongation were needed at the scapula of the reaching hand to inhibit retraction and elevation at the shoulder. Activities such as bubble popping with a feather duster were effective in encouraging Kristy to reach with her hand at shoulder height. As the shoulders become stronger, the feather duster can be replaced with a Nerf bat, and later with a glitter wand or weighted cardboard tube. Fly swatters, which come in a large variety of styles, weights, and shapes, are also useful for grading this activity.

In the initial months of therapy brushing and joint rotation were repeated approximately three times during the 90-minute therapy session. Withdrawal posturing of the hands and upper extremities diminished markedly. Eventually, brushing was done at the beginning of each session and just before Kristy entered the group program, which occurred during the last 30 minutes of each therapy session.

Step 3: Development of Control at the Arm and Hand

While Kristy was still on the floor and mats, work was done in quadrupedal posture to stabilize the forearm, wrist, and extrinsics of the hand. While supported in this posture, Kristy was slowly rocked forward and back, side to side, and diagonally. Movement from quadrupedal to sitting was done, with a diagonal weight shift, so that the weight bearing on the upper extremities placed the arms in a diagonal pattern.

In preparation for reaching while in the upright posture, activities were done to facilitate abduction of the scapula on the ribs and to allow the clavicle to move forward. A game of "row, row, row your boat" was played, with the therapist facing Kristy, holding her arms in a forward position, extended at the elbows. The therapist's hands are placed at the distal ends of the humerus. By having the child lean back as the therapist pulls gently forward, there is active freeing of the shoulder girdle. This can also be facilitated by placing one hand on the sternum and pushing back while pulling forward on the upper extremities (Boehme, 1988). Kristy enjoyed this rocking game and did it at home with her mother quite often. Kristy then appeared ready to attempt upper-extremity activities in the seated posture.

With Kristy seated at the table, support was provided by the therapist to facilitate reaching and inhibit scapular retraction. The therapist, sitting behind Kristy, placed her hands on the scapula or ribcage when Kristy was reaching, to assist with elongation at the shoulder. Support was also given on the opposite (nonreaching) side, to maintain stability and to keep the shoulder on that side from retracting.

Several activities were needed to facilitate a stronger grasp. Pressure was given to the midpalm area and combined with gentle wrist traction. The feather duster handle was rolled into Kristy's palm (distal to proximal) to facilitate grasp. Then Kristy was engaged in a game where she swatted small balls around on the table with the feather duster. Whenever she dropped the duster, it was rolled into her hand in the described manner, rather than just placing it back in her hand. As grasp strengthened, a serrated rhythm stick was also used for this activity. This could be pulled through Kristy's hand to stimulate grasp and provided more of a challenge than the feather duster since it was heavier. Games of tug-of-war were played with theratubing hooked into Kristy's fingers. Stability was given at the forearm for this game (Boehme, 1988).

Kristy enjoyed swinging in the net hammock in the prone position. By offering her thick theraband to pull up on, cocontraction patterns in the entire upper trunk were facilitated and grasp and wrist stability were improved. Kristy resisted the use of theratubing for this activity, and upon observation it did appear to pinch her skin when she pulled against it. There was no problem with tolerance for the theraband.

At this point in Kristy's therapy, work began on encouraging bilateral use of the upper extremities when seated. This was initiated with a peek-a-boo game, where Kristy held an 8-inch diameter hoop with both hands, looked through it, and played "peek." By using embroidery hoops, colored cellophane could be stretched across, so Kristy was encouraged to look at various toys and pictures through her colored window, which could be done successfully only by using both hands.

Kristy then advanced to a board game. Boards were prepared with animals, vehicles, and other small toys secured to them. Kristy was directed to place one of several sized rings over the objects, an activity which she enjoyed doing. As she became adept at placing rings over objects, Kristy was encouraged to put rings on a rhythm stick, which the therapist held at various angles. The rings were colorfully painted and had bells attached, which added to the interest level as well as giving them an unbalanced weight, which made manipulating them a challenge.

Work began on developing Kristy's radial-digital grasp. One-inch diameter pegs were used, with the therapist pulling the peg outward toward the ends of the fingers. Also used were the modified stamps and a golf ball maze. (This is similar to a marble maze but uses golf balls). Later Kristy advanced to a marble maze. Poking activities were also begun, to encourage isolated finger motion. Other games included putting 1½-inch washers through a slit in a coffee can, (the can and lid are painted like a clown; the child "feeds" the clown through the slit mouth), putting little people

(Fisher-Price) in vehicles and on a bus, and rolling small cars down a ramp. In each case stability was given at the shoulder, elbow, and wrist where needed. In addition, Kristy was encouraged to use both hands by alternating the position of the target object.

During this time Kristy began to show an interest in tactile input, running her hands over textured materials and into her mother's hair and hugging stuffed animals. Materials were offered that expanded her experience with tactile input, including theraputty, salt dough, commercial playdough, shaving cream, and vats of beans and rice to dig in. When working with the various dough-like materials, 1-inch and ¾-inch washers as well as large marbles were stood on end in the material to encourage a crude pincer grasp.

Currently Kristy is refining her ability to use thumb and digits to grasp. Finger feeding, recently introduced, is providing ample opportunity to practice her newly acquired skills.

Case 4: Ricky, 18 Months

Ricky, an 18-month-old boy, was diagnosed as having a mild right hemiparesis. Ricky was exposed to drugs prenatally, and his physicians felt that his hemiparesis and slight overall hypertonus were probably due to prenatal drug exposure. Ricky was born at term and was a very floppy baby.

Currently Ricky presents with overall slight hypertonus, which is seen most in the hips, right shoulder, right elbow, and right wrist. He will use both hands when reminded to but tends to ignore the right hand. He is walking with a slightly broad-based gait and shows fair balance responses. He is unable to tailor sit, probably due to tightness of the hip adductors and low back muscles. There are no limitations of passive range of motion in any joints. Ricky has a short attention span, and there are problems with frequent tantrums at home.

Ricky appears to have mild sensory loss on the right side, particularly in the right upper extremity. He enjoys vestibular input but is hesitant to try new activities. He appears to have motor planning problems that extend into the fine motor area. When in a noisy environment, he becomes more active and less compliant with instructions.

Step 1: Providing Sensory Input

Therapy began with an attempt to improve the sensory awareness in Ricky's limbs. While the loss appeared mainly on the right, sensory input was applied to both sides of the body, with the less involved side receiving the sensory input first. Various textured materials were attempted, with Ricky's attending responses used as a gauge of awareness. Ricky looked at his limbs when a rough cloth and the soapless scrub brush were used. He also enjoyed digging in a vat of dry pinto beans. Although not clinically defensive to touch, it was felt that Ricky was defensive to sound and light stimuli. Because of his affinity for the soapless scrub brush, it was decided to try heavy pressure brushing, with a careful monitoring of Ricky's muscle tone. Brushing began on the left lower extremity, proceeded up the leg to the left side of the trunk, to the left upper extremity, across the shoulders, on the right upper extremity, and down the right leg. Brushing was done without raising the brush. Joint compression was not done because of Ricky's hypertonus. Instead, the therapist used hip rotation, shoulder rotation, spinal rotation, and massage to the forearm and palm, spreading from the midpalm out to each side, to normalize tone and to assist development of the palmar arches (Boehme, 1988). No increase in tone was noted, and Ricky began to be more focused during therapy.

Step 2: Relaxation of Trunk Hypertonus with Activation of the Proximal Stabilizers of the Hand

Relaxation was accomplished with both rotation and weight-bearing activities. Ricky rolled up and down the hill, with the therapist facilitating trunk rotation as he went up against resistance. This was done by placing one hand on Ricky's hip as he rolled uphill, providing slight pressure to resist the rotation. The combination of rotation and shoulder compression equal to body weight helped to normalize the tone of the shoulder musculature. This is similar to the slow rolling technique of Farber (1974). A small ramp was placed at a right angle to the top of the hill, and small cars were lined up at the top. As Ricky rolled to the top, he could take a car and roll it down the ramp. This encouraged motor planning, and weight shift on the incline was required to reach and launch the cars. Other activities included rolling balls down the ramp, putting necklaces on a bear, and dropping large washers into a metal can (making a loud noise).

On the 36-inch therapy ball, Ricky went from a supine to a seated position with the therapist facilitating a rotary pattern. He played "hit the hanging balloon" in side-lying position, with weight bearing on the right elbow and forearm. Following this activity he was able to use the right hand to hit the balloon.

While prone on the ball Ricky continued to swat balloons and bubbles with various tools. Initially he was weight bearing on the right elbow, to relax the shoulder. Following this he leaned with the right hand on a table placed in front of the ball to play with pegs, blocks, and other manipulatives. Leaning on the right hand helped to lengthen the long finger flexors and to stabilize the wrist.

Step 3: Encouragement of Bilaterality in Preparation for Manipulative Tasks

One of the most important bilateral tasks for Ricky was creeping. This was done on flat ground, on inclines, and over uneven surfaces. Creeping surfaces were varied to supply additional tactile input to the hands. Since Ricky was applying pressure while creeping, the textured surfaces were well tolerated. Creeping obstacle courses were constructed, which included 6-foot square pillows filled with large lumps of foam rubber, inclines, foam wedges, inner tubes, ladders, wide balance beams, and bolsters.

Ricky needed to use two hands on most of the balance equipment in the clinic, which encouraged bilaterality. As he began ambulating, ball games were adapted to facilitate bilaterality. He was encouraged to hit a 3-inch foam ball with a hockey stick, a hula hoop, and a foam bat.

Contralateral skill with motor planning was accomplished by using equipment where Ricky could hold on with one hand and reach with the other. For example, Ricky can use a flexor swing, hold on with one hand, and pick up a beanbag off the floor with the other. A game is played where Ricky is swung on the flexor swing, and as he goes by a beanbag on the floor, he picks it up. As he goes by the deposit container, he drops the beanbag in. This can be done with various containers, including play basketball hoops. Initially, Ricky held on with his right upper extremity and picked up objects with his left hand. Eventually he was able to pick up some objects with his right hand as well. When he used his right hand to pick up the objects, however, Ricky needed to have the speed of the flexor swing slowed considerably.

Two-handed fine motor tasks were also encouraged at this time. Fine motor tasks were preceded by work on rotation at the shoulders with elongation of the right arm, relaxation at the elbow and wrist, and massage of the forearm and hand.

Following this, Ricky was encouraged to use his right hand as an assistive hand. Much could be done by simply not stabilizing toys too much for him. For example, Ricky loved to scribble and learned quickly to use his right hand to hold down the paper. Putting pegs into and out of a rubber mat pegboard requires the use of two hands, as do Legos, popbeads, pouring sand and water, and manipulating most pull-string toys, such as Mattel's See'n'Say. To secure stickers to paper, Ricky needed to peel them from their backing with his more dexterous hand while holding the backing paper down with his assisting hand. To put the sticker on the paper, he placed it with his left hand but had to use his right to secure it. This was a fun game for Ricky, which he carried over in his home program. Fine motor tasks were always preceded by a gross motor task requiring bilaterality, such as balancing on the ball, pushing himself in the net swing, creeping, or scooterboarding.

Currently Ricky is using a crude pincer grasp with the right hand and a fine pincer grasp with the left. He has mastered bilateral use of his hands where both hands are performing the same motion and can use the right as an assistive hand for activities such as holding down a paper. Tasks requiring the hands to perform different motions but work together (as in unscrewing a lid) are more difficult for him. These remaining needs help the therapist to decide where to go next in planning treatment for Ricky.

Case 5: Billy, 5 Years

Billy was diagnosed at age 1 year with cerebral palsy. He was further diagnosed as diplegic, having his main involvement in the lower extremities. He showed low tone in the trunk, with tightness or hypertonus of the hips, knees, ankles, and feet. He ambulated well with bilateral ankle-foot orthoses. He had been referred for therapy because he was showing delays in perceptual and fine motor skill development with poor pincer grasp and deficient eye-hand coordination.

Clinical observations of Billy during a fine motor-adaptive test showed the following.

- Deficient trunk stability: Billy needed to use distal support to remain upright at the table, leaning on one hand or the other. This limited his ability to use his hands and made it impossible for him to develop bilateral motor coordination without trunk support in sitting since one hand was always holding him up.

- Poor shoulder mobility and strength: Billy was unable to raise his hands more than a few inches from the support surface of the table, even when the therapist stabilized his trunk for him.
- Mild choreoathetosis was seen when Billy was attempting to copy forms.
- General weakness of the upper body: Billy was unable to pull himself along the floor by a rope and could not creep downhill without falling forward.

Billy enjoyed feeling textured materials. He appeared somewhat hyposensitive to touch. When allowed to explore a box of materials, he chose to rub his hands with a stuffed animal and a loofa sponge. He enjoyed running strips of silk, taffeta, and corduroy material through his fingers. He was also eager to play in wet sand, playdough, and glop (a wet but nonsticky material that is highly stimulating to the hands and fun to manipulate; see Appendix B for recipe). His mother reported that he was "always rubbing his hands on things." At the same time, Billy had difficulty manipulating objects and appeared to have poor sensory guidance for hand movement. When his hands were placed under a shield, he could not tell the therapist which finger was touched or pulled. His response to a sharp point was diminished in comparison with other children his age. The therapist concluded that Billy was not processing input from the tactile system very well.

Step 1: Developing Sensory Awareness

Therapy began with sensory awareness activities. Billy was encouraged to dig with his hands into vats of beans, rice, and popcorn to find buried objects. At first he was not able to feel things buried in the materials. Eventually he began to find larger items, and gradually smaller items were found. He played with various kinds of doughs to stimulate both tactile and proprioceptive receptors. Salt dough could be formed into geometric shapes using templates. This not only stimulated the sensory receptors in his hands but also provided the opportunity to work on Billy's delayed form perception.

Vibration was used to facilitate sensory perception in the hand. Jellyroll pans were spread with colored salt or beans. A vibrator was used as a wand to write or draw in the materials in the jellyroll pan. The colored salt was Billy's favorite and again afforded an opportunity to work on visual perception skills. (Colored salt was made by pouring salt onto a paper plate and then scraping a piece of colored chalk through it until ground; the ground colored chalk was then mixed with the salt.) Making the colored salt was also an interesting activity for Billy, which required the use of his two hands working in a contralateral pattern, as he held down the plate with one hand and scraped the chalk in the salt with the other. Rubbing the chalk over the gritty salt is an interesting tactile experience. Another way of introducing vibration to Billy's hands was through the use of the Squiggle Pen, which is commercially available in most toy stores. The pen vibrates and writes in tight circles as the child uses it.

Step 2: Developing Stability in the Trunk and Shoulders

While performing the preceding activities, a variety of positions were tried. Much of the activity was done while prone, with Billy lying on a wedge. This position provided stability of the trunk and facilitated cocontraction at the neck and shoulders. Some of the activities were done in a sitting position, with the therapist behind Billy providing stability at the trunk and shoulders. The best hand function appeared to occur when the therapist placed one hand on Billy's ribcage to support him on one side, while placing the other hand on Billy's scapula to assist reaching and forward movement. The hand placed on the ribcage was there to provide stability for the opposite side to pull against. When doing hand activity, Billy (and many other children) had difficulty stabilizing one side of his body so that the other side could move against a stable point. By providing this stability, Billy could manipulate the tactile materials more easily and could begin to work on upper extremity functions while doing this preliminary, but important, sensory work.

Several activities were attempted to improve Billy's trunk strength and improve upper trunk, neck, and shoulder cocontraction. Scooterboarding was attempted but discontinued when it produced an excessive amount of extensor hypertonus in the lower extremities. Three activities produced the best results.

The first was resisted rolling, where Billy rolled up an incline padded with egg crate foam padding to provide additional tactile input. A game was created wherein Billy carried an object up the incline as he rolled, with the goal for the object to be located at the top of the incline. Since Billy enjoyed puzzles, the game was usually played by having the puzzle base at the top of the incline and the puzzle pieces at the bottom. Billy would begin at the top, roll down to get a piece, and roll back up to put it into the puzzle.

Second, Billy enjoyed lying prone in the suspended net hammock. While in the hammock, Billy could push himself, picking up objects such as beanbags to throw into a goal. When the beanbags resembled small basketballs, soccerballs, and footballs, Billy was eager to play the game he called "slamdunk." Initially Billy would push himself with one hand followed by the other because he was unable to lift both hands from the support surface simultaneously. This was probably due to poor shoulder cocontraction. Later, when shoulder stability improved, he was able to push off from the floor with both hands.

Another activity involved the use of theratubing while Billy was prone in the net. The therapist would hold the two ends of a long strand of tubing, and Billy would hold the loop at the center with both of his hands. He was not able to hold on for very long at first since the resistance of the theratubing was too great for him. A cardboard tube slipped onto the theratubing kept the tubing from pinching Billy's fingers in the early stages of this activity (rubber hose, cut into 6-inch lengths, can also be slipped onto the theratubing to make a handle). Eventually, as Billy's upper-extremity strength improved, he was able to hold on for up to 3 minutes without resting. The rapid movement of the net and the resistance of the theratubing appeared to facilitate cocontraction of the shoulders and neck.

Third, Billy was able to swing himself while inside a suspended inner tube. Billy would place his head, arms, and upper trunk inside the tube and lie on the tube with his chest. The tube was standard tire size and suspended high enough so that Billy was not quite standing upright but leaning forward a little. As Billy ran forward, centrifugal force brought his feet off the ground, and he was airborne. To stay in the tube, however, he had to use shoulder depressors and upper trunk stabilizers; otherwise he would fall forward or backward or his arms would come up and out of the tube. At first Billy was able to orbit only part of the way around before putting his feet down. Eventually, he was able to orbit several times. He was also able to control the swing sufficiently to swing and kick a ball that was rolled to him.

Step 3: Working on Hand Skills

Billy began to show a great interest in manipulative and perceptual activities. It was decided that the areas of wrist rotation, bilateral and contralateral control, and eye-hand coordination needed special attention. Activities done in each area included a visual perceptual component whenever possible.

In the area of wrist rotation it was noted that Billy usually substituted humeral rotation for forearm rotation. With Billy lying prone over a wedge, the therapist could stabilize the humerus at the distal end so that Billy would have to use forearm rotation to manipulate a toy. One activity that worked well was using peel and press activity boards, where pictures can be made by putting pieces of plastic on a background board. Several commercial varieties of the toy are available, and Billy particularly enjoyed making scenes with his favorite television cartoon characters. Another successful activity involved making colored salt pictures. Clear 3-ounce plastic cups were used. Billy was given several containers of colored salt. He would scoop salt up from a chosen color with a small cup or spoon and pour it into one of the 3-ounce cups. As he used different colors, layers would form and be quite attractive. Since the cup was small, he was quickly successful in making a multilayered container. The movement required to do the pouring was carefully graded forearm rotation.

As Billy began to show more active rotation at the forearm, activities moved to the table. Initially the therapist continued to stabilize the humerus to prevent substitution of humeral for forearm rotation. Gradually the therapist's hold of the distal end of the humerus was phased out. Other activities that stimulated rotation were using a cooking baster to put colored water onto rice paper for a picture, playing with various art doughs, Etch-A-Sketch, Marble Maze, and lacing cards. (Lacing cards can be very boring, but when the concept of lacing is used to make gifts or holiday decorations, motivation increases greatly.)

Activities to improve bilateral and contralateral control were begun on the gross motor level. Many of the activities used to promote trunk and neck stability (such as pushing in a suspended net hammock) also require bilateral use of the upper extremities. In addition, Billy used the Whiz Wheel, in which the child sits between two large wheels, each of which has a handle on it. To go straight ahead, the hands are moved together; to turn, the hands must work in opposition (one hand goes forward, and the other does not). Because Billy sat in the Whiz Wheel with his knees and ankles flexed, he could go very fast without stimulating extensor or adductor hypertonus in the lower extremities. Also used during this time was a Roller Racer, which is available at most commercial toy stores. This toy is also one in which the child sits, but in this case the child holds onto handle bars and moves them from side to side to propel the Roller Racer forward. Billy also learned to use the Sit'n'Spin, which involves quite a bit of contralateral control.

These activities were followed up with activities that required more refinement of bilateral or contralateral hand skill. Most could be done in either the seated or standing position. One activity, which requires shoulder stability as well, is a game called shadowing. The therapist sits facing the child and places her hands at the level of the child's shoulders, palms facing the child. The child is asked to place his hands up to hers but with an inch or two of air space between their hands. As the therapist moves her hands, the child must "shadow" her hands. Billy's therapist began with simple bilateral patterns and gradually worked into contralateral movements, some of which required Billy to cross the midline, first with one hand and then with both hands. Other activities included hitting a hanging ball while holding both ends of a paper tube, hitting the ball with both hands inside a large sock, catching beanbags while holding onto a large plastic bottle with both hands, catching a ball while holding a wicker basket with both hands, balloon volleyball, Loopie (Southpaw Enterprises; see Appendix A), and field hockey on the carpet around traffic cones. Several commercial tabletop games were used. One favorite featured an alien planet landscape with several 2-inch diameter hoops, suspended at various heights above the landscape. Billy had control of two handles that produced puffs of air which would then direct the height and movement of a Styrofoam ball. The challenge was to move the ball around the landscape, going through the hoops, and landing the ball safely on the docking bay. It is helpful to have a variety of such games in the therapy clinic.

As Billy gained better shoulder control, activities were introduced that were designed to improve eye-hand coordination and wrist control. As the activities began to demand finer control, ability to move the fingers while stabilizing the thumb and ability to move the fingers against a stable palm also improved. A large supply of papers and foils, in a variety of textures and thicknesses, were used to make collages and mosaic pictures. Billy could tear them with his fingers or punch them out with paper punches. Included were construction paper, sandpaper of various weights, foils, paper lace, and wrapping papers. One of Billy's favorite games was paper chase, which is played with another child. The children face each other on opposite sides of the playing field. On each side are balls made of crumpled paper (the number of balls varies with the number of children playing).

The object of the game is to get all the balls onto your opponent's side. A good figure-ground activity, it also teaches motor planning. But perhaps most important for Billy's fine motor therapy was that he was the one who made all of the crumpled paper balls. A variety of pincer tools were collected, from spring-loaded barbecue tongs to tweezers, and games were invented with these. A popular game was dinosaur digging, with plastic bones hidden in sand. To combine hand strengthening with a visual-motor and form perception activity, a clay tray was made for Billy to write in. With Billy's help, firm plasticene clay was pressed into a jellyroll pan, to make a smooth writing surface. The therapist would trace rhythmic patterns for Billy to copy, and he would press them more firmly into the clay with a wooden stylus. Other activities that were explored for their manipulative value were pipe cleaners, Wiki-Stix (Kapable Kids; see Appendix A), and Geo-boards (with various thicknesses of rubber-bands providing a graded approach to the task).

When Billy began a new activity, he would often show a less mature pattern of control. For example, he might lean on the table with one hand or use humeral rotation rather than forearm rotation. At such times the therapist would again provide the needed stability of proximal joints so that less mature patterns would be inhibited, and more mature patterns of stability would emerge. It was always useful to do a gross motor warm-up with the suspended net hammock, Whiz Wheel, or another piece of equipment before beginning a new fine motor activity. Eventually, as Billy became stronger in the trunk and shoulders, less mature patterns were used for only the most challenging upper extremity tasks.

· · ·

The preceding case studies cannot possibly cover the range of challenges most client populations present. It is hoped that the reader will also find useful information in the references provided. The best source of ideas to make therapy exciting and fun for the children will, of course, be the children themselves.

ACKNOWLEDGEMENTS

I wish to thank my colleagues for their assistance: Katie Richardson, O.T.R., who provided valued editorial support, and Susan Leech, M.A., O.T.R., who did the illustrations. A special thank you goes to the families and children of the Ventura County Easter Seals Infant Development Program; they provide both the wisdom and reason for doing what we do.

REFERENCES

Boehme, R. (1988). *Improving upper body control: An approach to assessment and treatment of tonal dysfunction.* Tucson, AZ: Therapy Skill Builders.

Farber, S., & Huss, A. (1974). *Sensorimotor evaluation and treatment procedures for allied health personnel.* Lafayette, IN: Purdue University Press.

Finnie, N. (1975). *Handling the young cerebral palsied child at home.* New York: E.P. Dutton.

Wilbarger, P. (1990). *Personal communication.* Workshop on Sensory Defensiveness, Ventura County Easter Seals Society.

A

Index of Suppliers

American Printing House for the Blind, Inc.
1839 Frankfort Avenue
P.O. Box 6085
Louisville, KY 40206-0085

Kapable Kids, Toys For All Children
P.O. Box 250
Bohemia, NY 11716
This catalogue is the source for the book, *Mudworks*, which contains more than 100 recipes for art and manipulative dough materials. *Wiki-Stix* and several other manipulatives are also found in this catalogue, as well as switches and switch toys.

Pratt Medical, Inc.
404 N. Fourth Street
Olathe, CO 81425
This is the source for the Joe Cool thumb splints. They are made of neoprene and come premade, ready to adjust to a custom fit.

Southpaw Enterprises, Inc.
800 W. Third Street
Dayton, OH 45407-2840

TherAdapt Products, Inc.
17 W. 163 Oak Lane
Bensenville, IL 60106
This is a resource for the bolster chair, as well as several other tables and chairs that are modular and highly adjustable for use with a wide range of sizes from infancy to school age.

B

Recipe for Glop

Glop, which also goes by the names *Gorp* and *Slime,* is wet without being sticky. It stores indefinitely in a sealed container or bag and is a delight to children. It does not stick to clothing or carpets and dries to a powder that is easily vacuumed up.

Ingredients: White glue
Water
Borax (real borax, not Borateem)

Directions: Mix 1 cup water and 1 cup white glue.
In separate container, mix ⅓ cup water and 1 tsp. borax together.
Add glue mixture and borax mixture together. Stir thoroughly with wooden spatula or spoon. Knead with hands (yes, hands) until thoroughly blended.
(Experts tell me that an additional amount of borax and water should be added if the glop doesn't set up. Color may be added at this time using food color or dry tempera.)

16

Hand Function in the Down Syndrome Population

Sandra J. Edwards   Mary K. Lafreniere

PHYSICAL CHARACTERISTICS

GRASP AND MANIPULATION

CLINICAL IMPLICATIONS

ASSESSMENT
Child's Strengths
Vision
Atlantoaxial Instability
Grip Strength and Hand Measurement
Fine Motor Skills
Muscle Tone

TREATMENT
Positioning
Sensory Stimulation
Areas Needing Special Consideration
Objectives and Activities

The understanding of hand function in individuals with Down syndrome (DS) must be based on a knowledge of anatomic differences and variations in manipulation skills seen in this population. People with DS have a variety of complexities in relation to anatomic, physiologic, and psychosocial development when compared to the non-DS population.

PHYSICAL CHARACTERISTICS

The physical characteristics of the hands of individuals with DS differ in several ways from the hands of the non-DS population. The DS person's hand is approximately 10% to 30% shorter than the normal hand, often appearing small with relatively short fingers (Benda, 1969; Smith and Wilson, 1973). A normal hand at birth contains 27 bones and 18 intrinsic muscles; however, the DS hand may consist of only 23 bones at birth (Erhardt, 1982; Benda, 1969). The development of ossification centers may frequently be delayed and irregular in the DS population. It was noted in a majority of these infants that, although the capitate and hamate (two of the seven carpal bones) are present at approximately 6 months of age, they are often very small (Benda, 1969). After 4 years of age the development of ossification centers becomes more accelerated, and by the age of 15 most individuals with DS have developed a complete set of carpal bones and further growth has ceased (Benda, 1969).

The hands in the DS population consist of bones that are slender and short and have poor calcification (Benda, 1969). The fifth digit may be curved inward, due to the anomaly of the middle phalanx, which may be either very small or absent altogether. The distal phalanges of all the fingers, as well as the entire thumb, appear short and hypoplastic. Also the thumb may often be set at a lower position than normal (Figure 16-1) (Benda, 1969). Hypermobility of the joints and depressed muscular tone are two additional traits commonly identified with the DS population (Esenther, 1984).

According to Benda (1969), another common characteristic of the DS hand is the convergence of the main hand lines (numbered 2 and 3) into what has been termed the four-finger line or transverse palmar crease (Figure 16-2). The occurrence of a

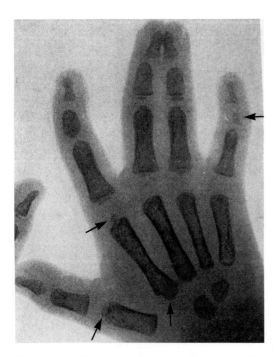

Figure 16-1. X-ray of the hand of a 3-year-old child with DS; bone age is only 6 months. Note the general shortness and delicacy of the bones, deficiency of calcification, and the rudimentary middle phalanx of the fifth digit. Only two carpal bones are present and the epiphysis of the radius is missing. In this particular photograph digits 3 and 4 are syndactyl; however, this is not frequently seen in the DS population.

(From Benda, C. E. [1969]. *Down's syndrome: Mongolism and its management.* New York: Grune & Stratton. p. 64.)

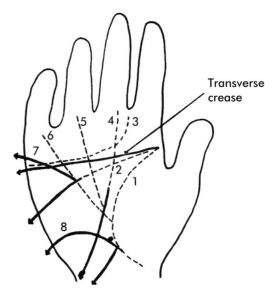

Figure 16-2. Transverse palmar crease.

(From Benda, C. E. [1969]. *Down's Syndrome: Mongolism and its management.* New York: Grune & Stratton. p. 34.)

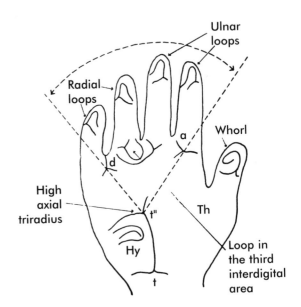

Figure 16-3. Dermatoglyphics of Down syndrome hand.

(From Benda, C. E. [1969]. *Down's Syndrome: Mongolism and its management.* New York: Grune & Stratton. p. 34.)

transverse palmar crease is seen not only in the hands of individuals with DS but also in a certain percentage of normal hands as well. The epidermal ridges and configurations on the plantar side of the hand, known as *dermatoglyphics,* frequently show characteristic deviations in the hands of the DS population with particular significance in the loop patterns on the right palm (Figure 16-3). The critical point of the triradius (or meeting place of three lines) is normally at an angle of 56 to 57 degrees; however, in the majority of hands of those with DS, the angle was found to be greater than 57 degrees (Figure 16-3). According to Cummins (Benda, 1969), these permanent patterns are formed by the third and fourth fetal months of life. The slight increase in transverse palmar crease as well as positive dermatoglyphic patterns seen in the DS population suggest to some researchers that there is a possible genetic implication (Benda, 1969).

According to Cowie (1970), the palmar grasp reflex of children with DS persists approximately 2 to 9 months longer than in those without DS

(until an estimated 4 to 10 months of age). It is theorized that, if the palmar grasp reflex of a normal infant were inhibited by higher cerebral function, then the slow cessation of the reflex in infants with DS may reflect an impairment of higher cerebral function that may later become clearly recognized as a mental deficiency (Cowie, 1970). The delayed cessation of both palmar and plantar reflexes is an example of the retardation of neuromotor development in individuals with DS.

A study of hands of the non-DS population showed a significant correlation between the length of a digit and the palmar pinch strength of that digit (Ager et al., 1984). The researchers concluded that the width of the palm was the single most important independent variable relative to strength and that the lateral pinch strength could be most accurately predicted. They stated that it was important to study both grasp and pinch strength since these variables could most accurately reflect the actual use of the hand, and, therefore, norms for these measures should be formulated and made available. Such information would allow therapists who evaluate children with congenital and traumatic hand problems to have a valid basis from which to determine normal and dysfunctional strength and ultimately to establish sound treatment goals.

A change in or interruption of any one of the anatomic components of the hand can affect the functional use of that hand. Chapter 2 presents a thorough review of the intricate interdependence and balance of the muscles, bones, and joints of the hand and a discussion of the importance of the delicate interplay between various anatomic structures. Included in the discussion is a description of the significance of the arches of the hand and their effect on function. Flatt (1972) states that grasp depends on the integrity of the mobile or longitudinal archs. If dysfunction of an identified joint occurs, the integrity of the arches is interrupted and may result in compromised hand function. The prehensile function of the hand depends on the integrity of the kinetic chain of bones and joints extending from the wrist to the distal phalanges. Interruption of the transverse and longitudinal arch systems formed by these structures contributes to instability, deformity, or functional loss at a more proximal or distal level.

Many interesting questions regarding hand function may arise when one considers the anatomy of the DS population. In the normal hand the proximal transverse arch has the capitate as its keystone, allowing it to remain reasonably fixed and provide stability. However, in the DS hand the capitate is often small and slow to develop, possibly compromising functional stability. The correlation between anatomic deficiency and hand instability has yet to be studied in the DS population. However, if several carpal bones are missing, small, or slow to develop in the DS population, the question arises as to the effect of these differences on the integrity of the hand and the effect on function.

Weakness of the intrinsic muscles of the hand can contribute to decreased function, which ultimately affects the arch system (see Chapter 2). The hypotonicity seen in the DS population may also contribute to functional problems with hand skills. Some studies have shown that over time grasp and prehension in the DS population eventually mature to normal, non-DS levels (Thombs and Sugden, 1991; Moss and Hogg, 1981). This may be due to the eventual development of the carpal bones and the added stability they provide for normal hand function.

GRASP AND MANIPULATION

A study of anatomy alone is not adequate for effective evaluation of hand function. Upper-extremity movement and manipulation as well as sensation, vision, hearing, motor planning, and organization make evaluation of hand motion much more complex and functionally based than anatomy alone.

Previous studies have outlined grip categories for normal hand function (Elliot and Connolly, 1984). Moss and Hogg (1981) propose that knowledge of grip classifications is required to better understand manipulation, which may reflect overall development. A valuable classification of the qualities of hand manipulation comes from Elliot and Connolly (1984). These authors provide a useful taxonomy of the manipulation of objects, distinguishing between digital, prehensile, and palmar grip patterns. They stress that palmar grips secure objects in the hand by maintaining them in contact with the palm. The digital (manipulative) patterns allow the object held in the digits to be manipulated within the hand itself. Their taxonomy provides a way of describing the dynamic actions of the hand in manipulating objects and has potential value to occupational therapists for assessment and prognostic purposes. This provides a system of identifying both hand development and functional deficits. The detail of digital movements described in this classification allows for a clearer description of a subject's abilities in the performance of manual tasks.

The ability of individuals with DS to grasp and manipulate objects has been observed by researchers as being notably different from that in the non-DS population. In a study by Cunningham (as reported in Thombs and Sugden, 1991), 12 infants with DS and 12 infants without DS were videotaped until they were able to have palmar contact and/or grasp an object. In comparing the two groups the author discovered that the infants with DS were slow to reach accurately and lacked adjustments during reaching. They were observed to have a lower percentage of hand adjustments in relation to the size and shape of the objects, suggesting that they were not using visual feedback in the same manner as the other infants. In addition, the DS population was less likely to manipulate and explore the qualities of the object once the object was in the hand. These observations suggested that there were qualitative differences in the development of children with DS, not simply a delay.

This observation is supported in a study by Cole et al. (1988). They looked at the excessive grip forces used by children with DS and questioned possible deficits in the sensorimotor mechanism associated with grasp force control. In their study several objects were covered with different textures (such as satin and sandpaper). The study found that there were aberrations in the control of the grasp forces. Although the grip in the DS population was similar to the grip of individuals without DS, the DS population displayed an inability to adapt grip forces to changes in the friction of object surfaces. The excessive grip forces observed in those with DS may indicate a general strategy in grasping where an increase in force compensates for a specific inability to adapt the grip force to critical object characteristics. The difference in grip force is not thought to be due to weakness or hypotonia but to a generalized deficit in sensory information for motor control. One reason for this sensory deficit could be that the skin of a person with DS may have impaired mechanical aspects of sensory transduction. The skin often becomes thick, dry, and rough with increasing age. There is an increased incidence of xerosis, ichthyosis, and palmar keratinization. Such characteristics may inhibit some of the sensation of the hand.

The results in the Cole et al. study reflect a general deficit in sensorimotor integration. This is observed most clearly in tasks dependent on somatosensory information, such as postural regulation and hand control. The influence of these deficits on day-to-day motor functioning of DS individuals may be quite subtle, as in the production of excessive grip forces. Pain sensation is intact in those with DS, so damaging grip forces probably do not occur. Therefore, with protective pain sensation setting an upper limit, grip forces may be adjusted by means of increased dependence on visual estimation of an object's weight or frictional

characteristics and by visual monitoring during grasp and manipulation. To circumvent the ill effects of increased grasp force, subtle changes in grasp may occur, such as an increased incidence of gross grasps vs. finer prehension to distribute the grip forces throughout the hand. Such a compensation may interfere with dexterity and promote the impression of clumsiness in individuals with DS (Cole et al., 1988).

Thombs and Sugden (1991) found that there was a general increased use of precision, as opposed to power grips, with increasing age in the DS population, thus showing an almost linear progression of precision acquisition. The development of children with DS was found to be less predictable in the early years than in the later years. This is thought to be due to the processes involved in the control of a skill as opposed to factors such as body size and strength. These authors concluded that many developmental changes occur through natural transactions between an individual's resources and the specific demands of a task, suggesting that even further enhancement may be possible with specific forms of remediation.

Moss and Hogg (1981) observed non-DS individuals and those with DS and found that both groups showed increased mastery of skills with increasing age (specifically increased speed, sophistication of prehension, and consistency with performance). However, the children with DS demonstrated generally inferior acquisition of adult precision (prehension) as demonstrated by a persistence of the reverse transverse grip (Figure 16-4). Their infrequent use of digital grips may be due partly to anatomic and somatosensory factors, which may be relevant when designing manipulation teaching materials. The Moss and Hogg study was unable to show the path by which the level of competency was reached for either group, or at which point developmental trends ceased (Moss and Hogg, 1981). Continued research in this area is needed to better understand developmental progression for the DS population.

In a qualitative pilot study conducted by Lafreniere, Edwards, and Smith (1985) six children with DS ages 20 to 44½ months were administered specific sections of the Erhardt Developmental Prehension Assessment (Erhardt, 1981, 1982, 1983). What was observed supports similar findings outlined in this chapter. None of the children were able to achieve all of the highest skill levels as identified by Erhardt, even though the children were at least 5 months older than the identified age of mastery. All children showed inconsistency in

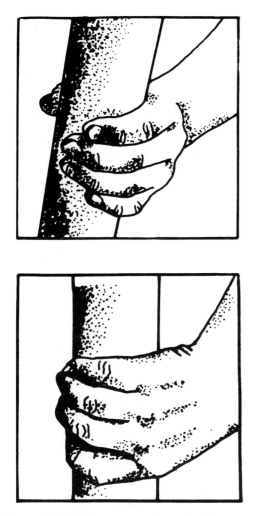

Figure 16-4. A, Transverse palmar grip. **B,**
Reverse transverse palmar grip.

(From Moss, S. C., & Hogg, J. [1981]. The development of hand
function in mentally handicapped and non-handicapped preschool
children. In P. Mittler, [Ed.]. *Frontiers of knowledge in mental
retardation: Social, educational, and behavioral aspects.*
Baltimore: University Park Press, p. 37.)

skill acquisition (inconsistent progression of sub-steps). The children completed tasks more frequently when using the right hand than when using the left. None of the children were able to attain a fine pincer grasp, only the lateral pincer grasp. The fifth, and occasionally the second, digit was frequently extended, and many were observed to use the reverse transverse palmar grasp. In general, skills decreased as more fine finger and wrist involvement were required. The results of this pilot study indicate delayed acquisition in manipulation skills for individuals with DS when compared to Erhardt's scale. Questions arise as to just how long such a delay in skill acquisition persists in this population.

Elliot and Connolly (1984) describe an apparent delay in motor performance of individuals with DS once verbal cuing for a task was terminated. The DS individual appeared to take more time to organize and initiate movements in the absence of verbal cues. These authors theorize that the slowed reaction times, when verbal commands are stopped, may be due to either difficulties remembering verbal cues or difficulty internalizing the previous verbal input so that it could be carried over into movement patterns.

In another study Hogg and Moss (1983) observed 50 children with DS (ages 15 to 44 months) and 50 children without DS (9 to 38 months) and found that there was no difference in their grip sophistication. In regard to development it was noted that both groups mastered the necessary manipulative subroutines (consolidated acts so well learned as to require minimal conscious attention) for effective execution of required grips. Differences were observed, however, in the rate of efficiency with tasks: those with DS displayed slower movement times. The authors hypothesized that this finding might be related to slowness in processing. This suggests that, if differences do arise in relation to manipulation in subjects with DS, the source may lie in the efficiency of organization, not with evolving specific behaviors of a given grip.

In summary, several studies have shown a delay in the development of hand manipulation skills in individuals with DS. Differences have been noted in relation to anatomy as well as possible cognitive influences on processing. Apparently the DS population eventually succeeds in the mastery of refined skills, showing an ultimate maturity. However, inconsistencies noted in the pathway to this ultimate maturity make assessment and treatment planning a challenge. An understanding of the complexities of anatomy and physiology is essential so that the clinician can become a skilled evaluator and therapist for this population. Continued research is needed in this area to further understand and formulate normative developmental pathways of hand function for the DS population.

CLINICAL IMPLICATIONS

The information regarding anatomy and manipulation skills outlined in this chapter may have significant impact in the planning and implementing of treatment by the clinician. Several beneficial suggestions for treating individuals with DS are outlined here.

The clinician should maintain realistic expectations of grasp and release abilities since these skills are noted to be inconsistent in the DS population. Difficulties with sustained grasp and the ability to hold and carry an object may have an impact on the performance of a variety of tasks. These tasks include holding onto a bottle during self-feeding and the ability to bring objects to the mouth for exploration. Inability to perform these tasks may influence oral-motor development. Treatment plans should include activities to stimulate oral-motor development with specific hand-to-face tasks.

The decrease in motor skills seen in individuals with DS may affect their level of social interaction. If objects, when presented to the individual, are not grasped, explored, and released, then the subject has a decreased interaction not only with the object but with the person presenting the object as well. A decreased ability to engage in playful interaction using objects may influence the DS individual's social development. Poor interaction with the environment may contribute to processing delays regarding the subject's relation to the world and to others.

Activities to improve overall muscle tone and improve eye-hand coordination should be incorporated in treatment planning. Tasks to improve eye-hand coordination should include objects that necessitate gross grasp and should eventually progress to smaller objects that require increased precision. Objects that help stimulate a variety of tactile sensory experiences should be provided, such as those differing in shape, surface texture, and weight. Enhancement of processing abilities may be achieved if the clinician reinforces the demonstration of specific motor tasks with verbal cues. To improve hand stability as well as ability to sustain a grasp, the clinician should introduce tasks that require pronation, supination, and wrist flexion and extension. These tasks ideally lead to consistent use of the transverse palmar grasp for writing. These ideas may prove helpful to the clinician when structuring intervention to improve prehension skills in the DS population.

ASSESSMENT

A thorough assessment of the individual with DS must be completed before treatment. This should include an assessment of the child's strengths as well as information about the child's vision and atlantoaxial stability. An evaluation of grip strength, hand measurements, fine motor abilities, and muscle tone must also be completed when focusing on hand function.

Child's Strengths

When completing an assessment, it is often easy to look for what is wrong with an individual. However, important assessment questions need to include: What are the strengths of the child with DS? What types of successes has the child had with hand function? What types of situations allow this child to succeed? It is already known that adaptations frequently need to be made to enhance success with hand function (Pueschel, 1987). Once the clinician understands the particular circumstances that provide success for an individual, adaptations to treatment can more easily be accomplished.

Vision

Special emphasis needs to be placed on the ophthalmologic examination of the child with DS because of the relationship of vision to eye-hand coordination. Whenever possible the examination should be done before the occupational therapy assessment. However, if the examination has not been done, then a recommendation needs to be made by the therapist to the parents or the caregiver to schedule an examination with a pediatric ophthalmologist who is able and willing to care for children with DS (Pueschel, 1987). The reason for the emphasis on this particular area is the frequency of ophthalmologic disorders and their potential impact on hand function. The frequency of ophthalmologic disorders found in one study of children with DS included 77% with refractive errors, most often myopia, 49% with strabismus, 35% with congenital nystagmus (horizontal, vertical, or rotary), and 20% with blocked tear ducts (Mumma, 1984). Knowledge of eye disorders is important to the occupational therapist working on hand function because of the relationship of vision to eye-hand coordination, motor and reflex development, and sensory and cognitive abilities.

Atlantoaxial Instability

Another important area to consider in children with DS is whether the child has atlantoaxial instability. This condition is defined as the shortest distance between the posteroinferior aspect of the anterior arch of the atlas and the adjacent anterior surface of the odontoid process. If the distance is 5 mm or more, the child is at risk: "It is important that atlantoaxial instability in individuals with DS be identified early because of its relatively high prevalence and its potential for remediation'' (Pueschel, 1987). According to Pueschel (1983) atlantoaxial instability is present in about 12% to 20% of persons with DS; however, the majority do not display symptoms. Although a cervical x-ray is necessary to diagnose the condition, knowledge of the symptomatic signs is important for the occupational therapist. The signs of atlantoaxial instability are hyperreflexia, a positive Babinski sign, ankle clonus, muscle weakness, abnormal gait, limited neck mobility, and a possible torticollis-like head tilt (Pueschel, 1987). The occupational therapist may observe the symptoms during a grip strength assessment or a sensory test. Children with symptoms usually require surgery. Children who are asymptomatic often do not require any intervention, but occupational therapists should show caution when engaging these children in activities such as somersaults, trampoline activities, and any other activities that might result in cervical injury.

Grip Strength and Hand Measurement

Grip strength is an important determinant of hand function because it can measure the degree of disability and can be used to document improvement resulting from treatment (Ager, Olivett, and Johnson, 1984; Pratt and Allen, 1989). Normative data for grip strength are not available for children with DS and are limited for the normal population of children as well. This lack of data makes it difficult to compare the average grip strengths between normal and DS children. However, a baseline measurement of grip strength is important to establish during initial assessment.

To measure strength, the Martin Vigorimeter* may be used instead of the Jamar Dynamometer because of the relative ease and comfort for a child-sized hand. The Jamar Dynamometer is designed for adults and is very large and heavy. It is difficult for the child with DS to place the entire hand around the device for optimal grip. The Martin Vigorimeter has a small bulb that can be comfortably squeezed by the child with DS. It is being used increasingly by occupational therapists who evaluate grip strength in children (Robertson and Deitz, 1988).

In addition to grip strength, occupational therapists need to measure hand size since several studies have found a linear relationship between hand width and grip strength (Ager, Olivett, and Johnson, 1984; Link, Lukens, and Bush, 1993). Methods of measurement have been outlined by Link et al. (1993). The measurement for the width of the hand can be accomplished by placing a ruler from the base of the second metacarpal to the base of the fifth metacarpal; another proposed method of measurement may be completed by placing the hand flat on a piece of paper and tracing the hand. Marks are then made on the tracing, identifying the bases of the second and fifth metacarpals. The distance between the two marks is then measured with a ruler.

Fine Motor Skills

The fine motor tests most often used by occupational therapists that can be used to assess children with DS are listed in Table 16-1. The tests have been divided into norm- and criterion-referenced tests.

A norm-referenced test makes a comparison to a preestablished standard, giving the subject a designated level of development. A criterion-referenced test shows sequence of development and therefore is more responsive to individual gains. Criterion-referenced tests are useful for evaluating children with DS because they assist in planning intervention and provide measures of outcome (Dunn, 1991).

The Bayley Scale of Infant Development has been used extensively for researching motor development in children with DS. It is in the "mental" section of the test that fine motor, along with language, cognitive, and perceptual items are administered.

The Erhardt Developmental Prehension Assessment provides extensive detail for the evaluation of the components involved in reaching, prehension patterns, grip, and finger control. The test contains finely graded items, providing sensitivity to identify delayed or abnormal behaviors. It has a lot to offer for assessing hand function, but the norms are established from the normal population and not from the DS population.

The Peabody Developmental Motor Scales have many items for the assessment of hand function, including grasp, hand use, eye-hand coordination, and manual dexterity. The test was also designed to assess gross motor function. The short form can be used for screening and the long form used for a more extensive evaluation.

*The Martin Vigorimeter, also known as the Hand Cynamometer Pinch Gauge and the Dynamometer Pinch Gauge Combination is available from Best Priced Products, Inc., P.O. Box 1174, White Plains, NY 10602.

Table 16-1. Fine motor tests to assess children with Down syndrome

TEST	AGE
Norm Referenced	
Bayley Scale of Infant Development	0-30 months
Gesell Preschool Test	2.5 - 6 years
Motor-Free Visual Perceptual Test	4 - 8 years
Peabody Developmental Motor Scales	Up to 7 years
Test of Visual Motor Skills	2 - 12 years
Bruininks-Oseretsky	4 - 14 years
Criterion Referenced	
Hawaii Early Learning Profile	Up to 3 years
Peabody Developmental Motor Scales	Up to 7 years
Brigrance Diagnostic Inventory of Early Development	Up to 7 years
Erhardt Developmental Prehension Assessment	Up to 6 years

Muscle Tone

Low muscle tone, or hypotonia, is the most frequently cited problem experienced by children with DS (Esenther, 1984). Studies report the incidence of hypotonia occurring at rates as high as 97.7% in this population (McIntire and Dutch, 1964), and other studies state that it occurs in 75% to 85% of the children with DS (Dmitriev, 1982). Hypotonia causes delays in motor development (Pueschel, 1984). Because of the high frequency of hypotonia and the relationship to motor development in children with DS, muscle tone needs to be assessed throughout the treatment process.

Experts seem to agree that muscle tone is best assessed from a composite of several measures. Most often these measures entail resistance to passive stretch, joint extensibility, muscle consistency, and antigravity posturing (Schumway-Cook and Woollacott, 1985). An item taken alone is unlikely to give an accurate assessment of muscle tone (Cowie, 1970). Bobath (1971) evaluated for the combined effects of tone and primitive postural reflexes by noting the adaptation of various muscle groups to change. One method described for observing muscle tone was termed *passivite*, which involves flapping the distal segments of the joints (Prechtl and Bientema, 1964).

In the last decade, efforts have been directed toward devising electronic instruments to quantify tone. An example of such an instrument is the Rouch Tonometer (1987), a hand-held instrument that quantifies muscle tone by using a simple palpation method.

It has been noted that the quality of muscle tone may be a predictor of overall motor development

(Reed et al., 1980; Cullen et al., 1981; Pueschel, 1984; Dmitriev, 1982). Because of the interdependent relationship of motor development, hand function, and muscle tone, an analysis of muscle tone could assist in determining the level of intervention required to improve hand function.

TREATMENT

The individual child with DS has many physical and mental challenges that have an impact on the intervention process of occupational therapy. Although hand function is the primary focus of this section, it is necessary to review briefly some of the neuropathology relative to DS.

Neuropathologic studies of the DS brain and vestibular apparatus have demonstrated areas of morphologic and neurologic abnormalities, including (1) decreased brain weight and smaller size cerebellum and brainstem (Crome, Cowie, and Slater, 1966); (2) incomplete myelination, reduction in the number of pyramidal neurons, and the abnormal organization of pyramidal neurons of the motor cortex and cerebellum (Harris, 1985); and (3) anomalies of the utricular space and the lateral semicircular canals (Igarashi et al., 1977). The retention of primitive reflexes, deficits in the autonomic postural control system, and generalized muscular hypotonia could result from such irregularities of the central nervous system (Cowie, 1970).

Behavior, auditory and visual perception, cognitive skills, and intellectual development all influence the intervention programs and need to be taken into consideration when planning treatment. Therapists need to be knowledgeable and skilled in behavior management, effective communication, and the appropriate use of visual and auditory cuing. In addition, the therapist needs to involve the family or caregivers since they are a necessary component of the planning and treatment program.

Positioning

When working with the child's hands, the child's body position and posture need to be assessed and monitored. The position of the head, shoulders, trunk, hips, knees, and feet require analysis and regulating before and during treatment. The neurodevelopmental theories of Bobath as well as reflex maturation are important to apply when positioning key joints. For example, if a child has a strong asymmetric tonic neck reflex at age 2 years, then a position to inhibit this reflex is necessary. For instance, instead of seating the child at a table and chair, place the child in a prone position over a roll, allowing symmetric use of the arms and hands.

Sensory Stimulation

Activities to stimulate specific sensory systems that can provide effective feedback to the child are important to incorporate into the treatment design. Therefore the results of a sensory integration assessment are necessary to identify areas of emphasis in the treatment program, such as proprioceptive, vestibular, and tactile systems. Activities that use a combination of neurodevelopmental and sensory integration have been effective with children in this population for improving fine and gross motor development (Edwards and Yuen, 1990). Ideas that may prove beneficial in stimulating the specific sensory systems are described here.

Proprioception

One method of providing proprioceptive input is to place a weighted sweatshirt over the arms and shoulders of the child. The sweatshirt is weighted by beans that fill the arms and body of the shirt. Another method for proprioceptive input is to have the child wear a weighted vest that provides additional stimulation to both the trunk and the shoulders.

Vestibular system

As mentioned earlier, hypotonia is prevalent in this population. Vestibular stimulation has been suggested to assist with the improvement of hypotonia (Ayres, 1972) and might be incorporated

within the treatment process. The amount and type of vestibular stimulation are most easily monitored when child-directed.

One way to integrate vestibular stimulation into treatment is to sit the child inside an inner tube that has been placed on a trampoline and ask the child to throw bean bags at a target. The task of throwing will address eye-hand coordination while the child's movements provide vestibular stimulation.

Tactile system

Due to skin changes of the hand, the child with DS may be particularly challenged in the interpretation of tactile sensation. Specific treatment ideas to enhance tactile feedback might include the following.

- Use shaving cream on a mirrored surface and encourage the child to draw using the whole hand or by isolating the index finger or thumb and finger. This activity can be used to develop bilateral hand function as well.
- Finger Jello (Jello that maintains its shape outside a container) is very appealing to children and can provide tactile input and assist with grasp and release development.
- Painting with chocolate pudding and finger paints can also accomplish hand function goals.
- The older child may be encouraged to roll out playdough and write in the claylike material with the finger.

Areas Needing Special Consideration

The child with DS may have difficulty with opposition because the thumb may be set lower on the hand and the phalanges of the thumb may be short. The fine pincer grasp has also been observed to develop more slowly (Lafreniere, Edwards, and Smith 1985). Therefore when selecting a toy to stimulate opposition and pincer grasp, ensure that it is the correct size and shape. The child can be encouraged to manipulate small objects if the therapist holds the child's thumb and index finger around an appropriate size object. Raisins and cereal can be used to facilitate the difficult fine pincer grasp. In addition, because visual feedback is not readily used by the child, observe whether he/she is focusing on the object (Thombs and Sugden, 1991). Toys with definitive texture may assist the child by providing increased somatosensory feedback; otherwise feedback may be limited by the thick, dry, skin characteristic of this population. For example, instead of using a smooth small ball, use a small textured ball or crumpled paper. Because both the proximal and distal transverse arches of the hand may be affected as well as the longitudinal arch, the child with DS has a challenge in accommodating objects of various sizes. It is important to introduce a variety of sizes and shapes, but in a calibrated method so that the child can develop a feedback loop that registers the fine motor experience. By using light pressure over the child's hand to convey the feeling of holding the toy and repeatedly using the word *hold,* the meaning of the work is gradually understood. Soon the child can be encouraged to pick up a small toy without assistance (Pueschel, 1990).

The child may choose to push objects with the palm of the hand rather than manipulating the object due to a combination of physical and sensory characteristics. A child who continues to prefer a palmar grasp can be stimulated to use a pincer grasp if an object is held out or handed to the child rather than placed on a table to be picked up. Extra practice and cuing to use the fingers may be necessary. Another idea to encourage pincer use is to place a glove with the finger and thumb tips cut out (or just the radial fingers and thumb) on the child's hand. Edible items such as pieces of crackers, fruit, and cereal can be used to encourage more frequent use of the pincer grasp so as to enhance eye-hand coordination and oral motor development.

As Pueschel (1990) indicates: "Young children with DS need extra cuing, stimulation, encouragement, guidance, and mediation to become engaged in manipulatory skills" (p. 144). This important point of extra cuing and stimulation is further suggested by a study of 229 children with DS where cognitive and motor skills were examined. The authors reported that this population seemed to take approximately twice as long as normal children to achieve a particular motor developmental level (Rauh and Rudinger, 1987). In addition to requiring repetition to develop motor skills, children with DS need to be assisted to explore objects manually as well as visually and to apply these experiences to cognitive learning.

Using both hands simultaneously and also transferring an object from one hand to another hand need to be practiced with the young child who has developmental delays. Some ideas for facilitating growth in two-handed activities is to play games like pat-a-cake. Hold the child's hands and clap them together while singing or listening to music. If the child starts to do the activity independently, gradually decrease your assistance. An additional idea for encouraging two-handed manipulation skills is to use a large ball, perhaps with a bell inside of it for additional auditory cues, or a large textured ball placed in between the child's hands. The therapist's hands can be placed on top of the child's hands to provide additional tactile input and to provide the feeling of holding firmly and with pressure. Demonstrate to the child the difference between grasp and release. In place of the ball, a colorful stick with a variety of textures can be used. Demonstrate how one hand alternately releases the grasp while the other hand maintains the grasp. This sequence of activities will often assist the child with the skill of transferring an object from one hand to the other.

The reverse transverse palmar grasp was observed at all ages in the DS population. The occupational therapist can encourage the use of the more mature transverse palmar grasp by putting the child's hand in the correct position and then holding his/her own hand over the child's to convey the feeling of holding firmly and with pressure. Using activities that require wrist motion along with the transverse palmar grasp, such as pouring water from a small pitcher, can help the child to experiment with the positions necessary to master the transverse palmar grasp.

Learning how to use the fingers independently rather than as a unit is an important goal. Isolating finger movements, such as poking, can facilitate learning how to let go of an object. Repeated demonstrations of how to open the fingers to allow the release of an object may be required. It is useful to have containers that motivate the child and/or give additional cues. Using metal containers that make a noise when the object drops can encourage the child to learn to let go of an object. Also, asking the child to hand a toy to the therapist requires the child to release the toy.

After the child has learned to grasp and release, throwing is the next sequence in hand development and assists with eye-hand coordination. A therapist must recognize that what develops normally in nondelayed children has to be demonstrated, encouraged, and practiced for the developmentally delayed child. The activity of throwing is often fun for the child and aids in the development of perceptual concepts, especially basic spatial relationships. Parents need to be cautioned that the child may not be able to distinguish between objects that can and cannot be thrown.

Objectives and Activities

Finally, the following outline is a sequential list of hand function objectives and activities that may be incorporated into treatment to enhance hand development of children with DS. As noted throughout this text, all objects and toys discussed in these activities must be of adequate size and shape for the child's hand. Activities 1 to 5 are for children with DS, approximate age range of 5 to 12 months; activities 6 and 7 are for children approximately 12 to 24 months.

1. Reach and grasp
   Objective: The child will reach, after making eye contact, and grasp the toy.
   Activity suggestions: The child needs to first visually register the object and then attempt to reach. Assist in turning the child's head if the child is unable to independently move the head to track effectively. If the child is unable to grasp the object, shape the behavior by curling the child's hand and fingers around the object. Reinforce the effort and attention to the task. Some suggestions for toys are beads, bells, and rings presented alone or suspended by a string. The child's position can be changed from prone to supine to sitting. The toy can be presented directly in front of the child, from the side, above the shoulder, and below or above the waist. Always encourage tracking along with reaching and grasping. Record grasp and hand use.

2. Reach and grasp from a container
   Objective: The child will independently reach and grasp an object from a container.
   Activity suggestions: The child is encouraged to first visually locate the object in the container and then to remove the object from the container. This step is repeated. Increase the difficulty by placing more than one object in the container and have the child reach and grasp. Change the container and objects for novelty. Encourage the child to manipulate each object. The more consistent the reinforcement the more successes the child will enjoy.

3. Transfer of an object
   Objective: The child will transfer an object from one hand to the other.
   Activity suggestions: Place an object on the table and allow the child to grasp and transfer the toy. If the child does not engage in this step, demonstrate the activity and shape the behavior by taking the child's hands through the sequence of steps. The transition from one hand to another may be encouraged by the introduction of yet another object(s) to be picked up.

4. Grasp, place, and release
   Objective: The child will look at an object, then grasp, place, and release it.
   Activity suggestions: Correctly position the child at a table and present one container with toys and one container that is empty. Elicit a game to place the toys in the empty container. The therapist may need to demonstrate and shape the activity initially. Make certain the child is looking at the object before reaching for it.

5. Grasping an object in each hand simultaneously
   (A child with DS between 8 and 12 months is ready to work on simultaneously picking up two small objects [Dmitriev, 1982].)
   Objective: The child will grasp an object in each hand simultaneously and manipulate them by either holding them or banging them together.
   Activity suggestions: The child will pick up two small, identical objects. The reason for using identical objects is to decrease the chance that one of the objects may seem more appealing to the child than the other and, consequently, the child will reach with only one hand. The toys need to be small enough to allow for complete grasp. Blocks about 1 inch square are recommended. If the child makes no effort to pick up the blocks, give physical assistance. Once the child has an object in each hand, encourage interaction of the two objects (such as banging them together).

6. Development of pincer grasp
   Objective: The child will use a pincer grasp to pick up an object using the thumb and forefinger.
   Activity suggestions: Small textured objects are important to use to give maximum sensory feedback: cloth-covered buttons, stones, cereal, and raisins

encourage the use of the pincer grasp (note: nonedible items are not appropriate for the child who still places objects in the mouth). The pincer grasp may be enhanced if objects are held up to the child vs. being placed on the table. This will discourage use of the palmar grasp.

7. Placing one object on top of another

   Objective: The child will pick up an object and independently place it on top of another.

   Activity suggestions: The child should be positioned correctly in a chair at a table of correct height. Encourage the child to grasp an object (such as a 1-inch cube) using a three-jaw chuck or a pincer grasp. Next, facilitate placing one object on top of another. Once again, this activity might need to be demonstrated and physically assisted initially. Engage the child's participation by making a game out of the task (build a tower). This activity requires good eye-hand coordination and precision.

The complexities of the DS population can pose an exciting challenge to the therapist. Many factors must be considered when assessing, designing, and implementing treatment for optimal enhancement of hand function. It is hoped that the information outlined in this chapter will prove beneficial to the therapist who assumes this rewarding challenge.

REFERENCES

Ager, C., Olivett, B., & Johnson, C. (1984). Grasp and pinch strength in children 5 to 12 years old. *American Journal of Occupational Therapy, 38,* 107-113.

Ayres, A. J. (1979). *Sensory integration and learning disorders.* Los Angeles: Western Psychological Services.

Benda, C. E. (1969). *Down's syndrome: Mongolism and its management.* New York: Grune & Stratton.

Bobath, B. (1971). *Abnormal postural reflex activity caused by brain lesions.* London: Heinemann Medical Books.

Cole, K. J., Abbs, J. H., & Turner, G. S. (1988). Deficits in the production of grip forces in Down syndrome. *Developmental Medicine and Child Neurology, 30,* 752-758.

Cowie, V. A. (1970). *A study of the development of mongols.* Oxford: Pergamon Press.

Crome, L., Cowie, V., & Slater, E. (1966). A statistical note on cerebellar and brainstem weight in mongolism. *Journal of Mental Deficiency Research, 10,* 69-72.

Cullen, S. M., Cronk, C. E., Pueschel, S. M., Schenell, R. R., & Reed, R. B. (1981). Social development and feeding milestones of young Down syndrome children. *American Journal of Mental Deficiency, 85,* 410-415.

Dmitriev, V. (1982). *Time to begin: Early education for children with Down syndrome.* Milton, WA: Caring, Inc.

Dunn, W. (1991). *Pediatric occupational therapy.* Thorofare NJ: Slack.

Edwards, S., & Yuen, H. K. (1990). An intervention program for a fraternal twin with Down syndrome: Case report. *American Journal of Occupational Therapy, 44,* (5), 454-458.

Elliott, D. (1985). Manual asymmetries in the performance of sequential movement by adolescents and adults with Down syndrome. *American Journal of Mental Deficiency, 90*(1), 90-97.

Elliott, J., & Connolly, K. S. (1984). A classification of manipulative hand movements. *Developmental Medicine and Child Neurology, 26,* 283-296.

Erhardt, R. P. (1982). *Developmental hand dysfunction: Theory, assessment, treatment.* Laurel, MD: Ramsco Publishing.

Erhardt, R. P. (1983). *Normal hand development: Birth to 15 months* (Videocassette recording). Laurel, MD: Ramsco Publishing.

Erhardt, R. P., Beatty, P. A., & Hertsgaard, D. M. (1981). A developmental prehension assessment for handicapped children. *American Journal of Occupational Therapy, 35,* 237-242.

Esenther, S. E. (1984). Developmental coaching of the Down syndrome infant. *American Journal of Occupational Therapy, 38,* 440-445.

Flatt, A. E. (1972). Restoration of rheumatoid finger joint function, III, *Journal of Bone and Joint Surgery 54A,* 1317-1322.

Harris, S. R. (1985). Genetic disorders in children. In D. A. Umphred (Ed.) *Neurological rehabilitation.* St. Louis: Mosby.

Hogg, J., & Moss, S. C. (1983). Prehensile development in Down's syndrome and non-handicapped preschool children. *British Journal of Developmental Psychology, 1,* 189-204.

Igarashi, M., Takahashi, M., Alford, B., & Johnson, P. (1977). Inner ear morphology in Down's syndrome. *Acta Otolaryngology, 83,* 175-181.

Lafreniere, M. K., Edwards, S., & Smith, D. (1985). *Hand manipulation skills of children with Down syndrome.* Unpublished graduate research. Western Michigan University, Occupational Therapy Department, Kalamazoo.

Link, L., Lukens, S. A., & Bush, M. A. (1993). *Spherical grip strength in children 3 to 6 years old.* Unpublished manuscript, Western Michigan University, Occupational Therapy Department, Kalamazoo.

McIntire, M. S., & Dutch, S. J. (1964). Mongolism and generalized hypotonia. *American Journal of Mental Deficiency, 68,* 669-670.

Moss, S. C., & Hogg, J. (1981). The development of hand function in mentally handicapped and non-handicapped preschool children. In P. Mittler (Ed.). *Frontiers of knowledge in mental retardation: Vol. I. Social, educational, and behavioral aspects.* Baltimore: University Park Press.

Mumma, P. (1984). *Ophthalmological concerns in Down syndrome.* Paper presented at the meeting of the National Down Syndrome Congress, San Antonio, TX.

Pratt, P. N., & Allen, A. S. (1989). *Occupational therapy for children* (2nd ed.). St. Louis: Mosby.

Prechtl, H., & Bientema, D. (1964). The neurological examination of the full term newborn infant. *Little Club Clinics in Developmental Medicine, No. 12.*

Pueschel, S. M. (1983). Atlanto-axial subluxation in Down syndrome. *Lancet, 1,* 1980.

Pueschel, S. M. (Ed.). (1984). *The young child with Down syndrome.* New York: Human Science Press.

Pueschel, S. M., Tingey, C., Rynders, J. E., Crocker, A. C., & Drutcher, D. M. (1987). *New perspectives on Down syndrome.* London: Brookes Publishing.

Rauh, H., & Rudinger, G. (1987). *Early development of Down syndrome children as assessed by the Bayley scales.* Poster Paper. Biannual Meetings of the International Society for the Study of Behavioral Development, Tokyo.

Reed, R. B., Pueschel, S. M., Schnell, R. R., & Cronk, C. E. (1980). Interrelationships of biological, environmental, and competency variables in young children with Down's syndrome. *Applied Research in Mental Retardation, 1,* 161-174.

Robertson, A., & Deitz, J. (1988). A description of grip strength in preschool children. *American Journal of Occupational Therapy, 42* (10), 647-652.

Roush, C. (1987). *The Roush tonometer for quantification of muscle tone.* St. Louis: Roush Scientific.

Shumway-Cook, A., & Woollacott, M. H. (1985). Dynamics of postural control in the child with Down syndrome. *Physical Therapy, 65* (9), 1315-1322.

Smith, D., & Wilson, A. (1973). *The child with Down's syndrome (mongolism).* Philadelphia: W. B. Saunders.

Thombs, B., & Sugden, D. (1991). Manual skills in Down syndrome children ages 6 to 16 years. *Adapted Physical Activity Quarterly, 8,* 242-254.

Glossary

affordances The perceptual features of objects, places, and events that enable particular functional actions.

anticipatory control The programming of action based on a mental representation of an object's properties that has developed through prior experience.

arches of the hand The musculoskeletal structures that allow the flattening and cupping of the hand. The arches are the **proximal transverse,** the **distal transverse,** and the **longitudinal.**

automatization; autonomous phase The stage of a learned motor skill when the action is carried out with minimal attention.

bilateral hold, cooperative An action in which one hand supports or stabilizes an object while the other hand explores or manipulates it.

bilateral simultaneous manipulation; complementary two-hand use An action in which both hands are performing different but complementary actions at the same time, as in bead stringing.

bilateral or two-handed hold, symmetric Holding objects with the two hands acting in unison.

central pattern generators Neural networks that interact in an organized manner to produce a motor act.

coincidence anticipation A form of anticipatory control in which movement coincides with an external event, such as catching a ball.

constructional skill The ability to perform the sequences of movement involved in producing two- or three-dimensional representations as in drawing or building.

constructional style vs. contoured style in drawing Refers to the execution of pictorial representations by the assembly of simple forms as opposed to beginning with a sketch of an outline.

disk grip (five-jaw chuck) A fingertip grip using the pads of all the fingers and the thumb, as on the lid of a jar.

dual motor systems Refers to the differentiation between central nervous system control of skilled distal movements such as those of the hand and the proximal movements of the limbs and trunk.

dynamic tripod grasp (pencil) Grasp in which the pencil is stabilized against the side of the middle finger by the pads of the thumb and index finger. Writing includes localized movements of the fingers and thumb as well as of the wrist.

executive function of the hand The use of the hand as a means of practical action on the environment, during which perceptual function is regulated by that which is needed to achieve the action.

eye-hand coordination The integration of visual perceptual information with the purposeful movements of the hand and arm.

feedback Sensory information that arises from movement.

fine motor coordination Use of small muscle groups for precise movements, particularly in object manipulation with the radial digits.

finger differentiation or individuation Controlled individual or isolated finger movements.

graphomotor skill The conceptual and perceptual motor abilities involved in drawing and writing.

grasp phase of reaching The phase of reaching for an object in which the hand is shaped in anticipation of the contact with the object.

grip The mechanical component of prehension; the hand configuration on the object during grasp.

grip force The pressure exerted on an object in the act of lifting and holding. In precision grasping, grip force is matched to object qualities such as weight, texture, and rigidity.

hand preference The consistent favoring of one hand over the other in the performance of skillful acts.

hand shaping The adaptation of the hand arches and the finger postures to the object's size, shape, and use in anticipation of grasp.

haptic perception Recognition of objects and object properties by the hand without the use of vision.

inferior or immature pincer grasp A grasp between adducted thumb and side of the index finger.

in-hand manipulation The adjustment of a grasped object within one hand while it is being held. Includes **translation, shift,** and **rotation** with and without stabilization.

in-hand manipulation with stabilization Manipulating one object with the fingers while holding one or more additional objects within the same hand.

intermodal perception The matching of objects or shapes that are perceived by one sensory modality, such as touch, to those which are perceived by a different sensory modality, such as vision.

intramodal perception Matching objects or shapes within a single sensory system, for example, matching one object explored haptically to another also explored haptically.

kinesthesia The conscious perception of the excursion and direction of joint movement and of the weight and resistance of objects.

lateral tripod grasp (pencil) Grasp in which the pencil is stabilized against the side of the middle finger, with the index finger pad on the pencil, and the thumb adducted with the thumb pad braced on the side of the index finger. Writing includes localized finger movements as well as wrist and arm movements.

motor functions of the two sides of the hand Refers to the differing functions of the ulnar (little finger) side and the radial (thumb) side of the hand. The primary function of the ulnar side of the hand is to hold, whereas that of the radial side is to manipulate.

multimodal exploration The simultaneous use of more than one sensory system in object exploration.

palmar grasp A whole-hand grasp in which objects are held against the palm of the hand by the fingers. The thumb may be active or passive.

palmar grasp (pencil) A grasp in which the pencil is positioned across the palm and held in a fisted grip.

perceptual activity of the hand Use of the hand as a perceptual system, in which motor activity is primarily exploratory and information seeking.

perceptual-motor skill The modeling of motor actions to the perception of objects, places, or events.

pincer grasp; pinch; fine prehension The grasp of an object with the index finger and thumb. Major types include **palmar pinch** (pad of finger to pad of thumb), **tip pinch** (using tips of both thumb and finger), and **lateral pinch** (thumb holding object against side of finger).

play An intrinsically motivating activity engaged in for its own sake.

play activity A therapeutic activity in which toys or games associated with play are selected by a therapist or teacher to achieve specific intervention objectives.

power grip A static grip applying force to an object to immobilize it in the hand.

precision grip The grasp of an object with the finger and thumb pads or tips. Precision grips may be static but often allow movement of the object by or within the fingers.

precision handling The dynamic or manipulative characteristics of precision grip used for in-hand manipulation and for the use of many tools.

prehension The voluntary act of grasping and manipulating objects with the hand.

preprogrammed movement/open loop movement A learned movement in which the entire motor pattern is programmed before the movement is initiated and which is not under sensory control during execution.

prereaching; prefunctional reach The more automatic movement of the very young infant's hand toward an object before voluntary reach has developed.

procedural or nondeclarative memory Memory for certain ways of doing things, for performing some act, for "knowing how." Includes sensory motor memory. A different memory system than **declarative memory,** which is the ability to "tell about" what one knows.

proprioception Sensory information about positions and movements of body parts from muscles, tendons, joints, and skin. Limb position sense and kinesthesia are forms of proprioception.

pyramidal tract Nerve fibers originating in the cortex that are essential for the skilled use of the hand, particularly the direct cortic spinal fibers, which pass from the cortex to the spine without a synapse.

quadrupod grip (pencil) Grip in which the pencil is held by three fingers and the thumb. May be static or dynamic.

radial digital grasp; inferior forefinger grasp Prehension of an object with the thumb, index, and middle fingers but with the object held proximal to the finger pads. Thumb may be in adduction or opposition.

radial palmar grasp An immature grasp in which the index and middle fingers and thumb press an object into the palm.

radial-ulnar dissociation; separation of the two sides of the hand The ability to perform holding functions with the ulnar fingers while manipulating objects with the thumb and radial fingers.

reflexive grasp The stereotypic closing of the hand on an object in response to tactile or proprioceptive information. Palmar grasp reflexes occur normally in early infancy and may persist in children with brain damage.

reverse transverse grip; radial cross palmar grasp (pencil) An immature pencil grip with the pencil positioned across the palm and the point projecting from the thumb side of the hand. The hand is fisted with the forearm fully pronated.

rotation An in-hand manipulation movement by which an object is turned or rolled in the fingers. **Simple rotation** turns an object partially, alternating direction, as in rolling a small ball of clay. **Complex rotation** turns an object 180 to 360 degrees, as in turning over a peg.

scissors grasp The prehension of small objects between the thumb and the lateral border of the index finger.

self-care activities The basic daily living activities of eating, dressing, bathing, and use of the toilet.

shift An in-hand manipulation movement that causes an object to move linearly on the finger pads, such as adjustment of a pencil to place fingertips near the point.

somatosensory Refers to the tactile and proprioceptive senses that contribute to the perception of objects and events as well as of the body and limbs.

squeeze grasp An immature grip in which an infant presses an object against the palm with total finger flexion. The thumb does not participate and force is not modulated.

static tripod grasp (pencil) Grasp in which the pencil is stabilized against the side of the middle finger and held by the pads of the index finger and thumb. The hand is moved as a unit by the wrist and forearm in writing.

stereognosis The recognition of familiar objects through touch.

three-jaw chuck A power grip of the fingertips. The object is held with the distal pads of the thumb, index, and middle fingers.

translation (1) A form of in-hand manipulation by which an object is moved in a linear direction between the palm and the fingertips. Includes the movement of an object from the palm of the hand to the fingertips (**palm-to-finger translation**), and the movement of an object from the fingertips to the palm (**finger-to-palm translation**).

translation (2) A form of precision handling of an object in which the object is moved toward and away from the palm by finger and thumb flexion and extension, such as threading a needle.

transportation phase; transport The phase of reaching that brings the hand to the target or moves an object through space.

visual-motor integration The coordination of visual information with movement. The term is often used to indicate the ability to copy geometric forms.

volition Action in which the achievement of a goal is seen as resulting from one's own activity.

voluntary controlled release Letting go of an object in a specific place and with timing that is appropriate for the specific task.

zone of proximal development A period of developmental maturation in which particular skills are within reach of a child.

Index